Osmosis

ANATOMY & PHYSIOLOGY ESSENTIALS

Edition 1.0

The Osmosis Team

2018

Copyright © 2017–2018 by Osmosis
ALL RIGHTS RESERVED

This book or any portion thereof may not be reproduced or used in any manner whatsoever without the express written permission of the publisher except for the use of brief quotations in a book review. For permission requests, email us with the subject "Attention: Permissions Coordinator," at the address below.

hi@osmosis.org

ISBN 978-1-947769-07-6

Osmosis
37 S. Ellwood Avenue
Baltimore, MD 21224
www.osmosis.org

Printed in Canada

Designed by Fergus Baird, Heidi Hildebrandt, Tanner Marshall, & Kyle Slinn
Copyedited by Fergus Baird, Andrea Day, Jessica MacEachern, & Malorie Snider
Cover design by Justin Ling & Vincent Waldman
Fonts: Roboto by Google Inc., Apache License, version 2.0
Written in Canada, Romania & the United States of America
SCP 10 9 8 7 6 5 4 3 2 1

Edition: 1.0.0

We'd like to thank our Osmosis Prime members, our supporters, the hundreds of volunteers who double check our facts and translate our videos, and of course, our viewers on YouTube. You all have played a huge part in helping us make the best learning experiences possible.

If you find any mistakes, let us know here:
osms.it/anatomyfeedback

Osmosis Team

Hillary Acer, BA
Fergus Baird, MA
Kaia Chessen, MScBMC
Sarah Clifford, BMBS, BSc
Laura Coscarelli, MA
Harry Delaney, MBChB
Evan Debevec-McKenney, BA
Rishi Desai, MD, MPH
Allison Dollar, BFA
Ursula Florjanczyk, MScBMC
Caleb Furnas, MA
Shiv Gaglani, MBA

Sam Gillespie, BSc
M. Ryan Haynes, PhD
Heidi Hildebrandt, MA
Matt Kaminski
Justin Ling, MD, MS
Kara Lukasiewicz, PhD, MScBMC
Casey Manning, BS
Tanner Marshall, MS
Samantha McBundy, MFA
B. Gil McIntire
Ashwin Menon, MS, MSEd, BE
Sam Miller, BA
Brandon Newton, BBA
Elizabeth Nixon-Shapiro, MSMI, CMI

Brittany Norton, MFA
Marisa Pedron, BA
Viviana Popa, MD candidate
Pauline Rowsome, BSc
Kyle Slinn, RN, MEd
Diana Stanley, MBA
Sean Tackett, MD, MPH
Vincent Waldman, PhD
Will Wei
Sidney Williams
Owen WIllis, MEd
Yifan Xiao, MD

AUTHORS

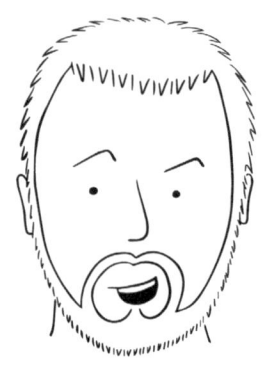

Fergus Baird
MA

Fergus is a copywriter, copy editor and textbook designer at Osmosis, and he dabbles in a little scriptwriting for the YouTube channel as well.

Before moving to Canada, Fergus lived in a small village in Scotland. He earned his Master's degree in English literature at Concordia University in Montréal, writing his thesis on history and the graphic novel. Prior to joining the Osmosis team, Fergus worked as a GIF curator, a movie subtitler, a meme master, and a ghost writer, and spent a year teaching elementary school kids in Japan.

When he's not eating or cooking elaborate meals for his friends, Fergus spends his spare time playing video games and the theremin, drawing strange pictures, and consuming horror media in all its gruesome forms.

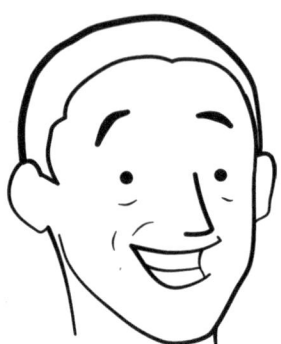

Rishi Desai
MD, MPH

Rishi is a pediatric infectious disease physician at Stanford University and serves as the Chief Medical Officer at Osmosis. He recently led the Khan Academy Medicine team, which put together a collection of videos and questions for students entering the health sciences.

With the help of his parents and teachers, Rishi completed high school and received his BS in Microbiology from UCLA by the age of 18. He completed his medical training at UCSF, pediatric residency at Boston Children's Hospital, and did an infectious disease fellowship at Children's Hospital Los Angeles. He earned his MPH in epidemiology at UCLA, and then spent two years chasing down infectious disease outbreaks for the Centers for Disease Control and Prevention, before beginning his work in online medical education.

In his spare time, Rishi enjoys watching his son torment the family dog, while eating nature's finest fruit—the raspberry!

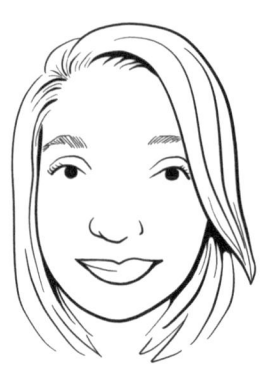

Jessica MacEachern
MA

Jessica MacEachern edits copy for Osmosis. She has an MA in Creative Writing from Concordia University in Montréal, Québec. She is a PhD candidate in English Studies at the Université de Montréal, as well as a part-time professor in Concordia's English Department.

Jessica studies feminist poetry—and occasionally writes it, too. She began her secondary education in psychology at the University of New Brunswick, where she received a student research grant to study sex differences in spatial cognition. As with her hero Gertrude Stein (the modernist poet who studied under the psychologist William James) these early pursuits in the scientific study of the mind continue to inform her creative explorations.

When she's not reading or writing, Jessica is likely pinned underneath her darling cat, Kitty—though this is generally true even if she has a book in hand.

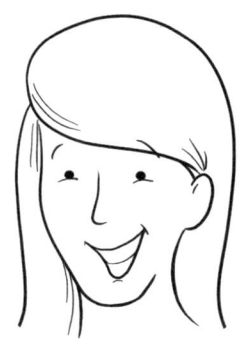

Brittany Norton
MFA

Brittany is a medical illustrator currently based in Santa Clara, California, who creates illustrations and animations for Osmosis.

Unable to choose between her passions for both art and biology, Brittany decided to pursue a degree in medical illustration at the Rochester Institute of Technology. Since graduating with her MFA, she has worked as a video illustrator for Khan Academy as well as a 3D medical modeler/animator for a patient education startup in Silicon Valley. She loves drawing all things anatomical and helping others understand complex concepts through the universal language of art.

When she's not working, Brittany can be found jamming out to Disney music, planning her next traveling adventure, or chasing down neighborhood dogs to pet.

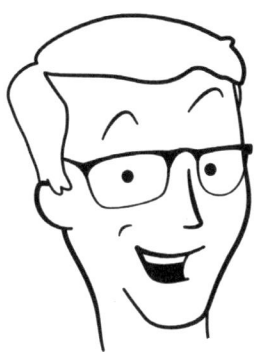

Kyle Slinn
RN, MEd

Kyle is a project manager and instructional designer at Osmosis. He wears many hats, such as managing volunteers and contractors, designing future projects, producing videos, leading internationalization efforts, and designing Osmosis's textbooks. A jack-of-all-trades. Before Osmosis, he worked as a project coordinator for Khan Academy Medicine, where he managed the creation of videos, questions, and text-based articles for MCAT and NCLEX-RN students.

Kyle also worked in the pediatric intensive care unit as a nurse at the Children's Hospital of Eastern Ontario, in Ottawa, Canada. He received his Bachelors of Science in Nursing from the University of Ottawa and holds a Masters of Education in Distance Education from Athabasca University.

With his free time, Kyle loves to go on adventures, hang out with friends, play board games, bake bread, and play musical instruments.

ACKNOWLEDGMENTS

Creating accurate content is really hard. Thousands of eyeballs will look at our work for years to come and inevitably we'll have missed something, or something will go out of date. What's nice about our way of producing content is we get a lot of feedback really fast. Within 24 hours of releasing a video we've meticulously crafted and reviewed, we get thousands of views. In the rare instance there's a mistake, our audience is always quick to use the comment feature to point out where we went wrong. Yep, we're listening! We read every single comment across all of our videos.

Whenever someone points out a factual inaccuracy, we update our video and rerelease it. Currently, YouTube doesn't allow editions of videos to exist. When we rerelease a video, we're effectively pulling the existing, well-established and easily searchable video out of circulation and putting a new, less searchable video in its place. There have been several times where our team has silently cried inside as we take down our most viewed video in the name of scientific accuracy. In the end, though, the result is that we can confidently say our videos (and textbooks) are factually accurate.

We'd like to thank the following people who have given us so much guidance as we've created our content.

Adeeb Aghdassi, MD	**Kelly MacKenzie**, MA
Jodi Berndt, PhD	**Lisa Miklush**, PhD, RNC, CNS
John Bloom, MD	**Kevin F. Moynahan**, MD
Bernadette S. de Bakker, MD, MS	**Nacole T. Riccaboni**, BSN, RN, CCRN-CMC
Armando Hasudungan Faigl, BBiomedSc	**Thomas M. Schmid**, PhD
Jennifer French, MEd	**Kathy W. Smith**, MD
Vanita Gaglani, RPT	**Eric Strong**, MD
Kristine Krafts, MD	**Todd W. Vanderah**, PhD

FOREWORD

"The human body is the most complex system ever created. The more we learn about it, the more appreciation we have about what a rich system it is." - Bill Gates

When we began medical school we were plunged into an immersive, seven-week anatomy course that not only provided us with knowledge about the form and function of the human body, but also gifted us with a sense of wonder and appreciation for our bodies. It is our hope that *Osmosis Anatomy & Physiology Essentials* will impart within you this same sense of appreciation.

The Osmosis Team decided to write this textbook with the goal of providing you an integrated foundation of anatomy & physiology. We combed through each physiological system and identified essential, high-yield information that you absolutely need to know to build a solid foundation for learning medicine, whether you are a budding surgeon or a practicing physician assistant.

While each organ system is unique, there are interdependencies and commonalities as well. The cardiomyocytes of the heart contract in a similar way to the skeletal muscle cells, and both are dependent on calcium that is stored in your bones and released by hormones from your parathyroid gland. Of course, you are also dependent on your gastrointestinal system to absorb that calcium in the first place, and your renal system ensures that you maintain the right levels of calcium. Each heartbeat relies on every other system to perform its role optimally. It is this interdependency that makes health much more than just the absence of disease, but rather the promotion of wellness. Making sure that each body system is performing at its best requires that you understand how they work interdependently.

The *Osmosis Anatomy & Physiology Essentials* textbook takes a deep look at how each of the 14 body systems function, with special additional chapters on how we perceive sights, sounds, and tastes. The textbook explores a range of core topics in physiology, from how the immune system is able to fight off infections, to how the reproductive systems ensures that we propagate our species. You will learn how these systems function from the cellular level all the way up to tissues and whole organs. By the time you have finished the 17 chapters of this book, you will have a solid foundation of how the entire human body functions to maintain homeostasis.

While you read through this book, we encourage you to make use of the powerful and comprehensive Osmosis learning platform to watch our exclusive Osmosis Prime-only anatomy and physiology videos and actively quiz yourself with tens of thousands of associated multiple choice questions and flashcards. Please visit www.osmosis.org and each chapter's URL headers to learn more!

Best wishes on your journey ahead,

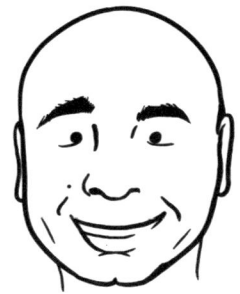

Shiv Gaglani
MBA
Co-founder & CEO

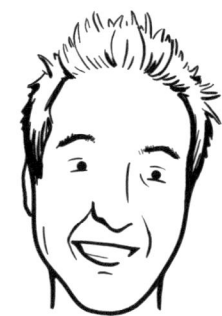

M. Ryan Haynes
PhD (Neuroscience)
Co-founder & CTO

CONTENTS

- 11   THE CARDIOVASCULAR SYSTEM
- 26   THE RENAL SYSTEM
- 36   THE RESPIRATORY SYSTEM
- 43   THE GASTROINTESTINAL SYSTEM
- 52   THE ENDOCRINE SYSTEM
- 67   THE IMMUNE SYSTEM
- 78   THE LYMPHATIC SYSTEM
- 87   THE HEMATOLOGIC SYSTEM
- 93   THE MUSCULAR SYSTEM
- 100   THE SKELETAL SYSTEM
- 110   THE INTEGUMENTARY SYSTEM
- 118   THE MALE REPRODUCTIVE SYSTEM
- 126   THE FEMALE REPRODUCTIVE SYSTEM
- 137   THE NERVOUS SYSTEM
- 148   THE EAR
- 155   THE EYE
- 162   THE TONGUE

APPENDIX

- 171   CREDITS
- 173   SOURCES
- 177   INDEX

THE CIRCULATORY SYSTEM

osms.it/cv_system

The **circulatory system** is also called the cardiovascular system, where cardi- refers to the heart, and -vascular refers to the blood vessels. The two key parts are the heart, which pumps blood, and the blood vessels, which carry blood to the body and return it back to the heart again. Ultimately, this is how nutrients like oxygen get pushed out to the organs and tissues that need them, and how waste like carbon dioxide (the main byproduct of cellular respiration) is removed **(Figure 1.1)**.

The heart is about the size of a person's fist, which makes sense: a bigger person has a bigger fist and, therefore, a bigger heart **(Figure 1.2)**. It's shaped like a cone, and sits slightly shifted over to the left side, in the mediastinum, which is the middle of the chest cavity, or thorax. The heart sits on top of the diaphragm, which is the main muscle that helps with breathing, behind the sternum, or breastbone, in front of the vertebral column, squished in between the two lungs, and protected by the ribs **(Figure 1.3; Figure 1.4; Figure 1.5; Figure 1.6)**.

SEROUS PERICARDIUM

If you look more closely, you can see that the heart sits inside a sac of fluid that has two walls, called the serous pericardium. The outer layer is called the parietal layer. It gets stuck tightly to another layer called the fibrous pericardium, which is made of tough, dense connective tissue, which holds the heart in place and prevents it from overfilling with blood. The inner layer is called the visceral layer, and it gets stuck tightly to the heart itself, forming the epicardium, or the outer layer of the heart. The cells of the serous pericardium, of both the parietal and visceral layer, secrete a protein-rich fluid that fills the space between those layers. This fluid is a lubricant for the heart, allowing it to move around a bit with each heartbeat without feeling too much friction **(Figure 1.7)**.

Figure 1.1

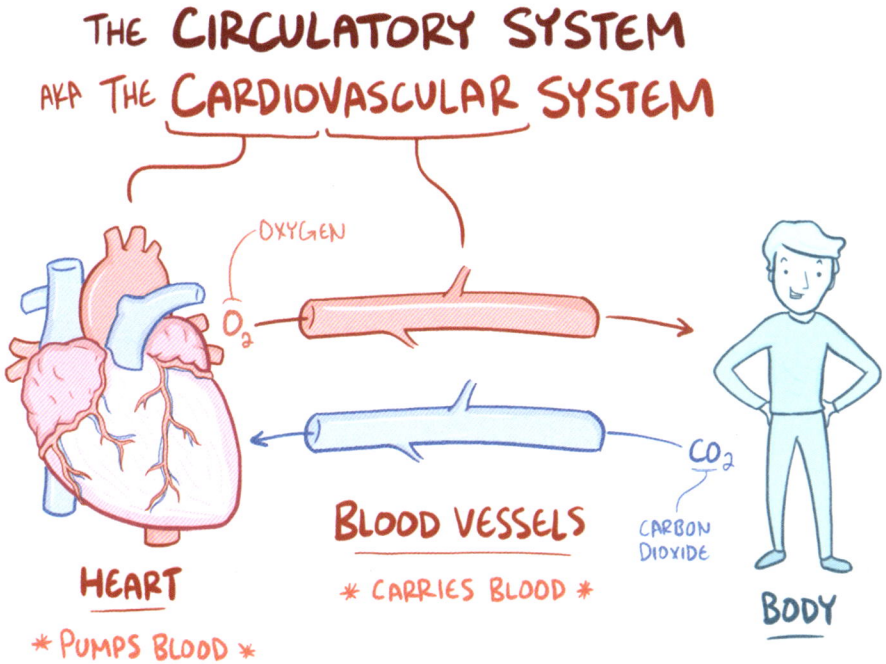

OSMOSIS.ORG 11

Figure 1.2

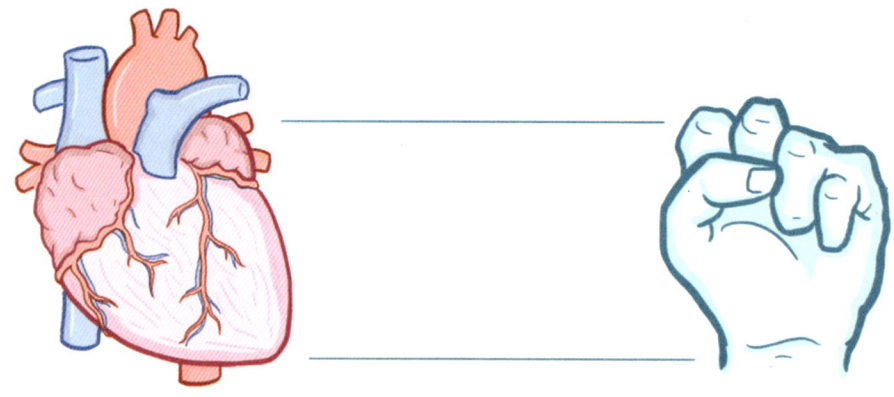

Figure 1.3

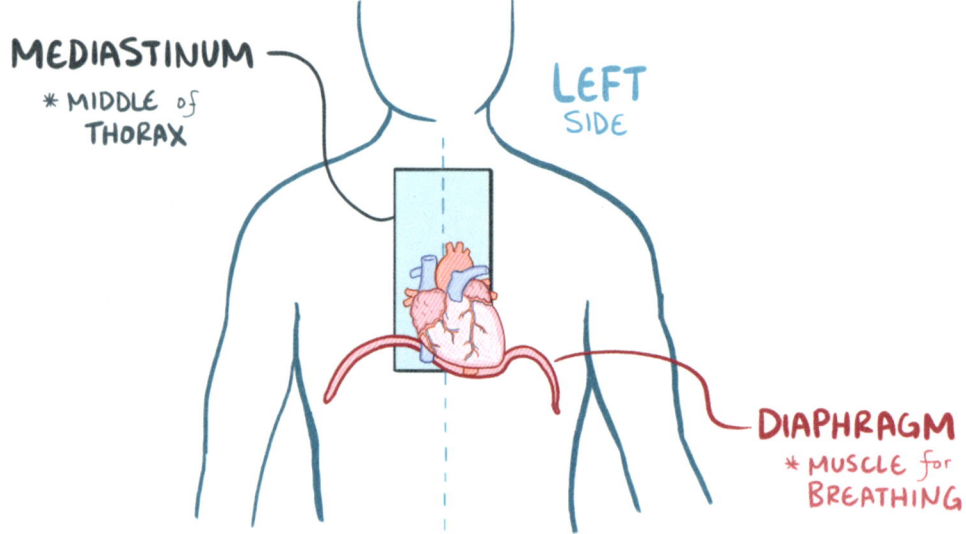

Figure 1.4

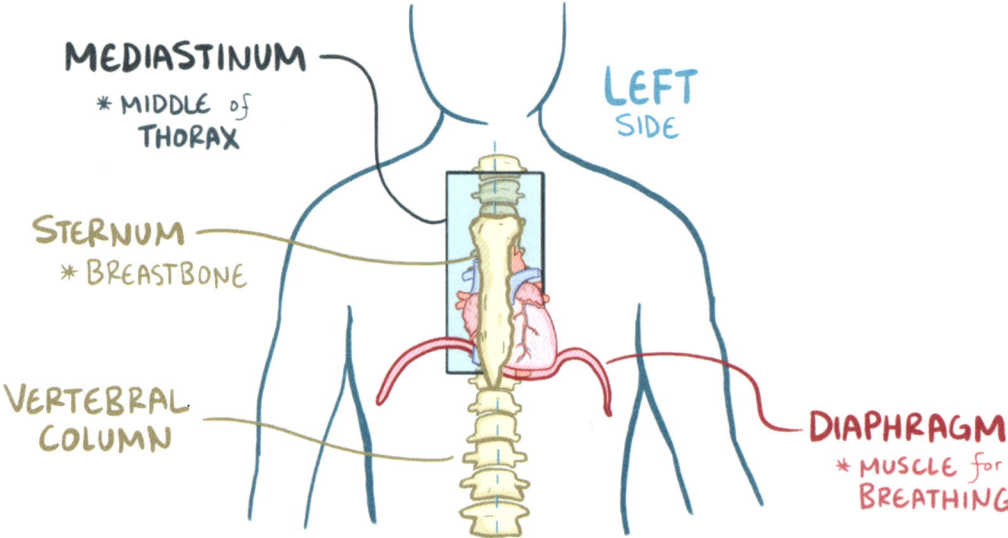

12   OSMOSIS.ORG

Chapter 1 The Circulatory System

Figure 1.5

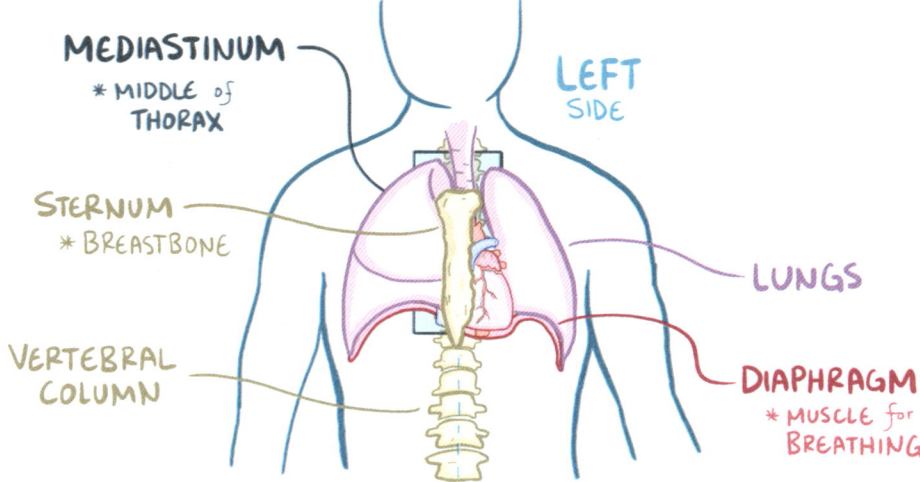

Figure 1.6

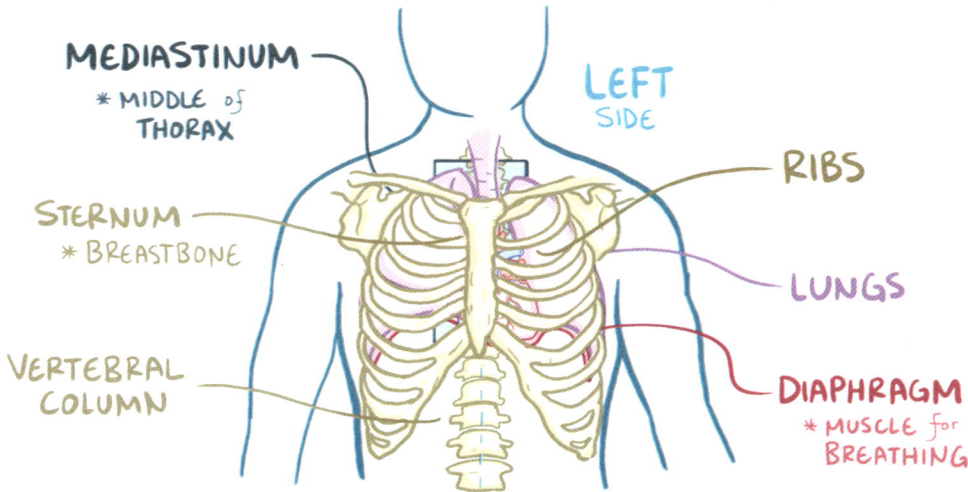

Figure 1.7

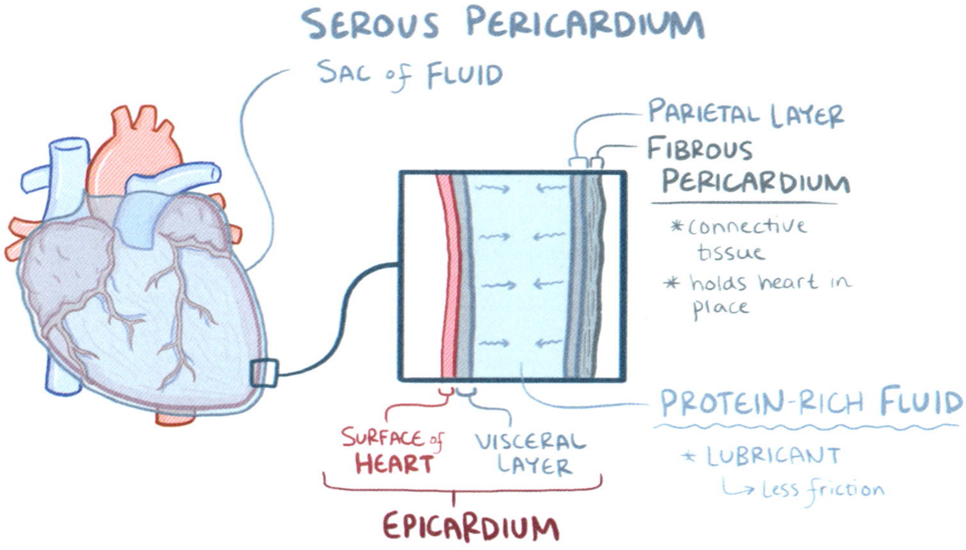

OSMOSIS.ORG 13

EPICARDIUM → MYOCARDIUM → ENDOCARDIUM

So, if we move from the outside to the inside of the heart, after the epicardium, we will find the myocardium, which is the muscular middle layer. This forms the bulk of the heart tissue, because these are the cardiac muscle cells that contract and pump blood. In addition to cardiac muscle cells, there are criss-crossing connective tissue fibers made of collagen. Together, they form the fibrous cardiac skeleton, which helps supports the muscle tissue. The myocardium also has dedicated blood vessels called coronary vessels. These lie on the outside of the heart and penetrate into the myocardium to bring blood to that layer, which needs a lot of energy in order to continue pumping blood. Finally, there's the innermost layer of the heart, called the endocardium, which is made of a relatively thin layer of endothelium—the same layer of cells lining the blood vessels. This endocardium lines the heart chambers and heart valves **(Figure 1.8)**.

PULMONARY CIRCULATION

Okay, so on the right side of the heart, deoxygenated blood enters via two different pathways. The first option is through the top, through a blood vessel called the superior vena cava. The second option is through the bottom, through a blood vessel called the inferior vena cava. Both pathways enter the right atrium (it's useful to know that "atrium" means "entryway.") Both vena cavae are veins which bring blood towards the heart. There's also a tiny third opening into the right atrium called the coronary sinus, which collects blood from coronary vessels returning from the myocardium **(Figure 1.9)**.

Now, all of that blood then goes through the first of two atrioventricular valves separating the atria from the ventricles. This first valve is the tricuspid valve, and it allows blood into the right ventricle. The tricuspid valve has three little flaps or "cusps." Each cusp looks kind of like a parachute because it has tiny little strings called chordae tendineae projecting from it. These tether the cusp to a small muscle called a papillary muscle. When the heart contracts, the papillary muscle keeps the chordae tendineae taut. This helps to prevent regurgitation of blood back into the atrium, allowing it to flow out the next valve **(Figure 1.10)**.

The contraction pumps the blood out the pulmonary valve and, like the tricuspid valve, the pulmonary valve has three cusps. It, too, prevents blood from going backwards. Unlike the tricuspid valve, however, the pulmonary valve doesn't have any of those chordae tendineae. Once the blood is past the pulmonary valve, it enters the pulmonary arteries, which carry the blood away from the heart to the left and right lung. You just need to remember that arteries start with "a" and carry blood "**away**" from the heart **(Figure 1.11)**!

Figure 1.8

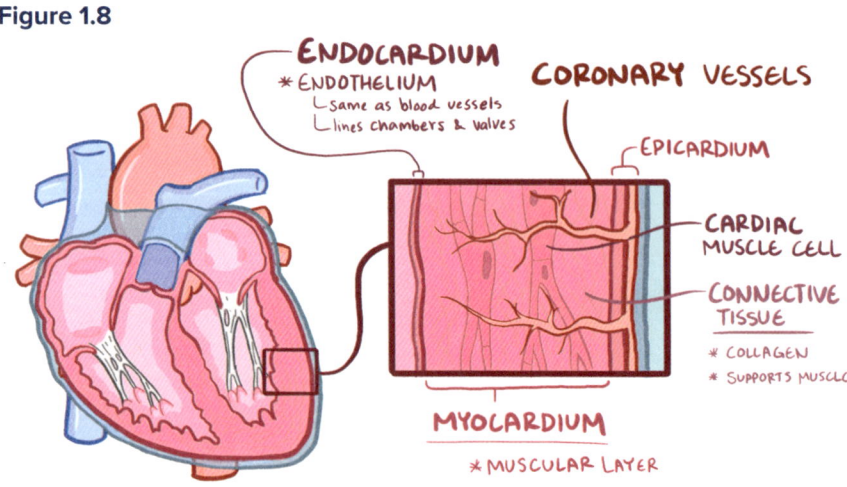

14   OSMOSIS.ORG

Chapter 1 The Circulatory System

Figure 1.9

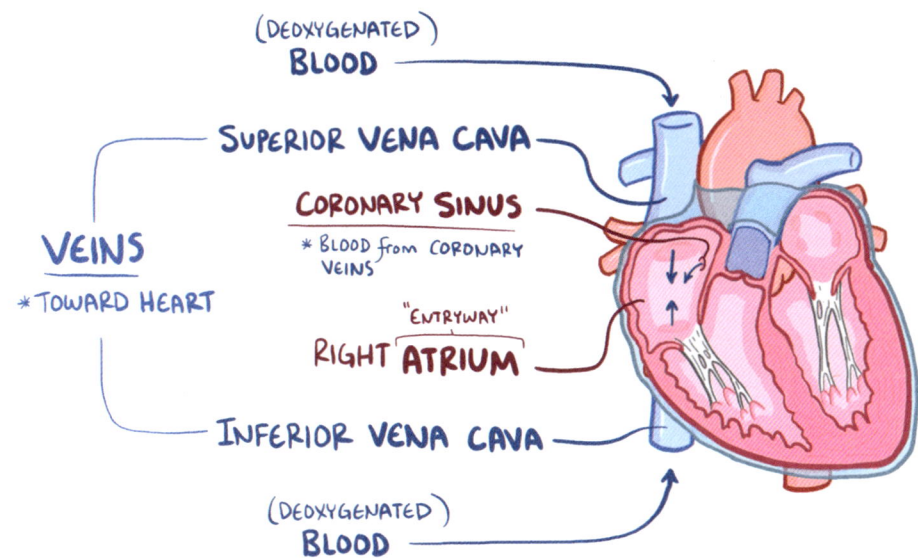

Figure 1.10

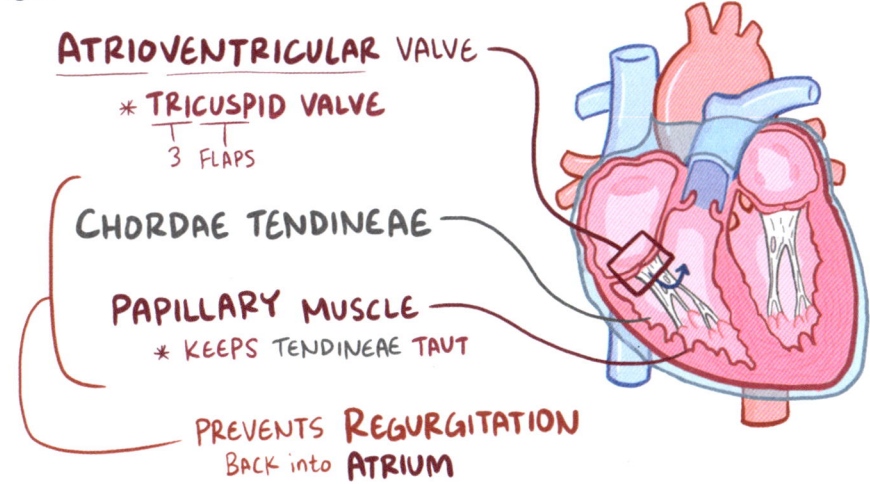

Figure 1.11

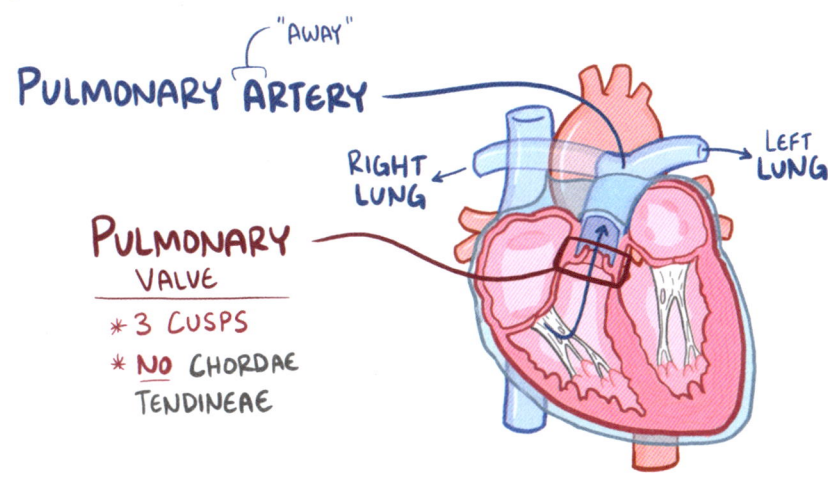

OSMOSIS.ORG 15

The blood goes from the pulmonary artery into a pulmonary arteriole, which is a bit smaller, and finally into a capillary, which is the smallest. In the lungs, the capillary lines up alongside a small sack of air called an alveolus (more commonly seen in the plural form, alveoli.) Up until now the blood has been loaded with carbon dioxide, which makes the blood look dark red rather than blue—which is how it's usually drawn and how we'll continue to draw it as such in order to remain consistent. Now, at this point in the journey, the carbon dioxide moves from the capillary to the alveolus and oxygen moves from the alveolus to the capillary, giving the blood that nice bright red color **(Figure 1.12)**.

In the blood, each red blood cell has millions of hemoglobin proteins and each of these hemoglobins can bind to four oxygen molecules. This means each red blood cell can carry millions of oxygen molecules when fully loaded! The oxygen-rich blood moves into a venule and then eventually into a pulmonary vein which dumps the blood into the left atrium. This entire trip—from the right ventricle of the heart, through the pulmonary artery, to the lungs, and back to the left atrium of the heart—is called pulmonary circulation **(Figure 1.13)**.

SYSTEMIC CIRCULATION

After entering the left atrium, the blood goes through the second atrioventricular valve, called the mitral valve, and into the left ventricle. The mitral valve has only two cusps or leaflets: one in front called the anterior leaflet, which is a little smaller; and one behind it called the posterior leaflet. Both of these have chordae tendineae projecting from them that tether the valve to papillary muscles in the left ventricle. Similar to the right side of the heart, the contraction prevents blood from going backwards **(Figure 1.14)**.

Finally, blood in the left ventricle gets pumped out through the aortic valve, which normally has three cusps, out to the aorta—the largest artery in the body. Just like in the lungs, the aorta branches into arterioles, which are smaller arteries, and finally into capillaries, which are the smallest. At this point, we've arrived at the organs and tissues. In the organs, the red blood cells line up alongside tissue cells and drop off oxygen and pick up carbon dioxide—basically the reverse of what happened with the alveolus in the lung. Loaded up with carbon dioxide, the blood turns that dark red color again, shown as blue in our illustrations, and starts the return journey to the heart: travelling through small venules and then larger veins. Now, the lower half of the body drains into the inferior vena cava, and the upper half drains into the superior vena cava, both of which dump blood back into the right atrium **(Figure 1.15)**.

Figure 1.12

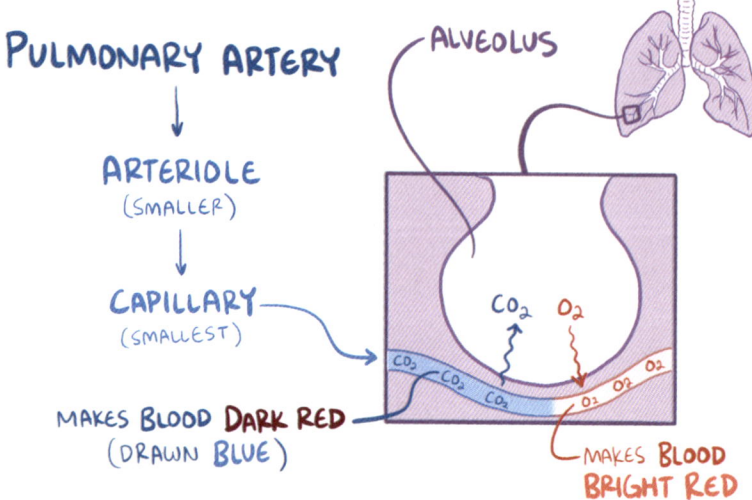

Chapter 1 The Circulatory System

Figure 1.13

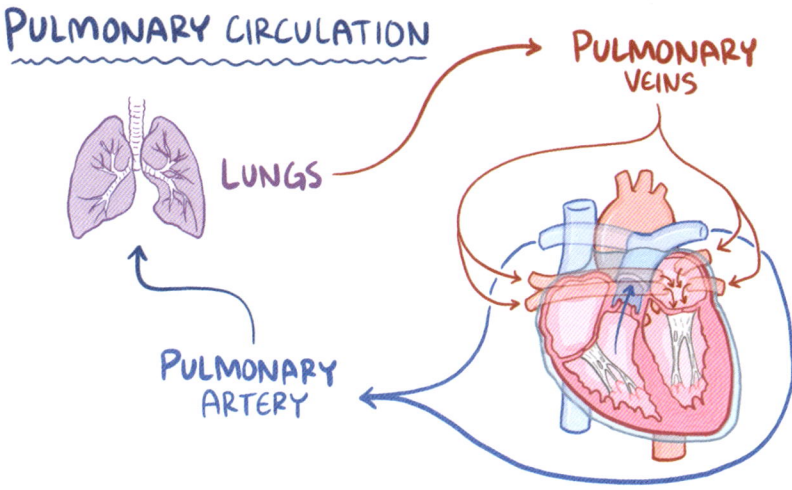

Figure 1.14

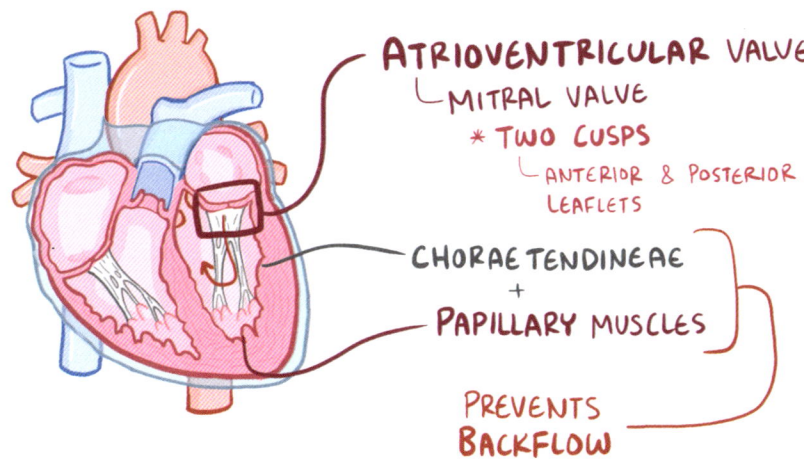

Figure 1.15

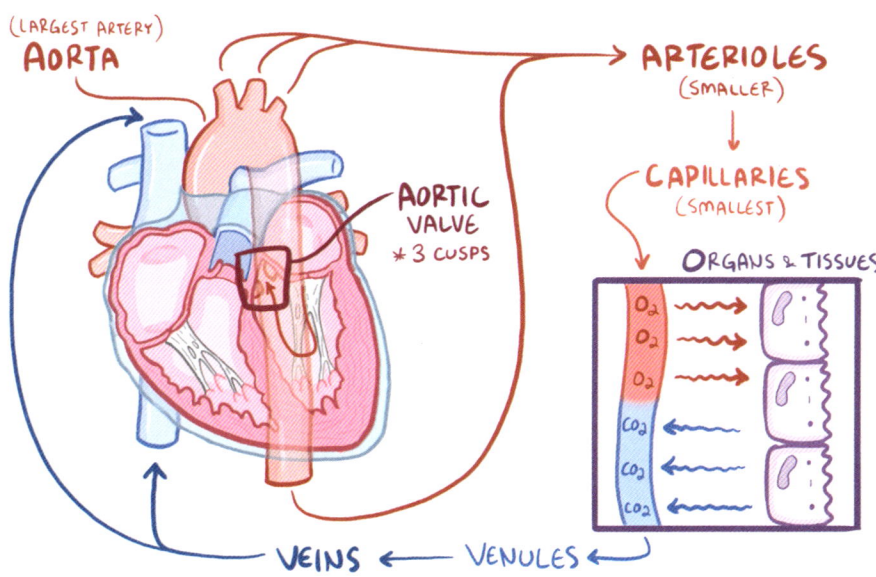

OSMOSIS.ORG 17

Figure 1.16

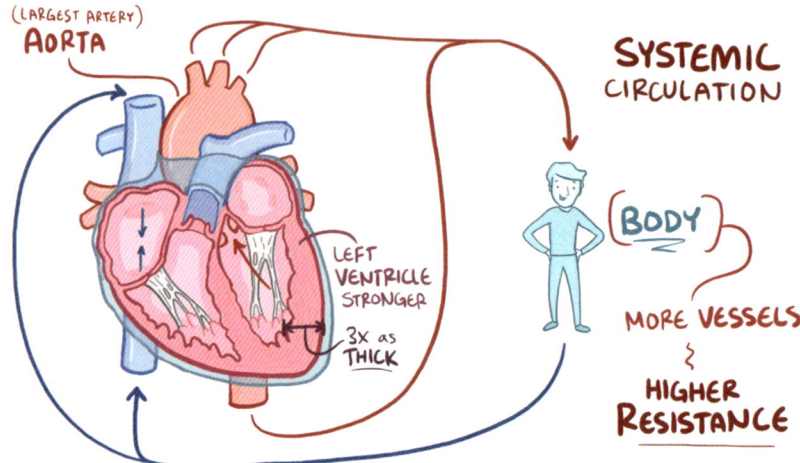

This trip—from the left ventricle of the heart, through the body, and back to the right atrium of the heart—is called the systemic circulation. Now, relative to pulmonary circulation, systemic circulation includes many more blood vessels, which means there's about a five times greater resistance to blood flow. Basically, it's a lot harder to pump blood through, even though it's the same amount of blood being pumped. Because of this difference, the left ventricle needs to be stronger, so the muscular layer of the left ventricle wall—or its myocardium—is three times thicker than the myocardium of the right ventricle **(Figure 1.16)**.

HEARTBEAT

Okay, so let's talk about that pumping. Every heartbeat sounds something like this: "lub dub, lub dub, lub dub." The first heart sound, that "lub," is called S1. The noise comes from the tricuspid and mitral valves snapping shut when the left and right ventricles contract, which happens at about the same time. Right after the S1 sound, the aortic valve and pulmonary valve open, allowing blood to be pushed out to the body. This period of time is called systole.

Next up is the second heart sound, that "dub," which is called S2. The noise comes from the aortic and pulmonic valves snapping shut to prevent blood from flowing backwards after it leaves the ventricles. This effectively ends the systole. Right after the S2 sound, the tricuspid and mitral valves open back up, allowing blood to fill the ventricles again. This period of time is called diastole. And that's it!

Each heartbeat can be broken into systole and diastole. So systolic blood pressure is the pressure in the arteries when the ventricles are squeezing out blood under high pressure, and diastolic blood pressure is when the ventricles are filling up with more blood under slightly lower pressure **(Figure 1.17)**.

CARDIAC OUTPUT & VENOUS RETURN

All right, let's simplify things. First, the amount of blood pumped out by either ventricle over a period of time is called the cardiac output. Second, the rate at which the veins return blood back to the atria is called venous return. Pretty easy to remember, right? Since the circulatory system is a closed loop, cardiac output and venous return are equal values **(Figure 1.18)**.

Okay, so let's use some numbers to make this a little more concrete. Let's say that about 70 ml are ejected per squeeze, with a heart rate of 70 beats per minute or 70 squeezes per minute. In this case, 70 × 70 is 4,900 ml per minute. This means the heart's pumping about 4.9 L per minute **(Figure 1.19)**.

Chapter 1 The Circulatory System

Figure 1.17

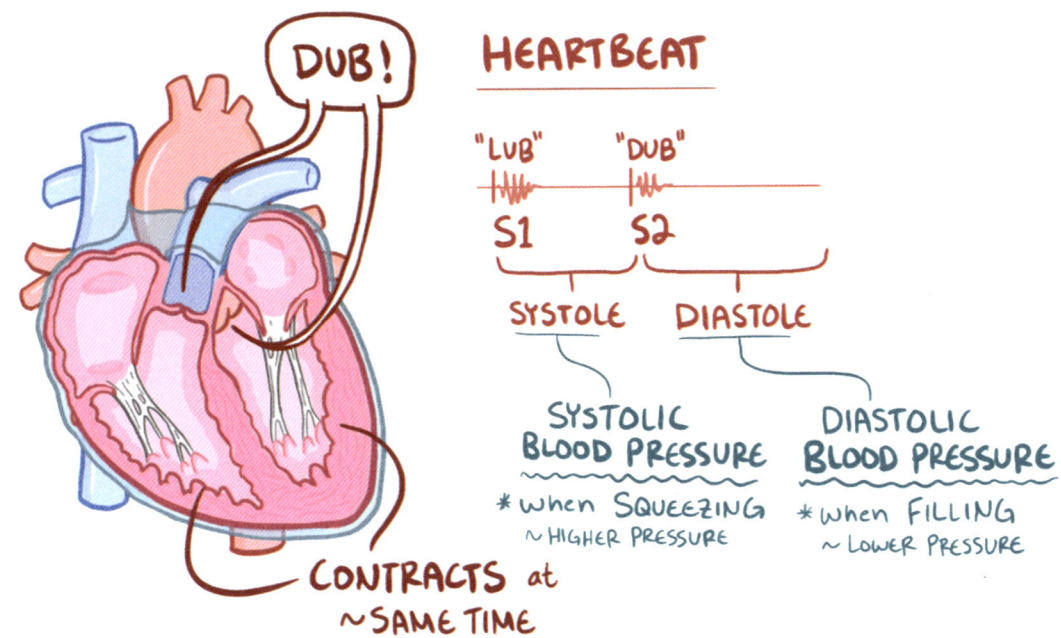

Figure 1.18

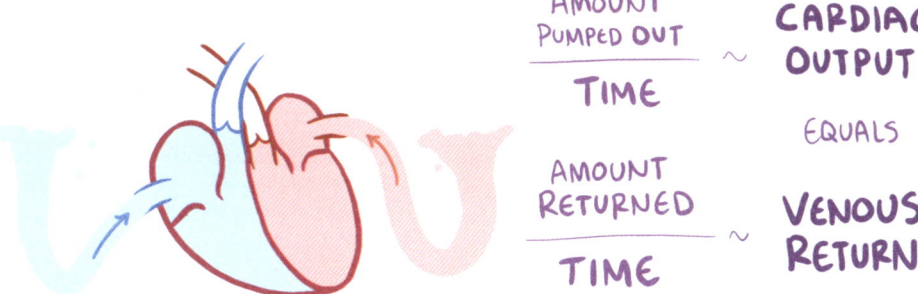

Figure 1.19

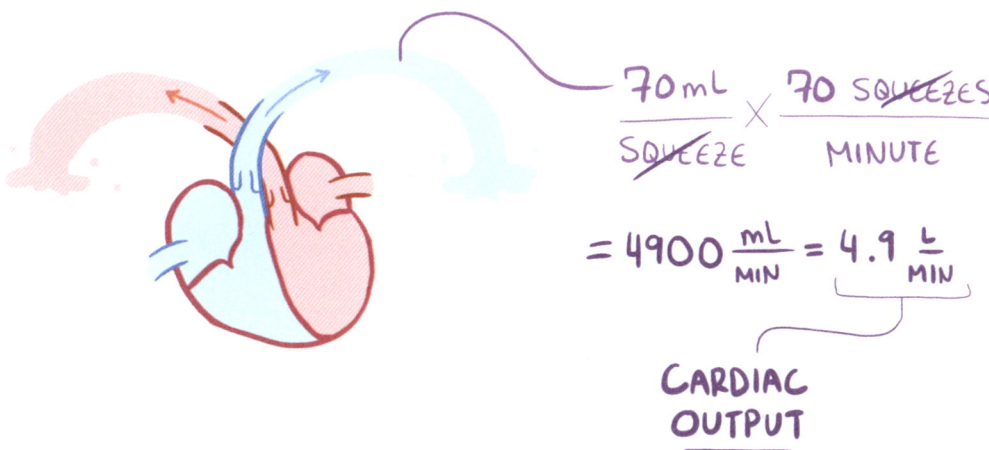

OSMOSIS.ORG 19

Now, in an average adult there's about 5 L of blood total in the body—which, just to be clear, is different from the cardiac output, or the amount pumped per minute, we just found. If we take this total volume of 5 L, 10% of that (or about 0.5 L) is in the pulmonary arteries, capillaries, and veins, which make up the pulmonary circulation. Meanwhile, another 5% (or 0.25 L) is in one of the four chambers of the heart itself.

Another 15% (or 0.75 L) is in the systemic arteries, travelling away from the heart, while yet another 5% (or 0.25 L) is in the systemic capillaries. The remaining 65% (or 3.25 L) is in the systemic veins returning to the heart **(Figure 1.20)**.

Now, where does all of that systemic arterial blood go? About 15% goes to the brain, 5% nourishes the heart itself, 25% goes to the kidneys, another 25% goes to the gastrointestinal organs, yet another 25% goes to the skeletal muscles, and the last 5% goes to the skin. These numbers can change—as they might during exercise, for example—but these figures should give you a general sense of things **(Figure 1.21)**.

So that was the systemic arterial blood, but you'll notice that there's a lot more blood in the systemic veins. That being said, arteries are generally lower volume while also being under much higher pressure. In contrast, veins are high volume, low pressure vessels. This explains why arteries and veins have different structures. For example, veins often have valves to help fight gravity and keep blood flowing in one direction back to the heart, whereas arteries don't need these valves because they're under such high pressure **(Figure 1.22)**.

BLOOD VESSELS

If we take a closer look at the blood vessels, we'll see they have three layers, also called "tunics" or coverings, that surround the vessel lumen—the hollow part of the vessel that contains the blood. The innermost tunic is the tunica intima, which includes the endothelial cells. These create a slick surface that minimizes friction for blood moving through. Next, there's the tunica media, or middle tunic, which is mostly made of smooth muscle cells and of sheets of elastin protein. Both the cells of the tunica intima and tunica media generally get the nutrients they need from the blood in the lumen. Finally, there's the tunica externa, or outside tunic, which is made up of loosely woven fibers of collagen protein that protect and reinforce the blood vessel and anchor it in place. The tunica externa also has nerve fibers, lymphatic vessels, and, in the biggest vessels, elastin.

Figure 1.20

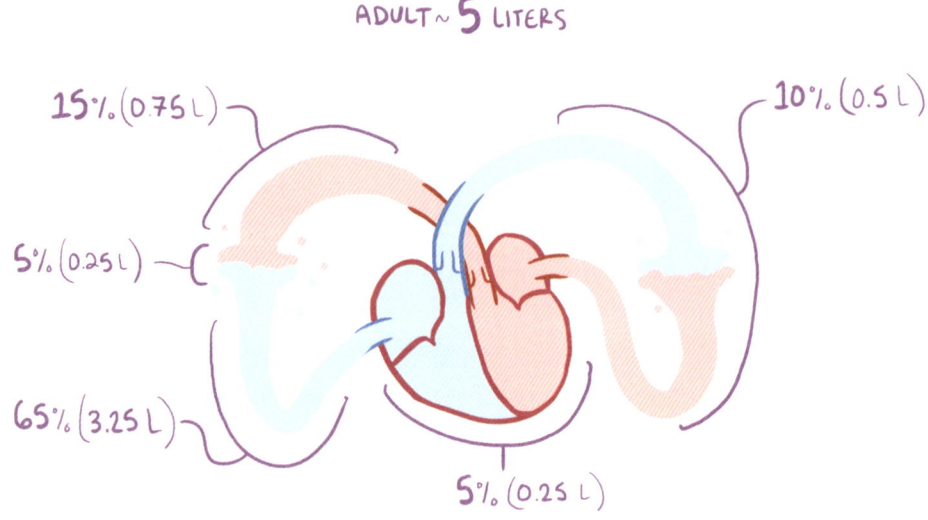

Chapter 1 The Circulatory System

Figure 1.21

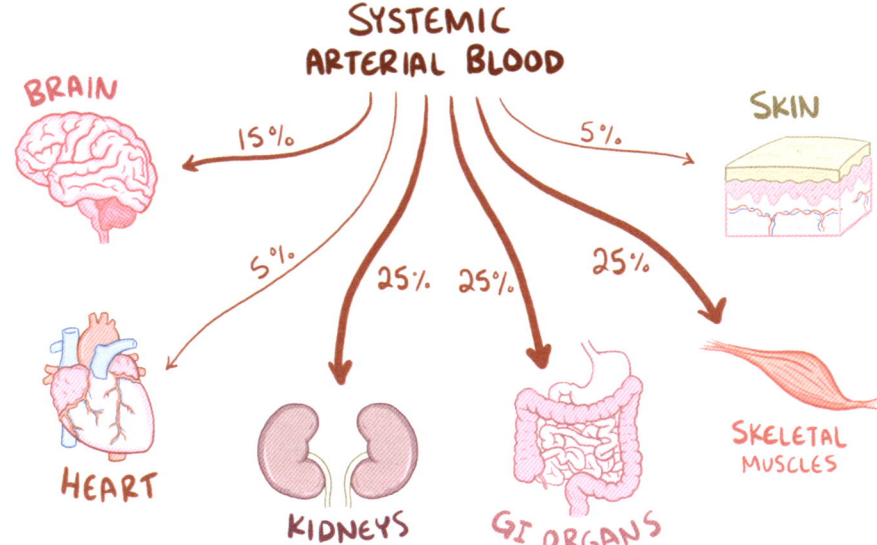

Figure 1.22

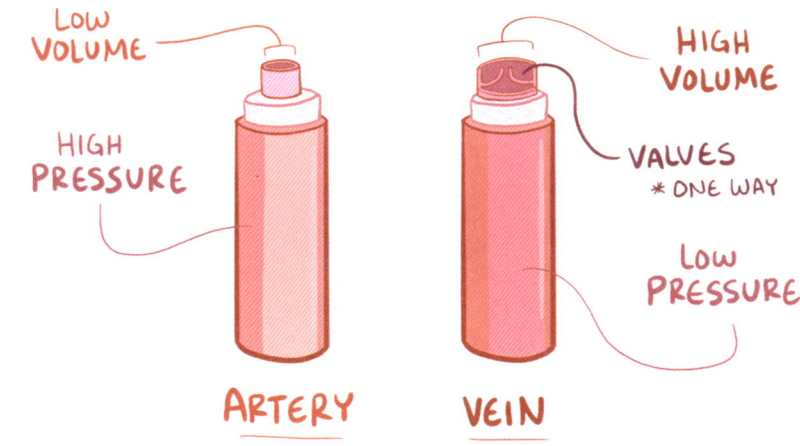

Figure 1.23

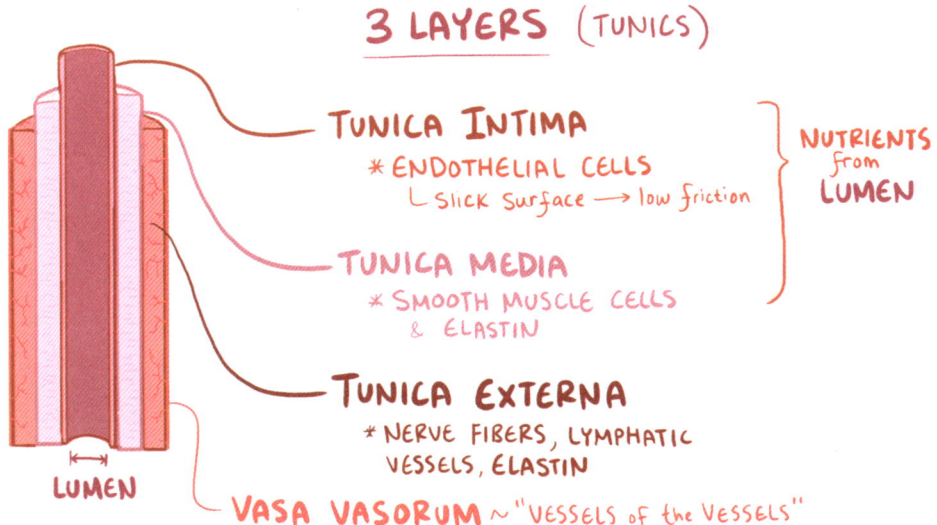

OSMOSIS.ORG 21

Want to know something really wild? Some huge vessels have a tunica externa that is so thick it needs its own blood supply! In these cases, there are tiny blood vessels—called the vasa vasorum, which mean "vessels of the vessels"—that creep along the tunica externa to bring nutrients to that layer of the blood vessel wall **(Figure 1.23)**.

If we take a closer look at the arteries, we'll find that the largest arteries are closest to the heart—the aorta, its main branches, and the pulmonary arteries. They have so much elastin in their tunica externa and media that they're also known as the elastic arteries. These arteries are really stretchy—think of spandex!—and this elasticity allows these arteries to keep their shape, as well as to absorb and even out the systolic and diastolic pressures **(Figure 1.24)**.

These arteries eventually branch into the arterioles, the smallest of the arteries. In the arterioles, the tunica media is bulky, and can contract in response to hormones and the autonomic nervous system. In a process called vasoconstriction, the lumen becomes much smaller, which decreases the amount of blood sent to the capillary beds and, ultimately, to organs or tissues. In contrast, there is also the process of vasodilation, during which the vessels relax, or vasodilate, and the lumen's diameter widens, increasing blood flow **(Figure 1.25; Figure 1.26)**.

These processes assist with temperature control, or thermoregulation. For instance, with the vasodilation of arterioles, blood flow increases and more heat is lost through the surface of the skin, lowering body temperature. In contrast, with the vasoconstriction of arterioles, blood flow decreases and less heat is lost through the skin's surface, raising body temperature **(Figure 1.27; Figure 1.28)**.

Figure 1.24

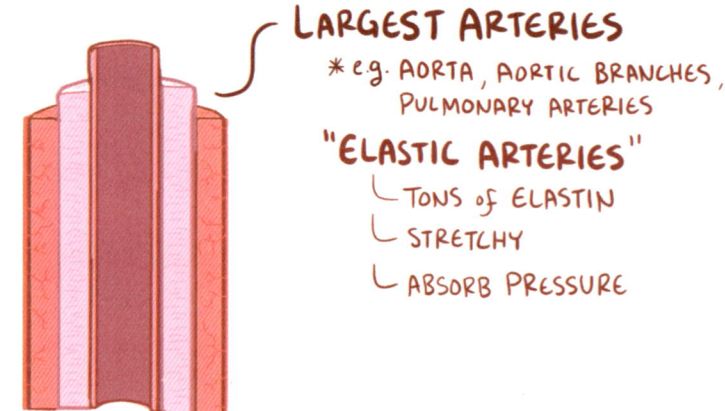

Figure 1.25

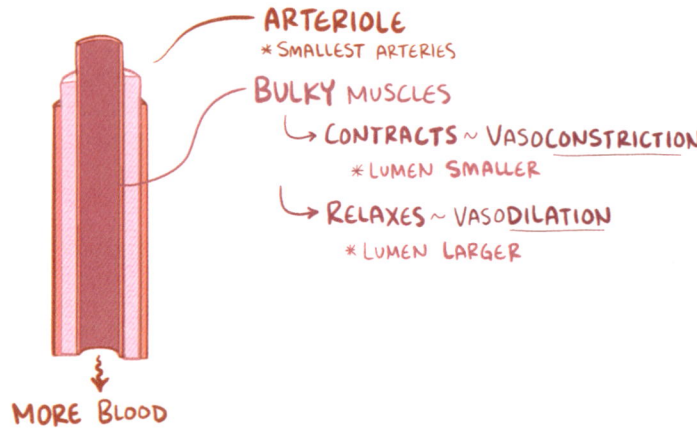

Figure 1.26

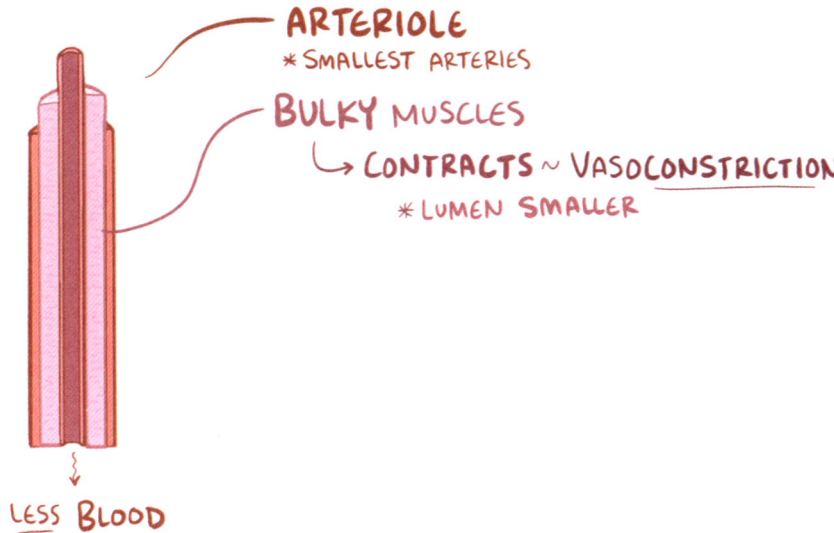

Figure 1.27

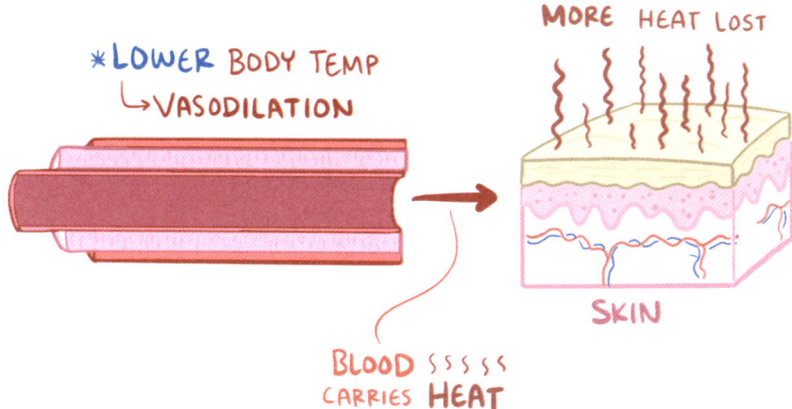

Figure 1.28

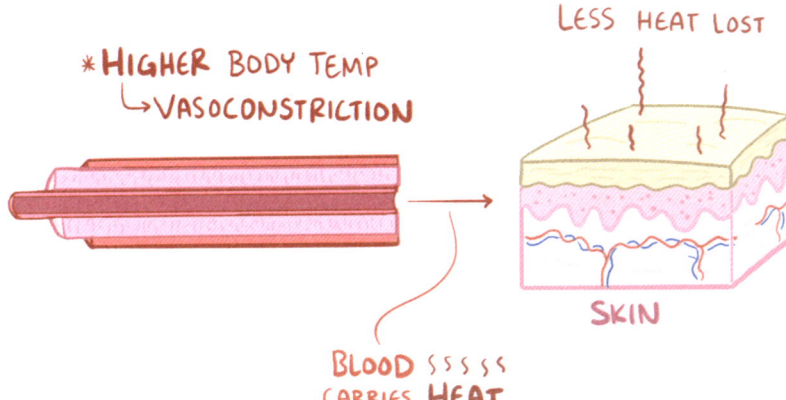

Finally, the capillary walls are generally only one cell thick. They are made up of just the tunica intima layer, with some larger vessels that also have a subendothelial basement membrane—a layer of protein just outside of the endothelial cells that provides extra support **(Figure 1.29)**.

In addition to allowing oxygen and carbon dioxide to flow back and forth, capillaries are also where nutrients like glucose are delivered. Capillaries are also where fluid can move out of the blood vessel and into the interstitial space—the space between the blood vessels and cells. Water-soluble substances, like ions, cross the capillary wall: either through water-filled spaces, called clefts, between the endothelial cells, or through large pores in the walls of fenestrated capillaries. Meanwhile, lipid-, or fat-soluble, molecules like oxygen and carbon dioxide can dissolve and then diffuse across the endothelial cell membranes. On the other end of the capillary bed, there's a venule. The arteriole and venule are usually directly connected by a vessel called the metarteriole **(Figure 1.30)**.

Whew—you made it! That's the end of the circulatory system!

Figure 1.29

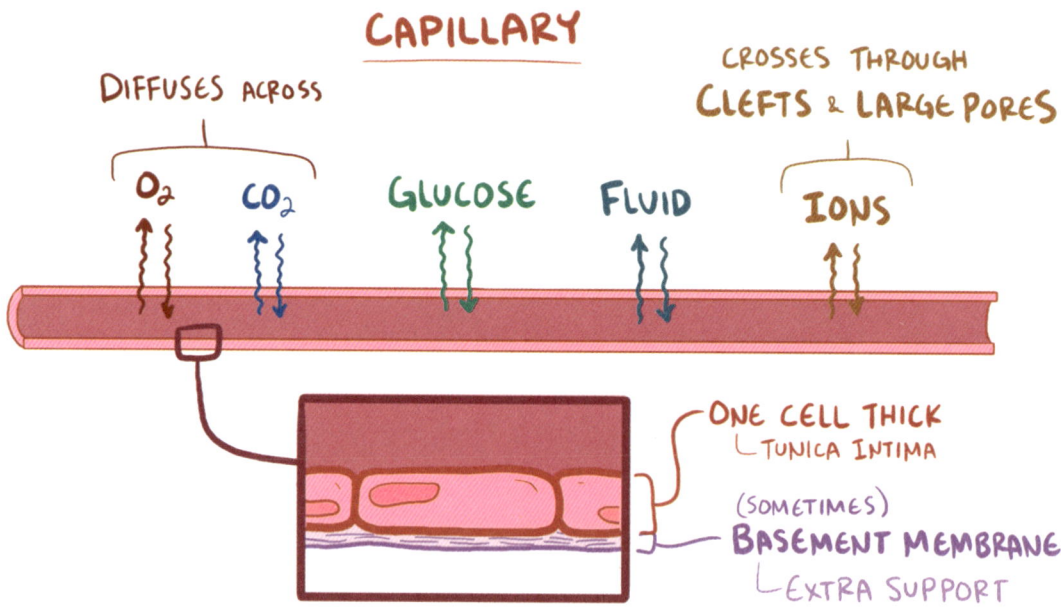

Figure 1.30

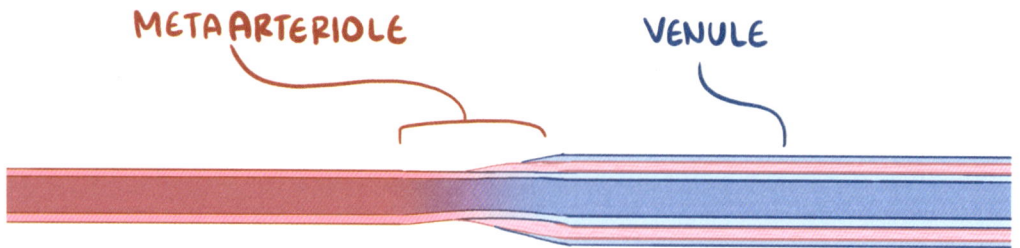

Chapter 1 The Circulatory System

SUMMARY

All right, as a quick recap, pulmonary circulation leaves the right ventricle, which delivers blood to the lungs, and then returns fresh oxygenated blood to the left atrium. At this point, the blood enters systemic circulation: starting with the left ventricle, which pumps blood to the body, until the deoxygenated blood returns to the right atrium. Then, it starts all over again **(Figure 1.31)**!

Figure 1.31

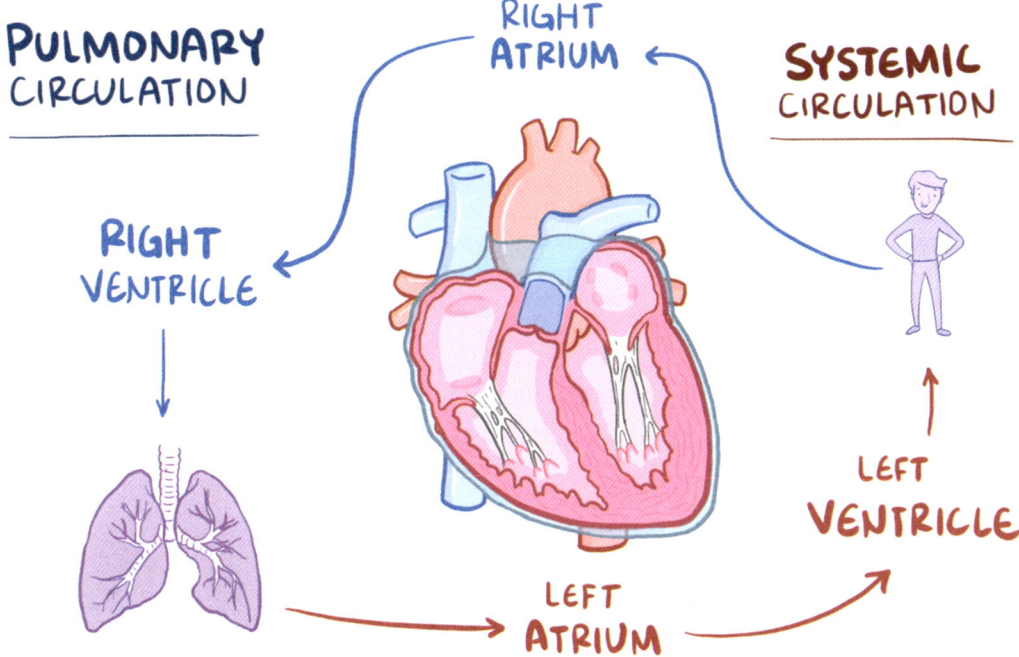

OSMOSIS.ORG 25

THE RENAL SYSTEM

osms.it/renal_system

The kidneys are the workhorses of the renal system, also known as the urinary system. These twin, bean-shaped organs clear harmful substances by filtering them out of your blood—you could think of them as a water purification plant that helps clean the drinking water for a city. They also regulate blood pH, volume, pressure, and osmolality, and also produce hormones.

The kidneys are located between the T12 and L3 vertebrae, and they're partially protected by ribs 11 and 12—the floating ribs **(Figure 2.1)**. The kidneys are roughly the size of a fist and are retroperitoneal, meaning they sit behind the peritoneal membrane alongside the vertebral column **(Figure 2.2)**. The right kidney is pushed down by the liver, so it sits slightly lower than the left kidney. In the middle of each kidney is an indentation that forms the renal hilum. This is the entry and exit point for the ureter, renal artery, renal vein, lymphatics, and nerves. The kidney is surrounded by three layers of tissue. On the outside is the renal fascia, which is a thin layer of dense connective tissue that anchors the kidney to its surroundings. The middle layer, the adipose capsule, is a fatty layer that protects the kidney from trauma. The deepest layer, called the renal capsule, is a smooth transparent sheet of dense connective tissue that gives the kidney its distinctive shape **(Figure 2.3)**.

Figure 2.1

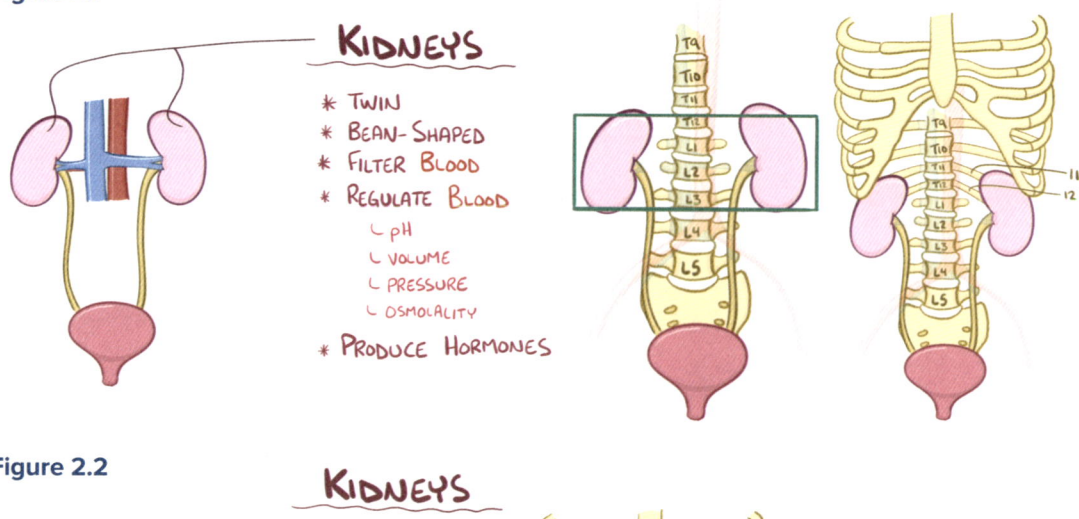

Figure 2.2

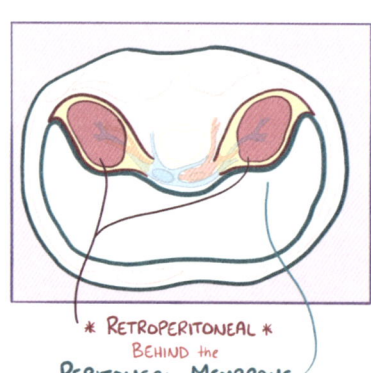
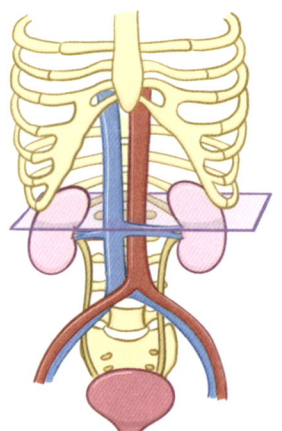

Chapter 2 The Renal System

If you take a cross-section of the kidney, there are two main parts: the inner portion and the outer rim. The inner portion is the renal medulla and the outer rim is the renal cortex. The medulla is made up of 10 to 18 renal pyramids. The base of the pyramids faces the renal cortex, and the tips of the pyramids—the renal papilla or nipples—point towards the center of the kidney. The renal papilla project into minor calyces, which join together to form major calyces, which funnel into the renal pelvis. Urine collects in the renal pelvis and then heads out of the kidney through the ureter.

The renal cortex can be divided into an outer cortical zone and an inner juxtamedullary zone. There are also sections of the cortex called renal columns, which extend down into the medulla separating the renal pyramids from one another. Each renal pyramid, as well as the renal cortex above, is called a renal lobe **(Figure 2.4)**.

BLOOD FILTRATION

So, an adult's kidneys filter about 150 liters of blood every day. If we assume that there are 5 liters of blood in the body, the entire blood volume gets filtered about 30 times a day, which is more than once every hour. Because of this, the kidneys account for a quarter of our entire cardiac output, which is the blood being pumped out of the left ventricle **(Figure 2.5)**.

To reach the kidneys, blood flows from the aorta into the left and right renal arteries. As these renal arteries enter the kidney, they divide into segmental arteries and then into interlobar arteries, which pass through the renal columns. They then divide into arcuate arteries, which travel over the bases of the renal pyramids, and then into cortical radiate arteries, which supply blood to the cortex. The cortical radiate arteries continue to divide, eventually forming afferent arterioles, which split into a tiny bundle of capillaries called the glomerulus. The glomerulus—plural glomeruli—is the site where blood filtration starts.

Interestingly, once the blood leaves these glomeruli, it does not enter into venules. Instead, the glomerulus funnels blood into efferent arterioles, which divide into capillaries a second time. These peritubular capillaries then reunite to become the cortical radiate veins, then the arcuate veins, then the interlobar veins, and finally the left and right renal veins, which connect to the inferior vena cava. This flow of veins is similar to that of the arteries, but in reverse. The only difference is that there's a segmental artery but there's no segmental vein **(Figure 2.6)**.

Figure 2.3

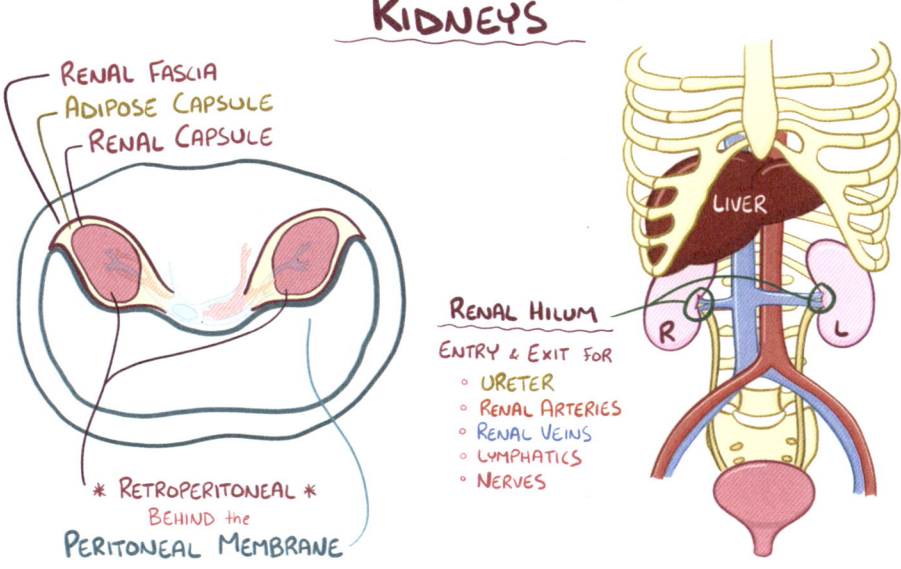

Figure 2.4

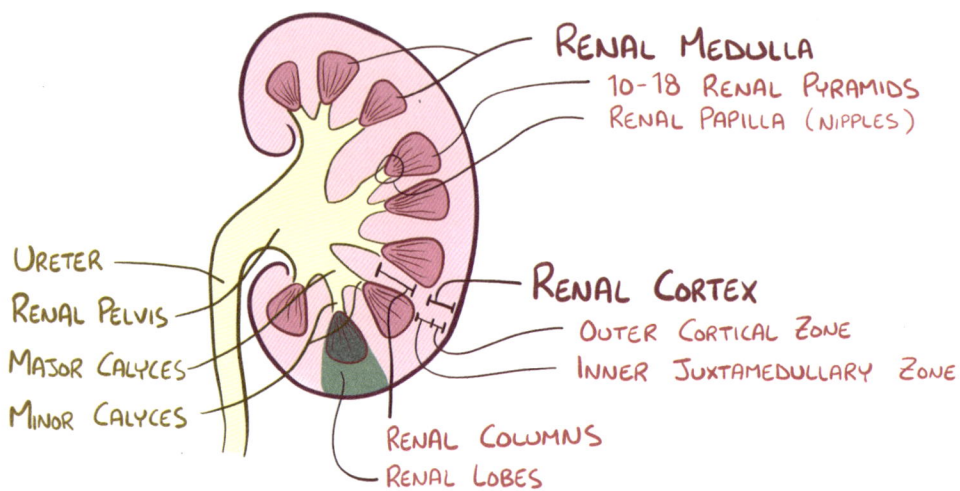

Figure 2.5

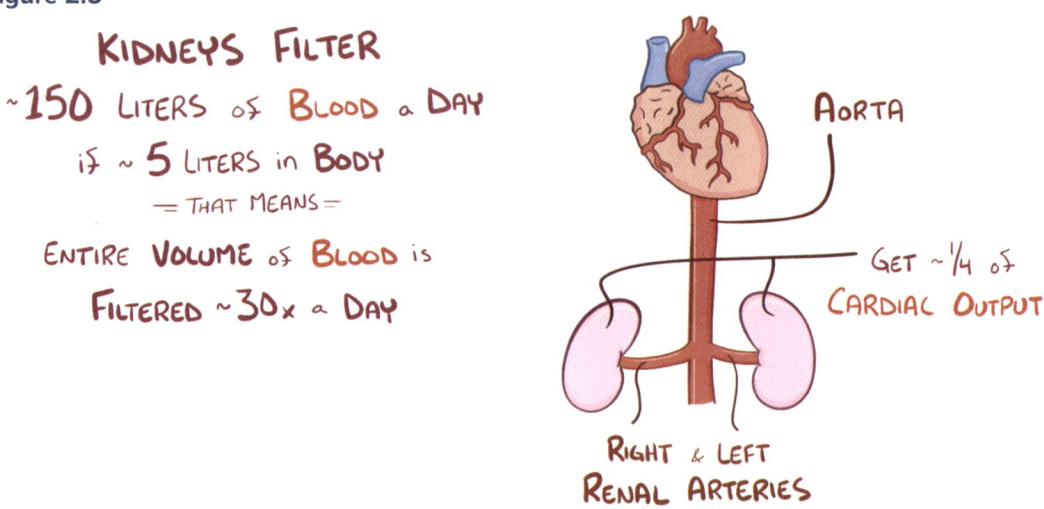

Figure 2.6

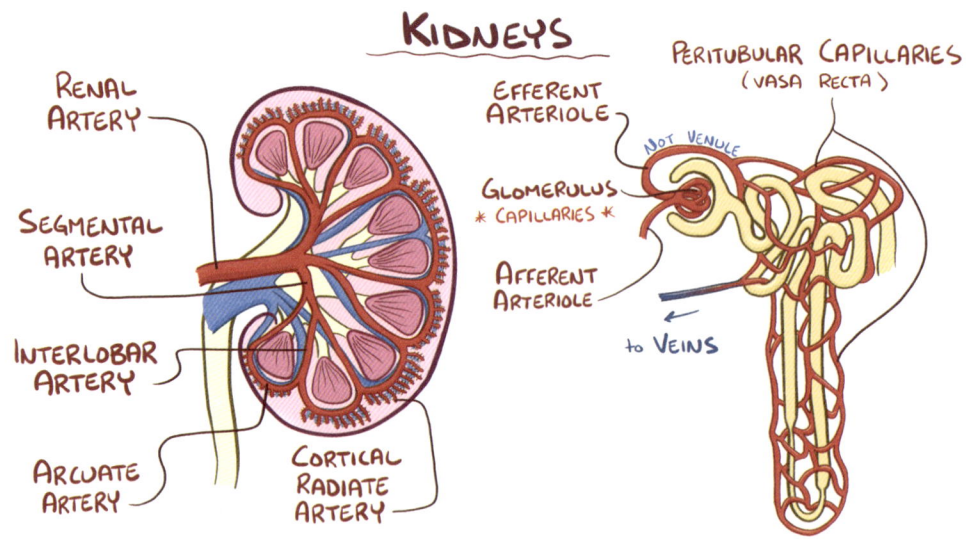

Chapter 2 The Renal System

Figure 2.7

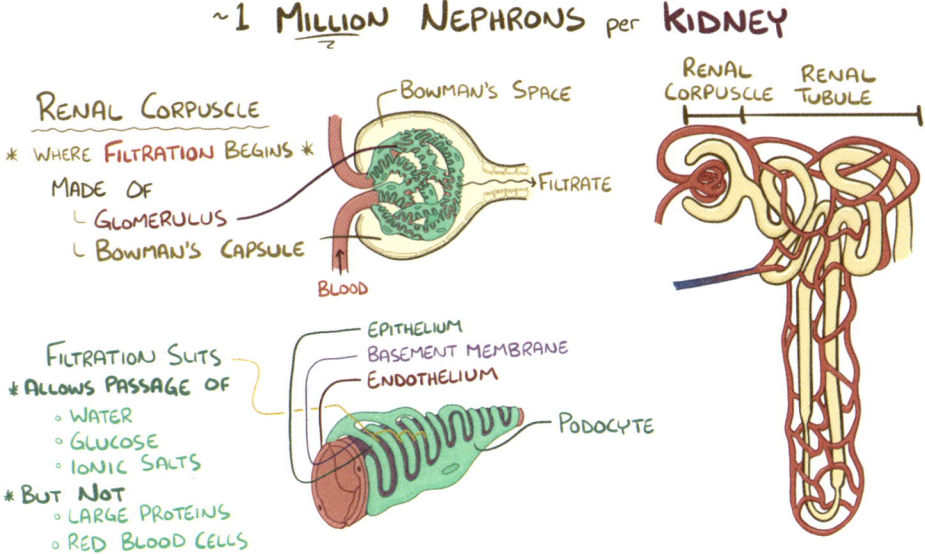

Figure 2.8

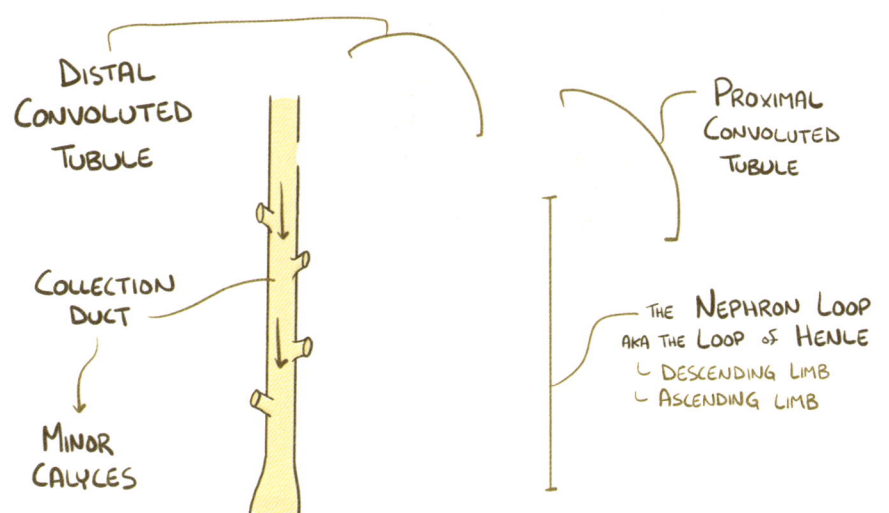

Figure 2.9

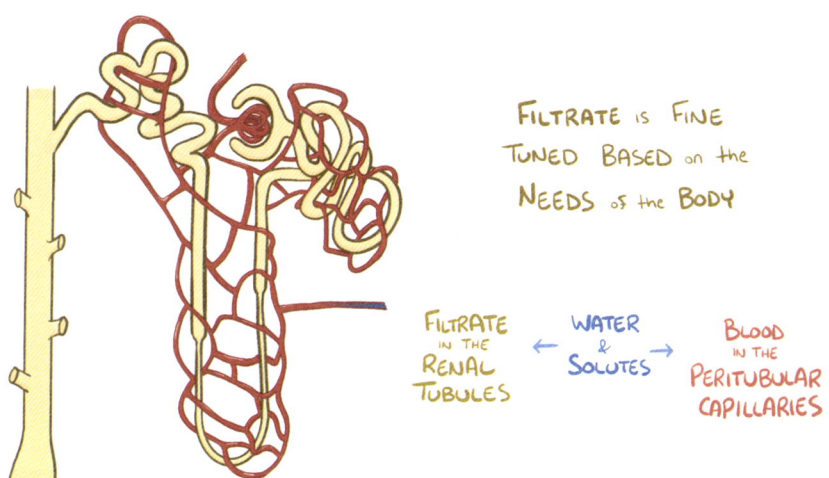

OSMOSIS.ORG 29

NEPHRONS

Within each kidney, there are about one million nephrons, and each nephron is made up of a renal corpuscle and a renal tubule. The renal corpuscle is where blood filtration starts. It includes the glomerulus, which is the tiny bed of capillaries, and the Bowman's capsule, which is the renal cells that surround the glomerulus.

As blood flows into the glomerulus, water and some solutes in the blood—like sodium—are able to pass through the endothelial lining of the capillary, move across the basement membrane through the epithelial lining of the nephron, and finally enter the Bowman's capsule of the nephron itself. At this point, it is called the filtrate. The epithelium of the nephron is made of specialized cells called podocytes, which wrap around the basement membrane like the tentacles of an octopus. Between these tentacle-like projections are tiny gaps called filtration slits, which act like a sieve allowing only small particles—such as water, glucose and ionic salts—to pass through while blocking large proteins and red blood cells **(Figure 2.7)**.

As the filtrate leaves the Bowman's capsule, it flows into the renal tubule, which is surrounded by the peritubular capillaries. The renal tubule itself can be divided into the following parts: the proximal convoluted tubule; the nephron loop—also known as the loop of Henle—which is made up of the descending limb and the ascending limb; the distal convoluted tubule; and, finally, the collection ducts, which ultimately send the urine to the minor calyces **(Figure 2.8)**. Here, the filtrate becomes fine-tuned based on what the body wants to keep versus what it wants to discard, with water and solutes getting passed back and forth between the filtrate in the lumen of the renal tubule and the blood in the peritubular capillaries **(Figure 2.9)**.

Each nephron has a unique region called the juxtaglomerular complex, which is involved in the regulation of blood pressure and the glomerular filtration rate—the amount of blood that passes through the glomeruli each minute. The juxtaglomerular complex is located in between the distal convoluted tubule and the afferent arteriole. There are three types of cells in the juxtaglomerular complex: macula densa cells, juxtaglomerular cells, and extraglomerular mesangial cells **(Figure 2.10)**.

Figure 2.10

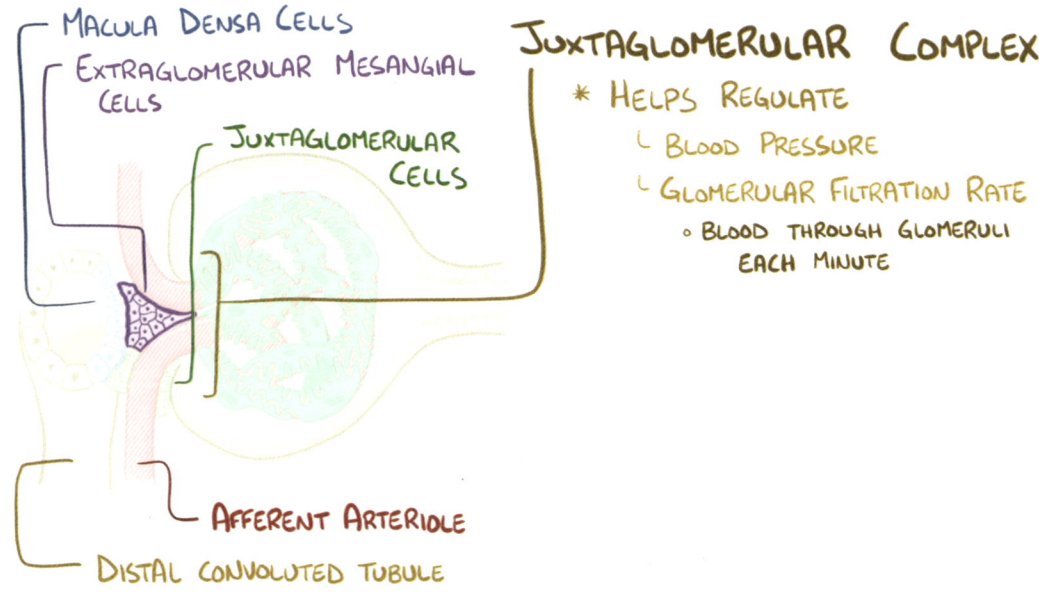

Chapter 2 The Renal System

Macula densa cells are located in the distal convoluted tubule and they can sense when levels of sodium and chloride are low. So, in the case of hypovolemia and hypotension, the macula densa cells sense the low sodium and chloride levels and send a signal to the juxtaglomerular cells, which are located in the wall of the afferent arteriole. The extraglomerular mesangial cells help with the signalling between macula densa cells and juxtaglomerular cells. The juxtaglomerular cells receive the signal. They also independently sense the low pressure in the blood vessels and secrete an enzyme called renin, which increases sodium reabsorption, which then helps raise the blood volume **(Figure 2.11)**. Renin also causes constriction of blood vessels, which helps raise blood pressure **(Figure 2.12)**.

Once millions of nephrons have each produced urine, it flows into the minor calyces, then the major calyces, and, finally, into the renal pelvis. From there, it goes down the ureter, which has a muscular lining, which helps to push urine along **(Figure 2.13)**. The ureter is inserted into the bladder at the ureterovesical junction at a sideways angle. This way, when the bladder becomes full, it compresses the openings to the ureter, preventing the backflow of urine. It's basically a one way valve that prevents urine from refluxing backwards from the bladder into the ureter **(Figure 2.14)**.

Figure 2.11

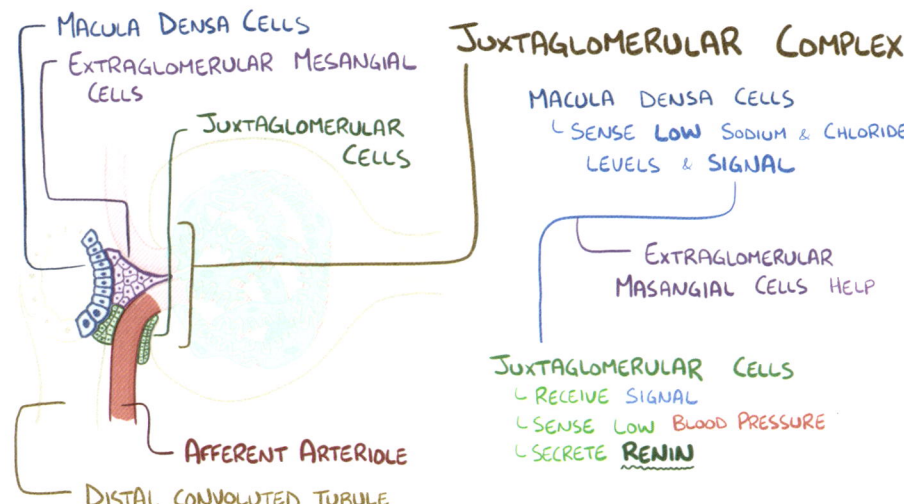

Figure 2.12

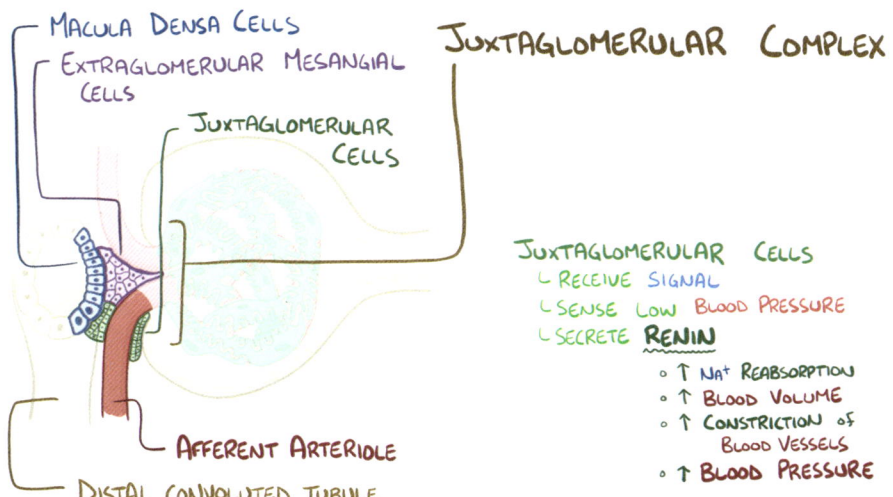

THE BLADDER

The bladder itself is like a balloon. Its muscular wall has many folds called rugae, which can contract when the bladder is emptied of urine and can expand when it is filled with urine. In the layers of the bladder wall is a mucosa layer with a transitional epithelium. This layer is stretchy, allowing for bladder distention while maintaining a barrier between urine and the body. In addition, there is a thick muscular layer called the detrusor muscle. It helps with bladder contraction during urination; it has a fibrous outer layer, the adventitia **(Figure 2.15)**.

In individuals who are biologically female, the bladder is in front of the vagina, uterus, and rectum. In individuals who are biologically male, the bladder is just in front of the rectum. On average, the bladder can hold around 750 millilitres of urine, or about the volume of a bottle of wine. This volume is slightly less in individuals who are biologically female because of crowding from the uterus, which is especially true during pregnancy **(Figure 2.16)**.

The floor of the bladder has a smooth triangular region called the trigone region, with two corners at the ureterovesical junctions and the third corner being the internal urethral orifice where the bladder meets the urethra. The trigone region is very sensitive to expansion and, once it stretches to a certain point, sends a signal to the brain—that it's time to pee **(Figure 2.17)**!

Figure 2.13

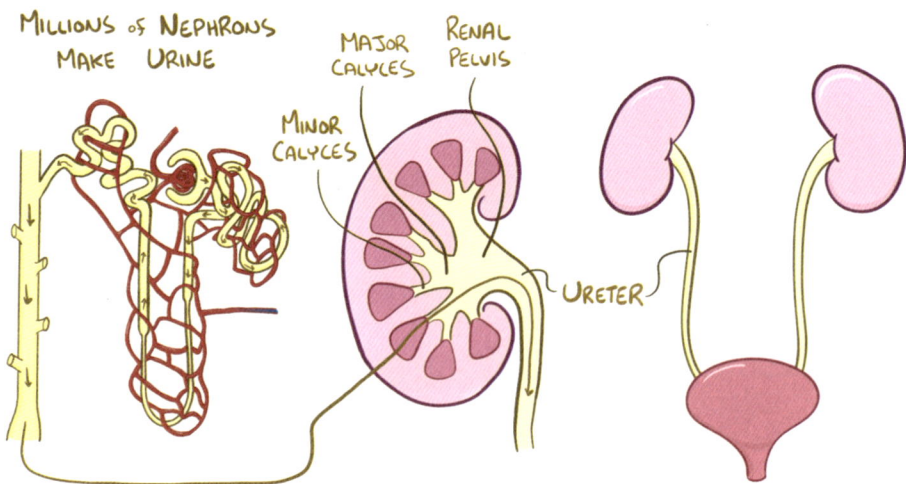

Figure 2.14

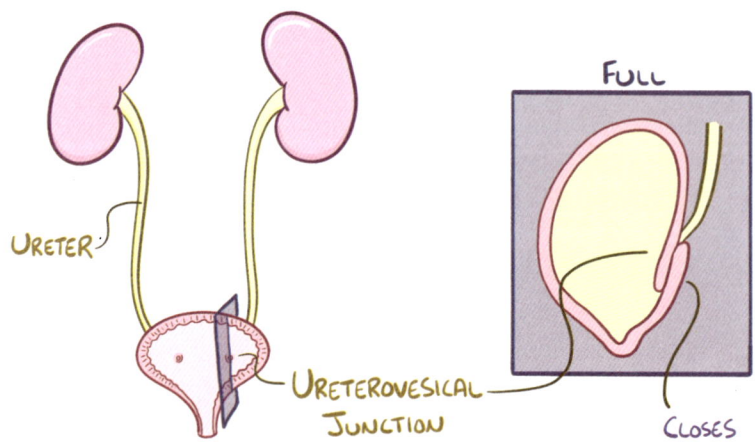

Figure 2.15

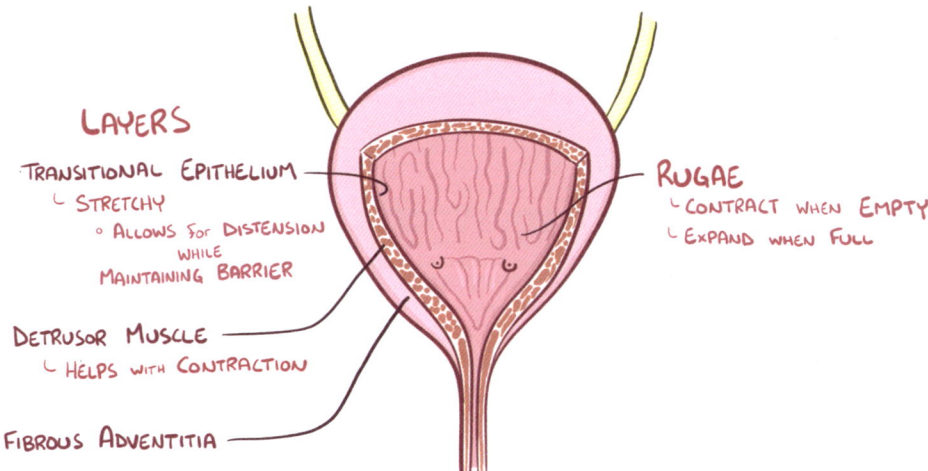

Figure 2.16

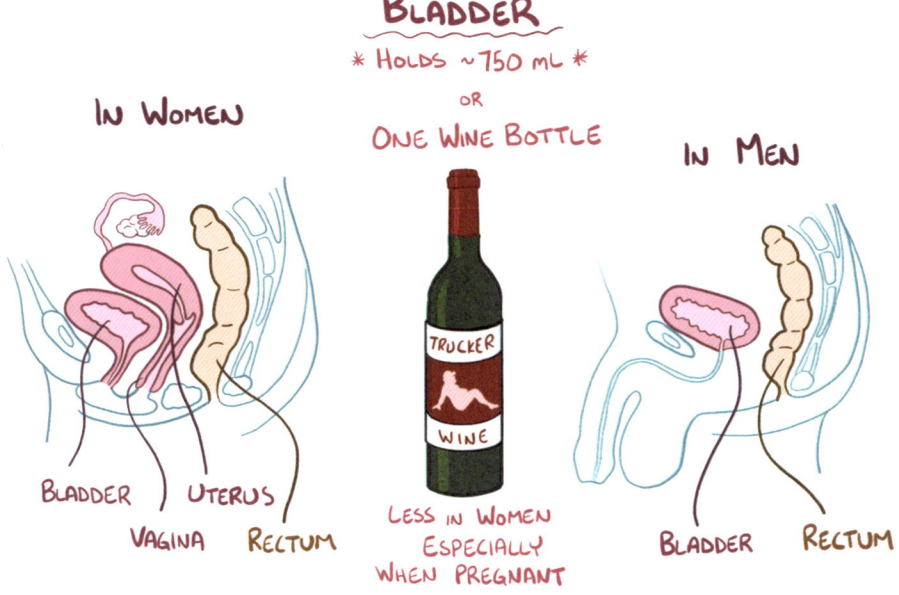

Figure 2.17

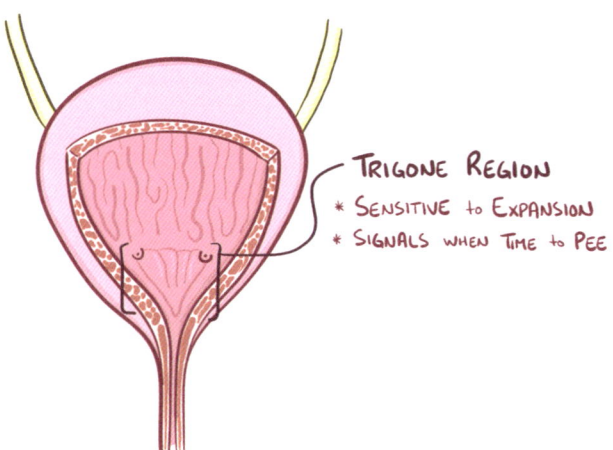

THE URETHRA

The urethra is a thin muscular tube that drains urine from the bladder, beginning at the internal urethral orifice and extending down to the external opening. In individuals who are biologically male, the urethra first passes through the prostate, where it is called the prostatic urethra; then it passes through deep muscles of the peritoneum, where it is called the intermediate urethra; and, finally, it passes through the penis, where it's called the spongy urethra. The male urethra is also used during ejaculation. In this case, however, semen enters into the urethra via the seminal vesicles. In individuals who are biologically female, the urethra runs through the perineal floor of the pelvis and exits between the two labia minora, above the vaginal opening and below the clitoris in an area called the vulval vestibule **(Figure 2.18)**.

Around the internal urethral orifice, the detrusor muscle thickens to form the internal sphincter. This involuntary sphincter is controlled by the autonomic nervous system and it keeps the urethra closed when the bladder isn't full. Additionally, there's an external sphincter, at the level of the urogenital diaphragm in the floor of the pelvis, which is under voluntary control. By contracting the skeletal muscles around the external sphincter, urination can be stopped voluntarily. This is called a Kegel exercise and it can be done to strengthen the pelvic floor.

Figure 2.18

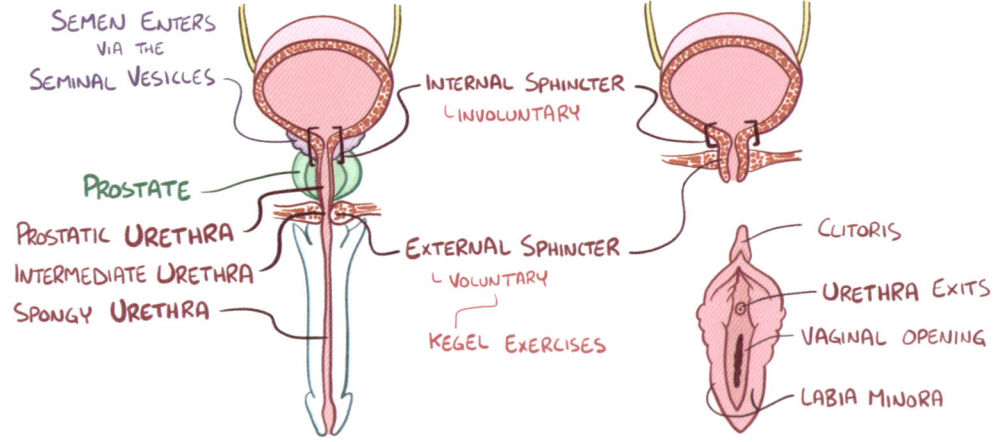

Figure 2.19

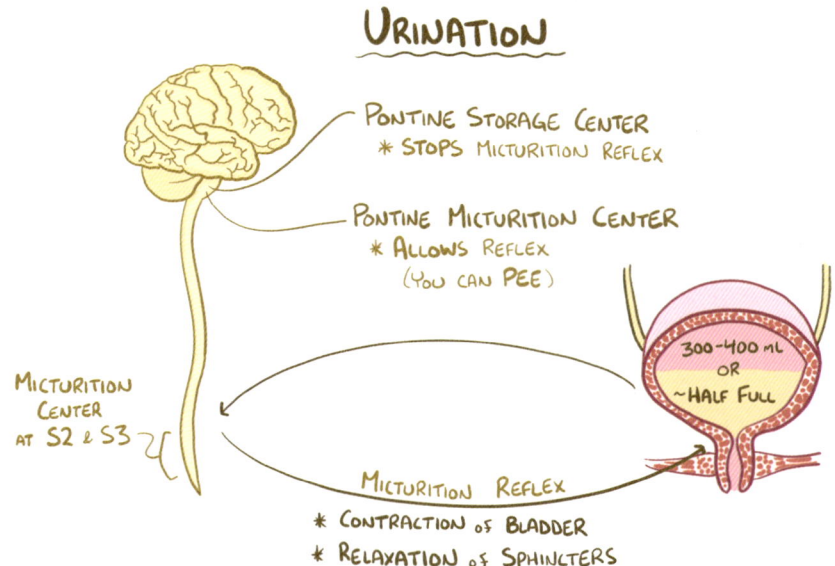

Chapter 2 The Renal System

URINATION

The act of urination involves close coordination between the nervous system and the muscles of the bladder. Once the volume of the bladder is greater than about 300–400 millilitres, basically when it's half full, pressure on the bladder walls increases and send signals to the urination or micturition center in the spinal cord, located at S2 and S3. This sets off a reflex arc called the micturition reflex, which causes contraction of the bladder and relaxation of the internal sphincter and external sphincter. Now, the pontine storage center and pontine micturition center are two areas in the pons part of the brain that help control urination. When you can't find a toilet and want to hold urine in, you activate the pontine storage center and that stops the micturition reflex. When you finally do find that toilet, and you're ready to urinate, the pontine micturition center is active and it allows the the micturition reflex to happen—and you can finally pee **(Figure 2.19)**!

SUMMARY

All right, as a quick recap, the kidneys' main function is to filter all of the body's blood about 30 times a day and to produce urine. The urine passes down through the ureter and into the bladder. As the urine collects in the bladder, it increases the pressure on the bladder wall and the micturition reflex is triggered. This allows the urine to flow through the urethra and out the body **(Figure 2.20)**.

Figure 2.20

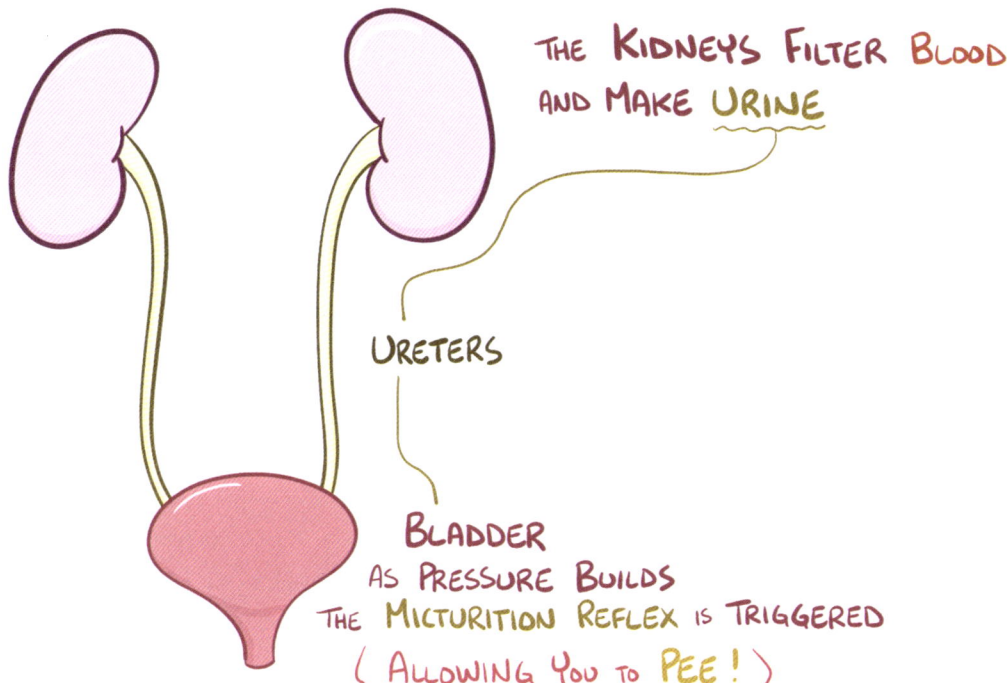

OSMOSIS.ORG   35

THE RESPIRATORY SYSTEM

osms.it/respiratory_system

The main job of the lungs is to facilitate gas exchange by pulling oxygen into the body and getting rid of carbon dioxide. During inhalation, the diaphragm contracts and pulls downward; at the same time, the intercostal muscles of the chest contract. Together, these contractions pull open the chest, giving the lungs space to expand as they suck in air like a vacuum. Then, during exhalation, these muscles relax again as the lungs push the air out and return to their normal size **(Figure 3.1)**.

INHALATION

When you breathe in, air flows through the nostrils and enters the nasal cavity, which is lined with cells that release mucus. This sticky, salty substance contains lysozyme, an enzyme that helps kill bacteria. Mucus-coated nose hairs at the entrance of the nasal cavity trap large particles of dust and pollen as well as bacteria, forming tiny clumps of boogers.

Figure 3.1

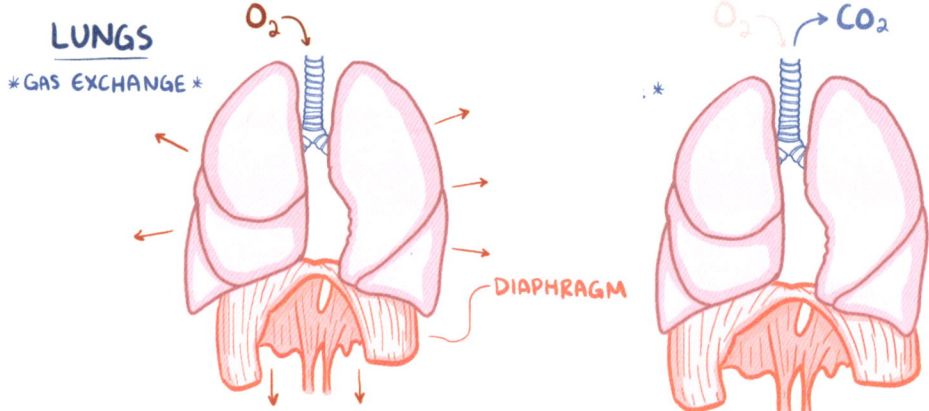

Figure 3.2

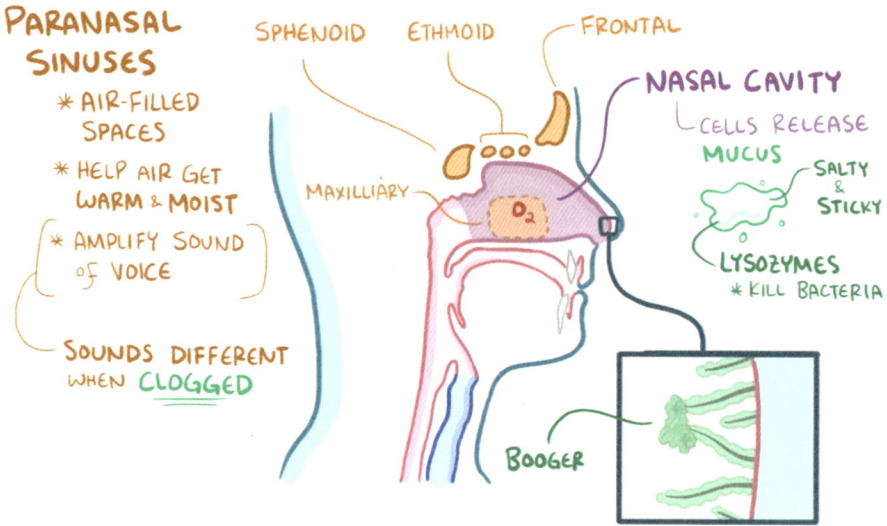

36   OSMOSIS.ORG

PARANASAL SINUSES

The nasal cavity is connected to four sinuses—the frontal, ethmoid, sphenoid, and maxillary sinus—which are air-filled spaces inside the bones surrounding the nose. Together, these four sinuses are known as the paranasal sinuses. They help inspired air circulate, giving it time to get warm and moist. The paranasal sinuses also act like tiny echo-chambers that help amplify the sound of your voice, which is why you sound so different when they're clogged with mucus during a cold **(Figure 3.2)**!

THROAT CAVITIES

So, this relatively clean, warm, moist air goes from the nasal cavity down into the pharynx or throat. The region connecting these two spaces is called the nasopharynx, while the part connecting the pharynx to the oral cavity is called—you guessed it!—the oropharynx. The soft palate (the softer portion of the roof of your mouth behind the hard part that you can feel with your tongue), and the pendulum-like uvula hanging at its end move together to form a flap or valve. This flap closes the nasopharynx off when you eat, preventing food from going up into the nasopharynx and coming out your nose. Finally, there's the laryngopharynx, the part of the pharynx that's continuous with the larynx or the voice box **(Figure 3.3)**.

Up to this point, food and air share a common path. But at the top of the larynx sits a spoon-shaped flap of cartilage called the epiglottis. The epiglottis acts like a lid, sealing the airway off when you're eating, so food can only go one way: down the esophagus, towards the stomach. If anything other than air enters the larynx, the cough reflex kicks it out **(Figure 3.4)**.

TRACHEA & BRONCHI

Now, when air makes its way into the larynx, it flows down through the trachea or the windpipe, which splits into the two main stem bronchi. The point at which the main stem bronchi split is called the carina; after they split, the bronchi enter the lungs. The right lung has three lobes: the upper lobe, middle lobe, and lower lobe. The left lung only has two lobes: upper and lower **(Figure 3.5)**.

To return to the bronchi, the right main stem bronchus is wider and more vertical than the left, which is why if you accidentally inhale something big that can't get coughed out (like a peanut), it's more likely to go into the right lung than the left. The mainstem bronchi divide into smaller and smaller bronchi. The trachea and the first three branch-offs of the bronchi (called generations) are all pretty wide, and are structurally supported by cartilage rings.

Figure 3.3

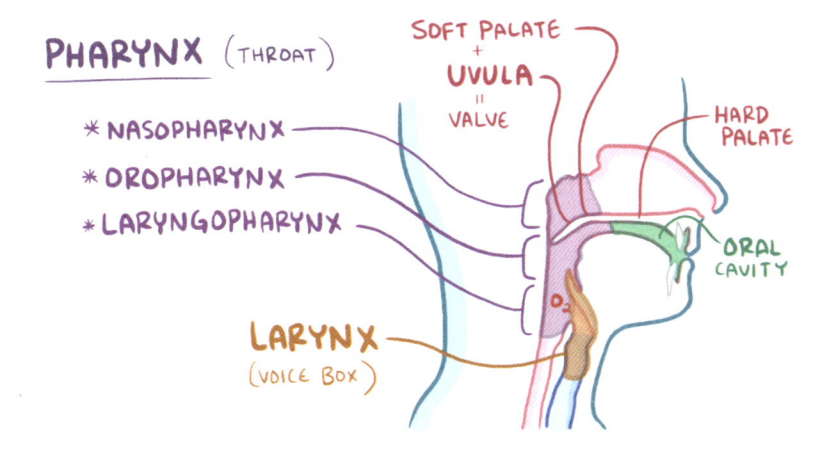

Figure 3.4

ESOPHAGUS → STOMACH

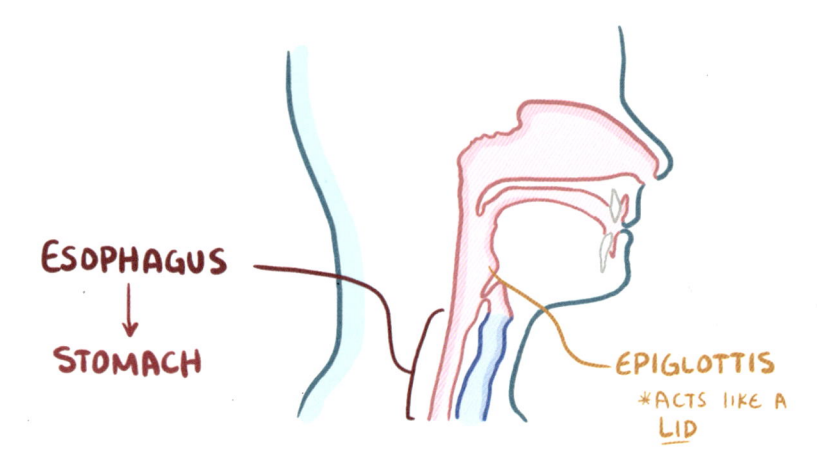

EPIGLOTTIS
*ACTS LIKE A LID

Figure 3.5

RIGHT MAINSTEM BRONCHUS
*WIDER & MORE VERTICAL

(WINDPIPE) TRACHEA

LEFT MAINSTEM BRONCHUS

RIGHT LUNG
* UPPER LOBE
* MIDDLE LOBE
* LOWER LOBE

LEFT LUNG
* UPPER LOBE
* LOWER LOBE

SMALLER BRONCHI

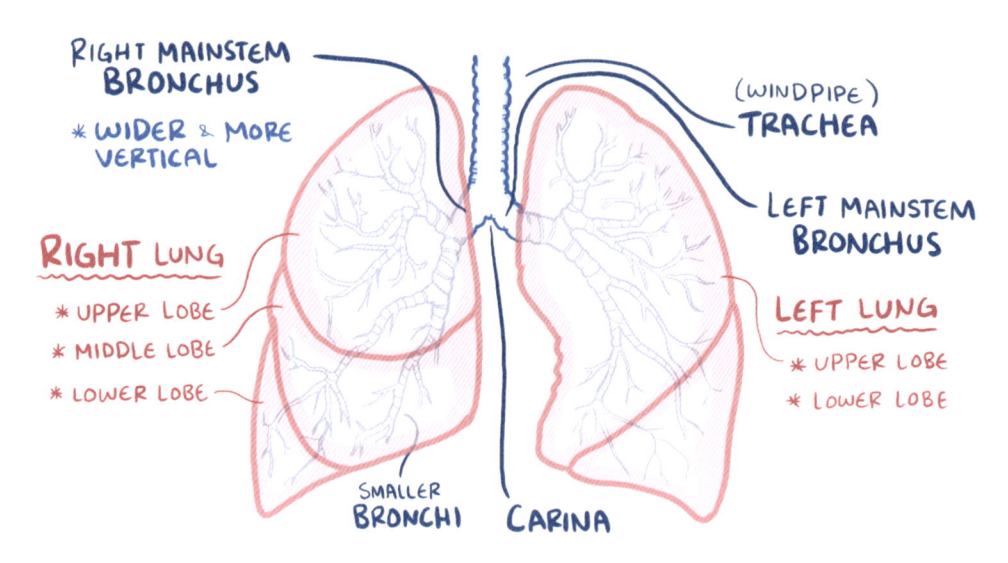

CARINA

Figure 3.6

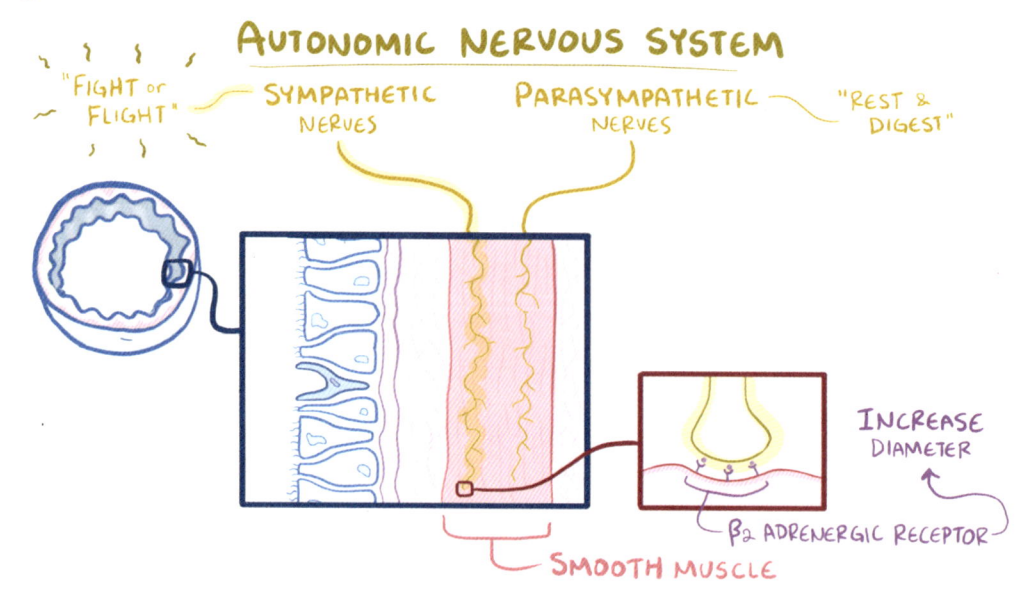

AUTONOMIC NERVOUS SYSTEM

"FIGHT or FLIGHT" SYMPATHETIC NERVES   PARASYMPATHETIC NERVES   "REST & DIGEST"

INCREASE DIAMETER

β2 ADRENERGIC RECEPTOR

SMOOTH MUSCLE

INNERVATION OF THE TRACHEA & BRONCHI

Taking a look at a cross-section chunk of the trachea and bronchi, there's also a layer of smooth muscle innervated by nerves from the autonomic nervous system. The autonomic nervous system is made up of two basic types of nerves: sympathetic nerves, which are involved in "fight or flight" mode (like running from a turkey), and parasympathetic nerves, which are involved in the "rest and digest" mode (like eating ice cream on the beach). Smooth muscle along the trachea and the first few branches of bronchi also contain beta-2 adrenergic receptors.

When you're running (from a turkey!) the sympathetic nerves stimulate those beta-2 adrenergic receptors and increase the diameter of the airways. However, those same airways also have muscarinic receptors; these can get stimulated by parasympathetic nerves, causing a decrease in the diameter of airways **(Figure 3.6)**.

MUCOCILIARY ESCALATOR

The large airways are lined mostly by ciliated columnar cells and a handful of goblet cells (so-called because they resemble a wine goblet or glass). The airways secrete mucus which helps trap foreign particles. The ciliated columnar cells beat rhythmically together, moving the mucus and any trapped particles from the airways towards the pharynx, where they can either be spit out or swallowed. This mechanism is known as the mucociliary escalator **(Figure 3.7)**.

BRONCHIOLES

After the first three generations of bronchi, the airways become more narrow. At this point, they're called bronchioles ("little bronchi") and these can stay open without the support of cartilage rings. Air is conducted through smaller and smaller bronchioles for about 15–20 generations; collectively, these are known as conducting bronchioles. These conducting bronchioles receive oxygenated blood from the bronchial arteries.

Figure 3.7

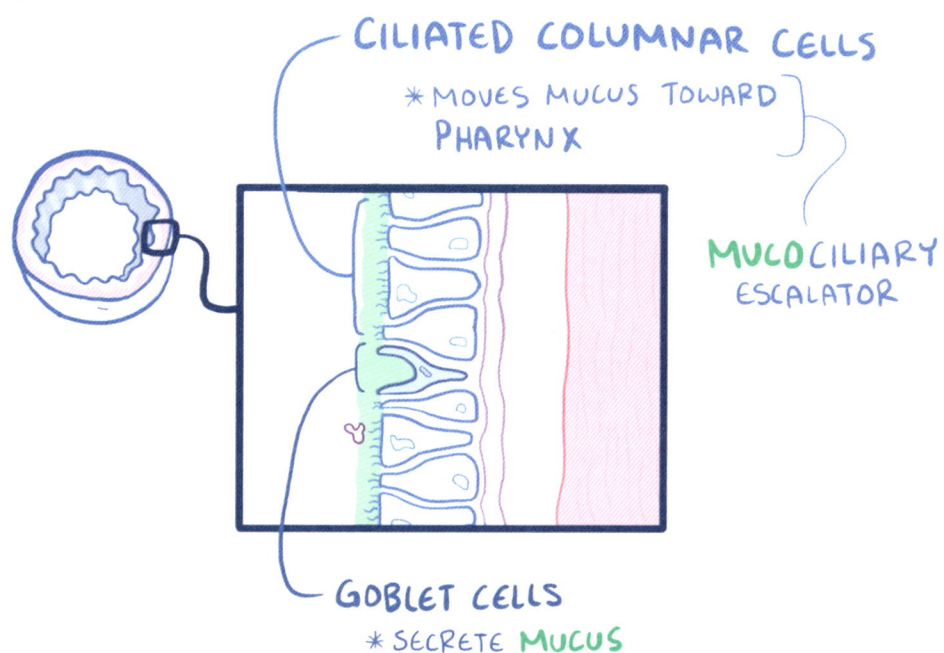

Like the previous generations, the walls of the conducting bronchioles are also lined by ciliated columnar cells and mucus-secreting goblet cells, as well as a new cell type called club cells (which, unsurprisingly, look like clubs). Club cells secrete glycosaminoglycans, a material that protects the bronchiolar epithelium. Club cells can transform into ciliated columnar cells, so they help regenerate and replace damaged ciliated columnar epithelial cells if needed **(Figure 3.8)**.

The last part of the conducting bronchioles are called the terminal bronchioles. Once the air has passed through the terminal bronchioles, it reaches the respiratory bronchioles.

Figure 3.8

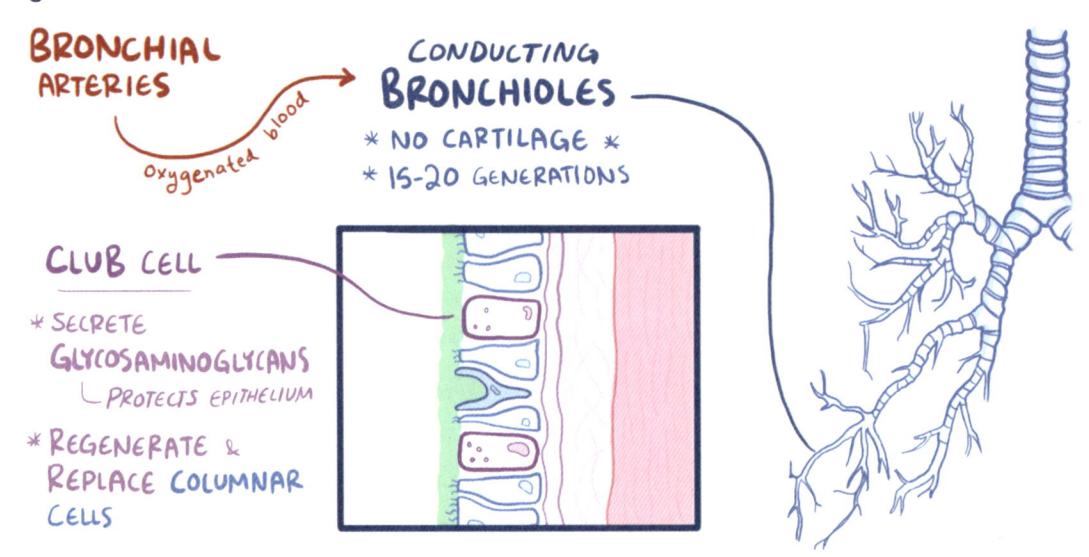

Figure 3.9

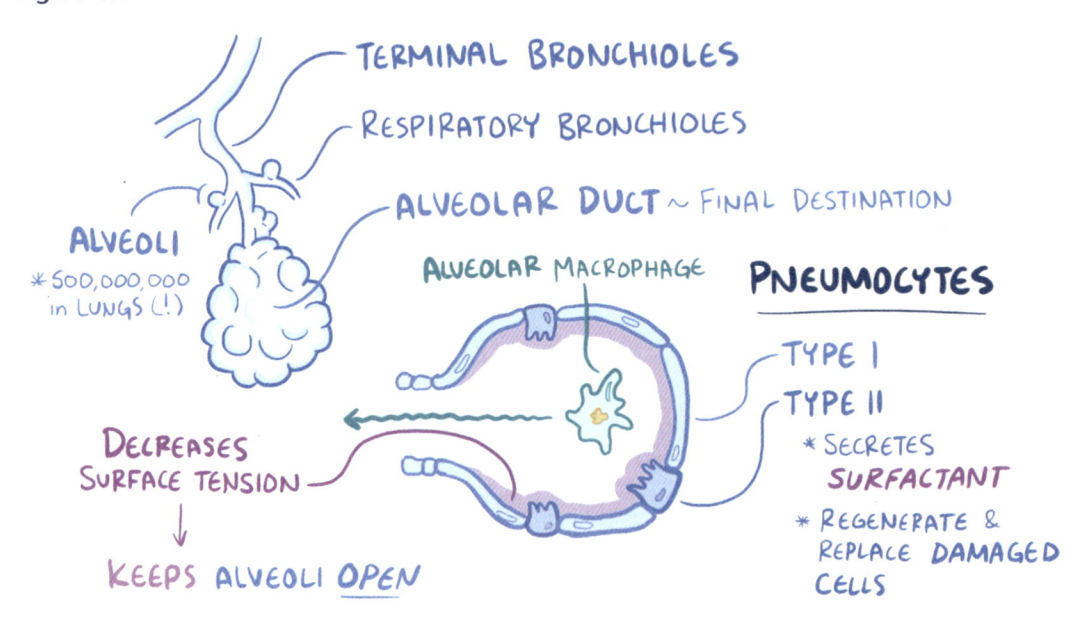

Chapter 3 The Respiratory System

ALVEOLI

Respiratory bronchioles are unique because they have tiny outpouchings budding off of their walls called alveoli. There are about 500 million alveoli within the lungs. The closer we get to the end of the respiratory bronchioles, the more alveoli there are budding off of them, until we reach a terminal point where there's nothing but alveoli. At this point the airway is called an alveolar duct rather than a respiratory bronchiole. This is the final destination of the inhaled air!

The alveolar wall has a completely different structure from the bronchioles. There are no cilia or smooth muscle cells; instead, the wall is lined by thin epithelial cells called pneumocytes. Most are regular pneumocytes (type I pneumocytes), but some, called type II pneumocytes, have the ability to secrete a substance called surfactant. Surfactant helps decrease the surface tension within the alveoli, keeping them open. Type II pneumocytes are flexible like club cells: they can transform into type I pneumocytes and help regenerate and replace damaged cells. Finally, if tiny particles ever make it deep into the lungs, tiny cells called alveolar macrophages are waiting there to gobble them up. The macrophages can physically move up to the conducting bronchioles. They're even capable of riding the mucociliary escalator all the way up to the pharynx to be coughed up or swallowed back down **(Figure 3.9)**.

BLOOD-GAS BARRIER

Free from particles, the inhaled air reaches the alveoli, where it's surrounded mainly by type I pneumocytes. On the other side of the pneumocytes are endothelial cells lining the capillary walls—which is where the blood is. This blood comes from the pulmonary arteries, carrying deoxygenated blood. The pneumocytes and the capillaries are glued together with a protein layer called the basement membrane. The alveolar wall, the basement membrane, and the capillary wall are all that separates the air from the blood; this is called the blood-gas barrier.

At this point, carbon dioxide diffuses out from the deoxygenated blood and into the air housed in alveoli, which then gets breathed out. Each time we breathe in, oxygen enters the alveoli and freely diffuses into the blood. That freshly oxygenated blood then heads off to the pulmonary veins, the heart, and then to the rest of the body's tissues **(Figure 3.10)**!

Figure 3.10

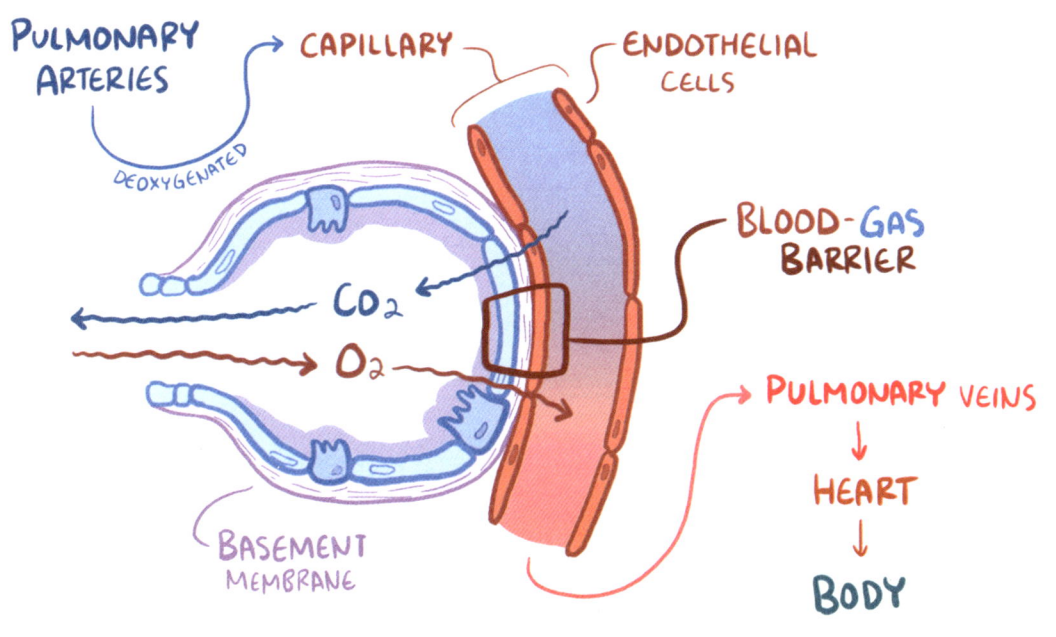

SUMMARY

All right, as a quick recap... The respiratory system facilitates gas exchange. Oxygen in the air is inhaled and makes it' way through the pharynx, larynx, trachea, large upper airways, conducting bronchioles, respiratory bronchioles, the alveoli, and finally the capillary to be sent to the body's tissues. Then, carbon dioxide makes the reverse journey to be exhaled out into the world **(Figure 3.11)**.

Figure 3.11

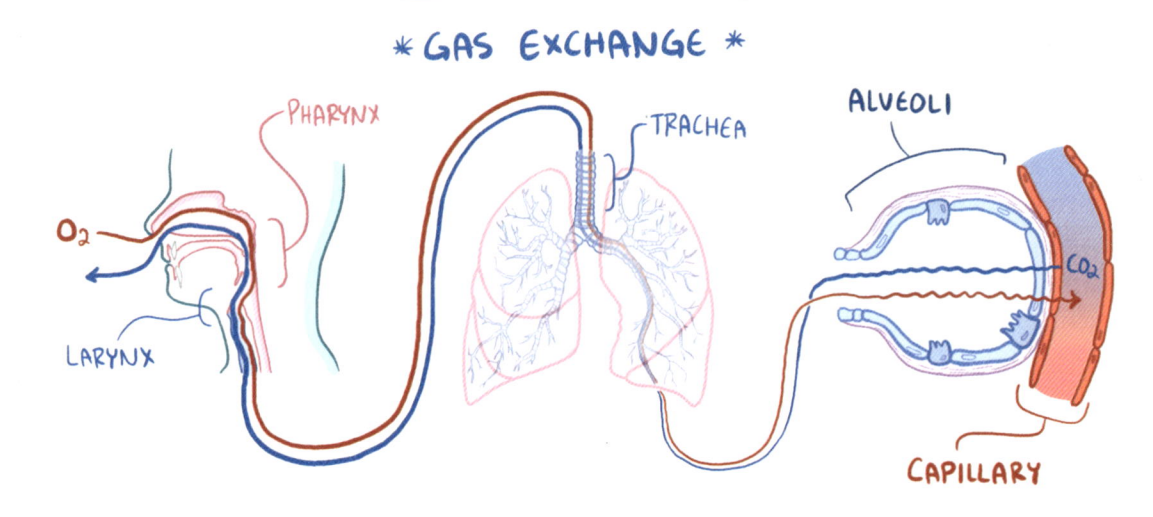

THE GASTROINTESTINAL SYSTEM

osms.it/gi_system

The gastrointestinal tract consists of a long tube, through which food travels, that runs from the mouth to the anus. It also includes a number of accessory organs which sprout off the sides of that tube. The gastrointestinal tract is made up of the mouth, pharynx, esophagus, stomach, small intestine, large intestine, and, finally, the anal canal. The accessory organs include the teeth, tongue, salivary glands, liver, gallbladder, and the pancreas **(Figure 4.1)**. The main job of the gastrointestinal system is ingestion (taking in food); digestion, (breaking it down into nutrients); absorption (pulling those nutrients into the bloodstream); and, finally, excretion, (getting rid of waste).

MOUTH → PHARYNX → ESOPHAGUS

All right, so let's say we eat a slice of pizza. The pizza goes in our oral cavity where we use our teeth to masticate, or chew, the food up into small fragments. These fragments get tasted and rolled around by the tongue, which is basically a huge muscle that lines the floor of the mouth. The roof of the mouth, which separates it from the nasal cavity, is made up by the anterior hard palate and the posterior soft palate. The anterior hard palate provides a hard surface for the tongue to mash food against and the posterior soft palate moves together, along with the pendulum-like uvula, to form a flap or valve that ensures the food flows downward—and does not, instead, travel up into the nose **(Figure 4.2)**.

At the same time, the salivary glands secrete saliva to lubricate the food. There are three sets of salivary glands: the sublingual, below the tongue; the submandibular, below the mandible; and the parotid gland, which is near the ear. The saliva secreted by these three glands helps to compact the food into a soft ball called a bolus. The saliva also contains salivary amylase, an enzyme that breaks long carbohydrates down into smaller sugars. Once the bolus of food is swallowed through the pharynx, it enters the esophagus. As the food is being swallowed from the pharynx into the esophagus, a spoon-shaped flap of cartilage, called the epiglottis, acts like a lid, sealing the airway. This ensures the food doesn't end up in the lungs **(Figure 4.3)**.

Figure 4.1

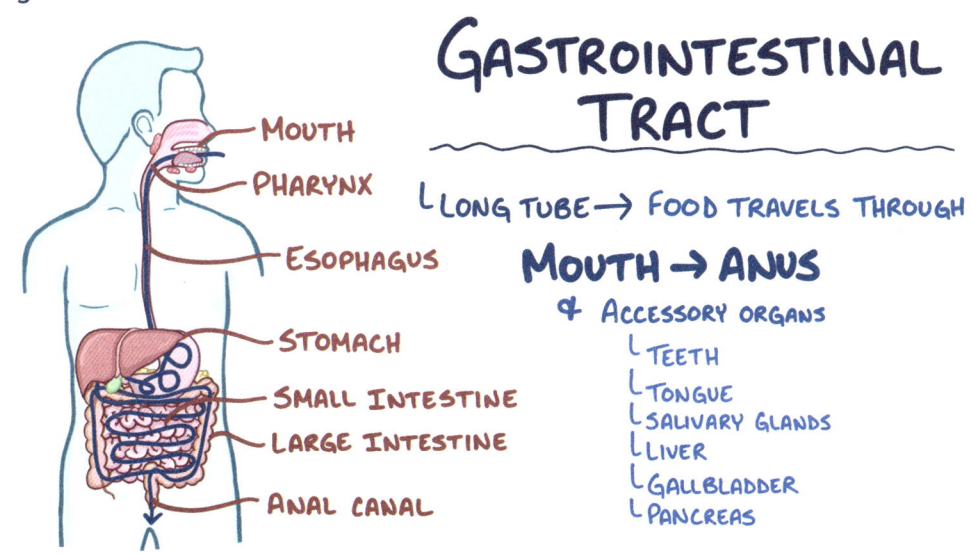

TISSUE LAYERS

Now, if we zoom in to a cross-section of the remaining gastrointestinal tract, anywhere from the esophagus to the anus, the walls are typically lined by the same four layers of tissue. The outermost layer is either the adventitia, a thick fibrous connective tissue, or the serosa, a slippery serous membrane.

Next is the muscularis externa, a smooth muscle layer, which contracts automatically, without you even having to think about it. If we look closer at this muscle layer, it's actually composed of two layers: an inner circular muscle layer and an outer longitudinal muscle layer. The inner layer is arranged in circular rings that contract and constrict the tract behind the food, which prevents the food from moving backward. The outer layer is arranged along the length of the tract and relaxes and lengthens, pulling the food forward.

Together, these inner and outer muscle layers perform peristalsis—a series of coordinated wave-like muscle contractions that squeeze the food bolus in one direction. In specific places along the tract, like the esophageal sphincter, the inner layer thickens, forming sphincters that prevent food passing from one part of the gastrointestinal tract into another. Also, between the inner circular muscle layer and the outer longitudinal muscle layer, there's a plexus—networks of nerves—which helps coordinate muscle contraction and relaxation. This is the myenteric plexus, also known as Auerbach's plexus. When activated, it causes smooth muscle relaxation **(Figure 4.4)**.

Now, surrounded by the muscularis externa is the submucosa, which consists of a dense layer of tissue that contains blood vessels, lymphatics, and nerves. Buried in the submucosa is a second plexus, the submucous plexus, also known as Meissner's plexus. It is responsible for helping to control the size of the blood vessels, as well as the secretion of digestive juices **(Figure 4.5)**.

And, finally, there's the inner lining of the intestine called the mucosa, which itself consists of three cell layers. The outermost layer of the mucosa is the muscularis mucosa or muscularis interna, and it's a layer of smooth muscle that contracts and helps break down food. The middle layer is the lamina propria and it contains blood and lymph vessels. Finally, there's the innermost epithelial layer and it absorbs and secretes mucus and digestive enzymes. This final layer is the layer that comes into direct contact with the food **(Figure 4.6)**.

Figure 4.2

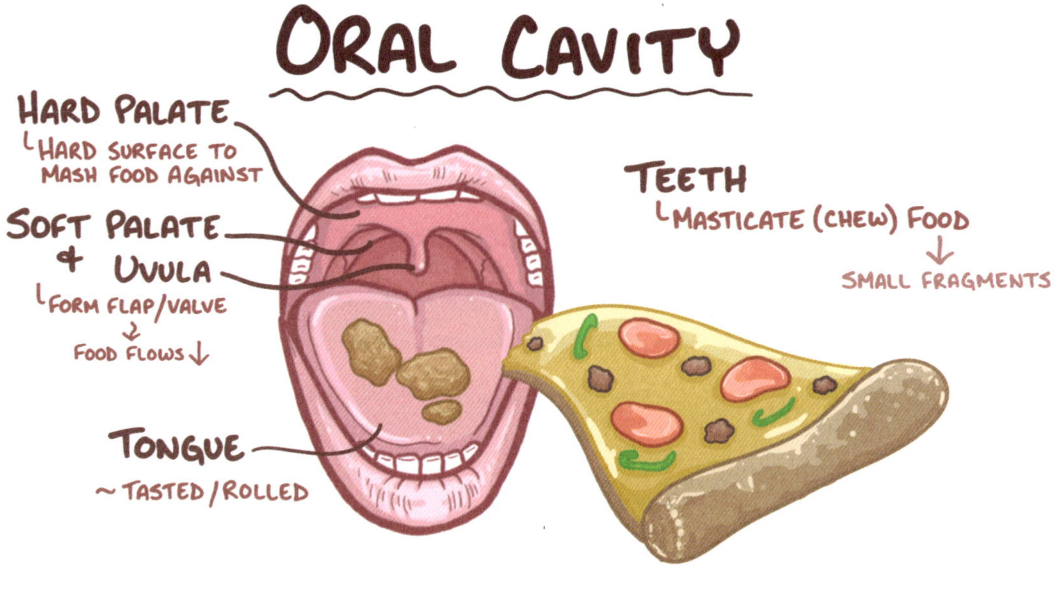

Chapter 4 The Gastrointestinal System

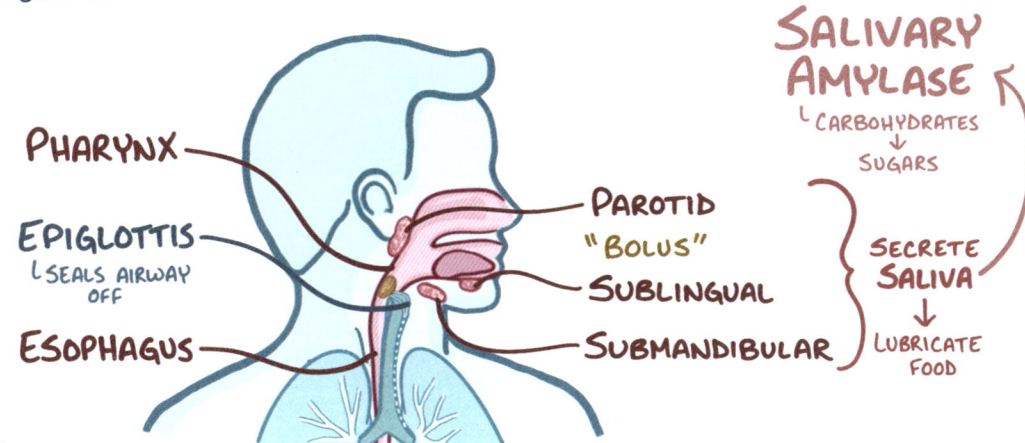

Figure 4.3

- PHARYNX
- EPIGLOTTIS
  - Seals airway off
- ESOPHAGUS
- PAROTID "BOLUS"
- SUBLINGUAL
- SUBMANDIBULAR

SALIVARY AMYLASE
- Carbohydrates → Sugars

Secrete Saliva → Lubricate Food

Figure 4.4

PERISTALSIS

* ESOPHAGEAL SPHINCTER
  - Circular layer thickens (sphincters)
  → Keep food from passing from one part of tract to another

MUSCULARIS EXTERNA
- Smooth muscle
- Contracts automatically
- ~ Inner circular layer
  - Contract / constrict behind food
- ~ Outer longitudinal
  - Relaxes & lengthens
  → Pulls food forward

MYENTERIC PLEXUS (Auerbach's plexus)
- Network of nerves

* RELAXATION

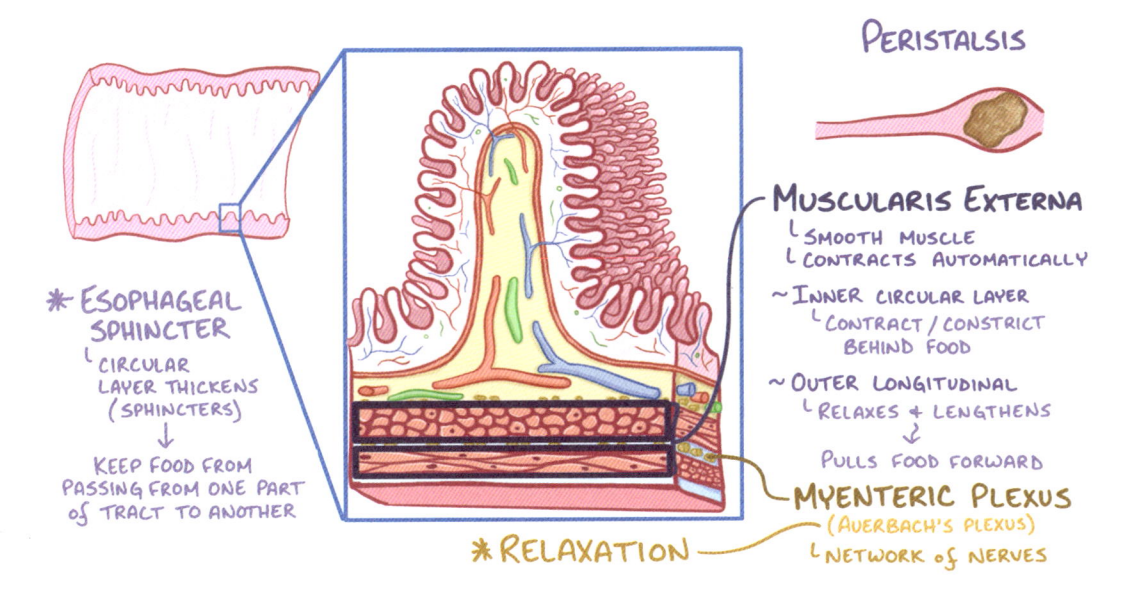

Figure 4.5

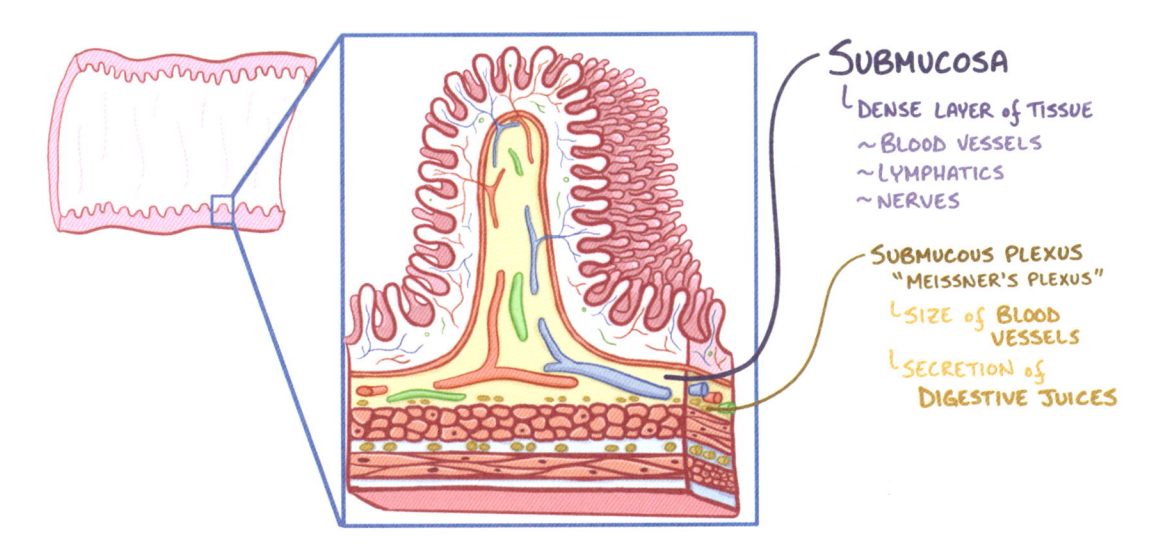

SUBMUCOSA
- Dense layer of tissue
  - ~ Blood vessels
  - ~ Lymphatics
  - ~ Nerves

SUBMUCOUS PLEXUS "MEISSNER'S PLEXUS"
- Size of blood vessels
- Secretion of digestive juices

OSMOSIS.ORG 45

Figure 4.6

MUCOSA

EPITHELIAL LAYER
└ ABSORBS & SECRETES MUCUS & DIGESTIVE ENZYMES

LAMINA PROPRIA
└ BLOOD & LYMPH VESSELS

MUSCULARIS MUCOSA (MUSCULARIS INTERNA)
└ SMOOTH MUSCLE
↳ BREAKS DOWN FOOD

THE STOMACH

Now, the esophagus has a particularly thick muscularis externa that propels the bolus of food down to the esophageal sphincter. The esophageal sphincter opens and allows the bolus to pass into the stomach.

In the stomach, there are four regions: the cardia, the fundus, the body, and the pyloric antrum. There's also a pyloric sphincter, or valve, at the end of the stomach, which closes while eating, keeping food inside and allowing the stomach to churn over and over again. To help with this churning, the stomach has an extra layer of oblique smooth muscle within its muscularis externa that allows it to contract and expand like a big accordion **(Figure 4.7)**.

The inner lining of the stomach has millions of tiny gastric pits that dive down to gastric glands. These glands contain a variety of secretory cells that produce gastric secretions. Gastric secretions are made up of the following: hydrochloric acid, which helps destroy any pathogens that may have slipped through the food; an enzyme called pepsin, which chops up proteins; mucus, which protects the stomach; and, water, which turns the bolus into a liquidy pulp called chyme **(Figure 4.8)**.

Figure 4.7

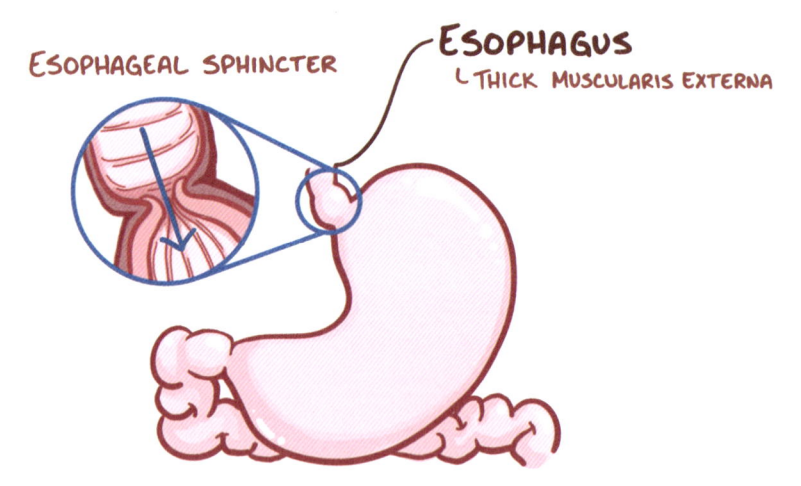

ESOPHAGEAL SPHINCTER

ESOPHAGUS
└ THICK MUSCULARIS EXTERNA

Figure 4.8

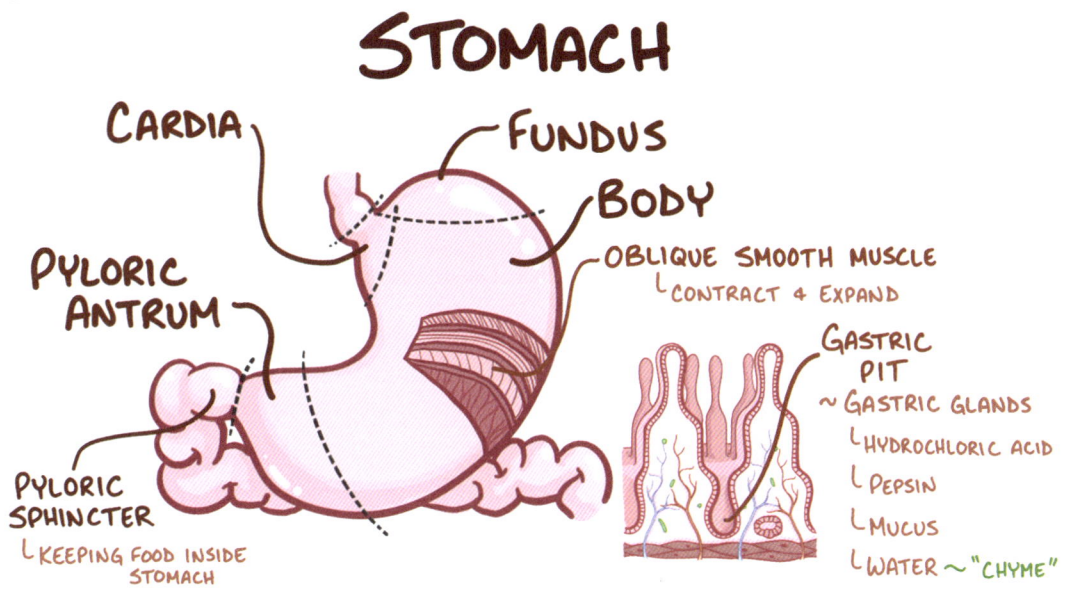

THE SMALL INTESTINE

Now, once the stomach is done, the pyloric sphincter opens, allowing the chyme to pass into the small intestine. The small intestine has three parts: the duodenum, the jejunum, and the ileum. Despite its name, the small intestine can be as long as 10.5 meters, or about 35 feet, with lots of tiny ridges and grooves, each of which projects little finger-like fibers called villi. In turn, each villus is covered in teeny tiny microvilli **(Figure 4.9)**. This means the small intestines include plenty of surface area for the absorption of nutrients. But almost no nutrient absorption can take place without the help of the trio of accessory organs: the liver, gallbladder, and pancreas.

Figure 4.9

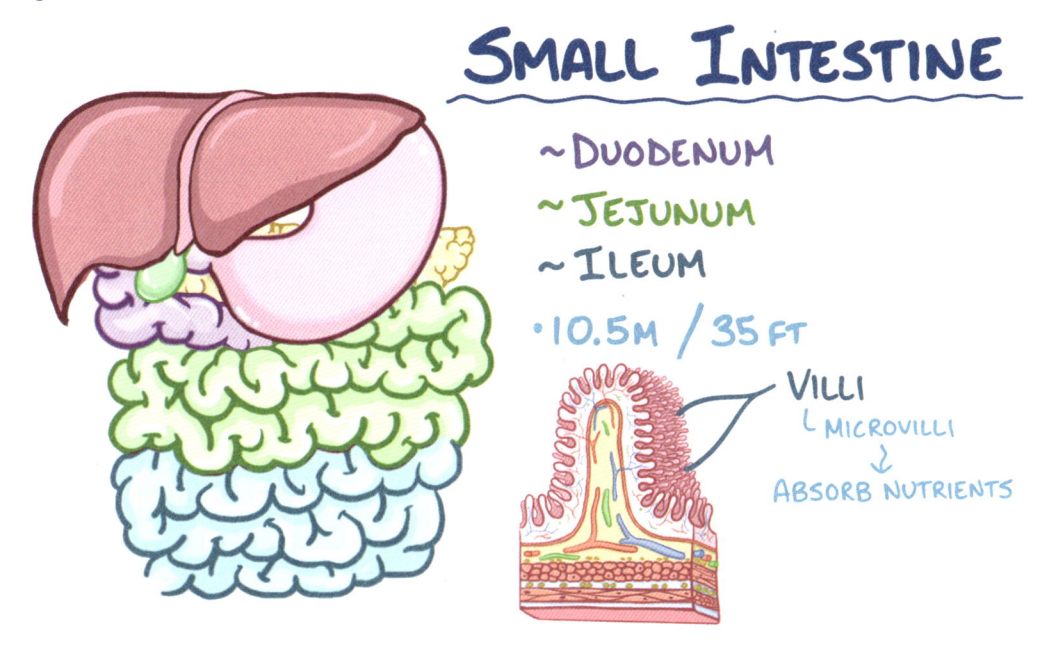

ACCESSORY ORGANS: LIVER, GALLBLADDER, & PANCREAS

First, the liver is a massive organ that sits under the right dome of the diaphragm, and it makes bile. If we return to the pizza slice, at this point the fats in the cheese are part of the chyme, and the chyme stimulates the enteroendocrine cells, or hormone-secreting cells, of the small intestine to secrete a hormone called cholecystokinin into the blood **(Figure 4.10)**.

The cholecystokinin makes its way to the gallbladder, the thin-walled, green sac snuggled up against the liver, and signals it to squeeze out some bile through the cystic and bile ducts into the small intestine. This is your gallbladder's job: to store and concentrate the bile that's made by the liver until the time comes to squeeze it out into the small intestine. That bile emulsifies the fat, essentially organizing it into small micelles, which are tiny bubbles of mixed lipids and bile acids. This process allows the fat to avoid clumping together, so the fat becomes easier to absorb.

This is where the pancreas comes in. The pancreas is a long, skinny gland about the length of a dollar bill, snuggled around the duodenum. Cholecystokinin stimulates acinar cells in the pancreas to secrete digestive enzymes that travel through the pancreatic ducts and into the duodenum. One enzyme is pancreatic lipase, which grabs the triglycerides hanging out in those micelles and breaks them down into fatty acids and glycerol. There's also pancreatic amylase, which breaks down carbohydrates into shorter oligosaccharides, and proteases, like trypsin, which cleaves proteins down into smaller peptides.

Now, to prevent the hydrochloric acid from the stomach damaging the intestinal mucosa, enteroendocrine cells secrete another hormone, called secretin, which stimulates the pancreatic duct cells to secrete water and bicarbonate. Bicarbonate helps neutralize the acidic chyme, and raising the pH in the intestinal lumen also helps digestive enzymes work more effectively. A generous amount of bicarbonate is also secreted by a number of glands lying in the submucosa of the duodenal wall **(Figure 4.11)**.

Figure 4.10

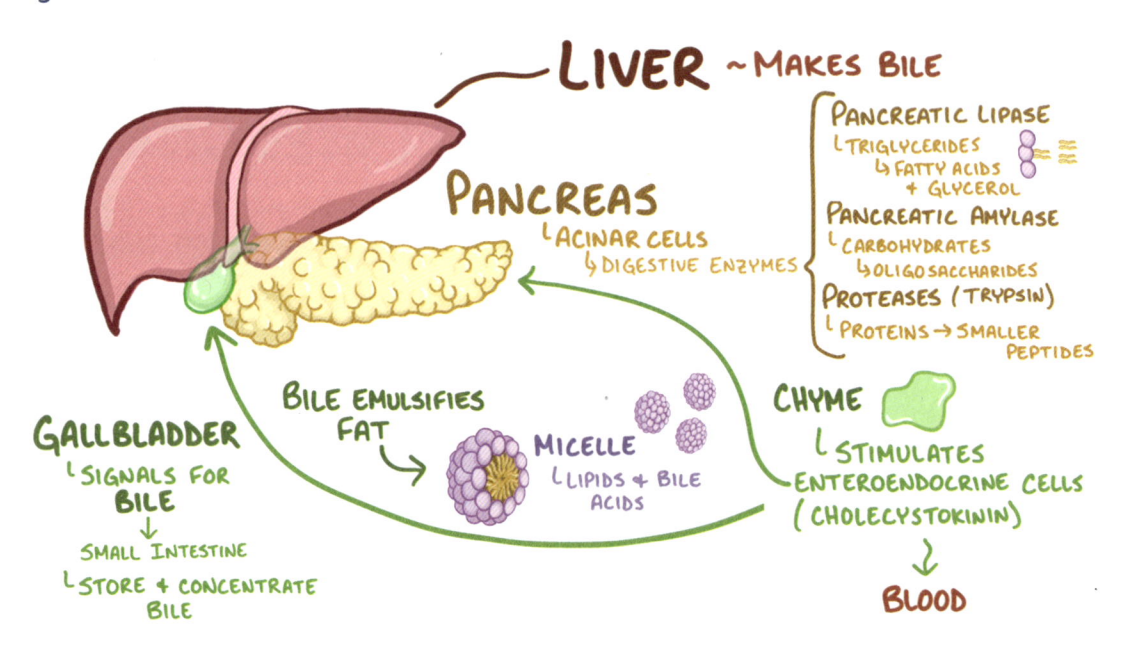

Chapter 4 The Gastrointestinal System

ABSORPTION

At this point, we're almost ready for absorption. Fatty acids and glycerol can easily pass through the small intestinal epithelial and into the lymphatics. But to help absorb sugars, there are special enzymes. These special enzymes can be found on the top surface, or the brush border of the intestinal cells, and they are called brush border enzymes. These are maltase, sucrase, and lactase, which break down the short chains of sugars called oligosaccharides into simple sugars, called monosaccharides. The monosaccharides include glucose, fructose, and galactose. Similarly, there are peptidases which break down peptide chains into single amino acids. The epithelial cells can absorb these nutrients into the bloodstream, and from there they travel to various tissues around the body **(Figure 4.12)**.

Figure 4.11

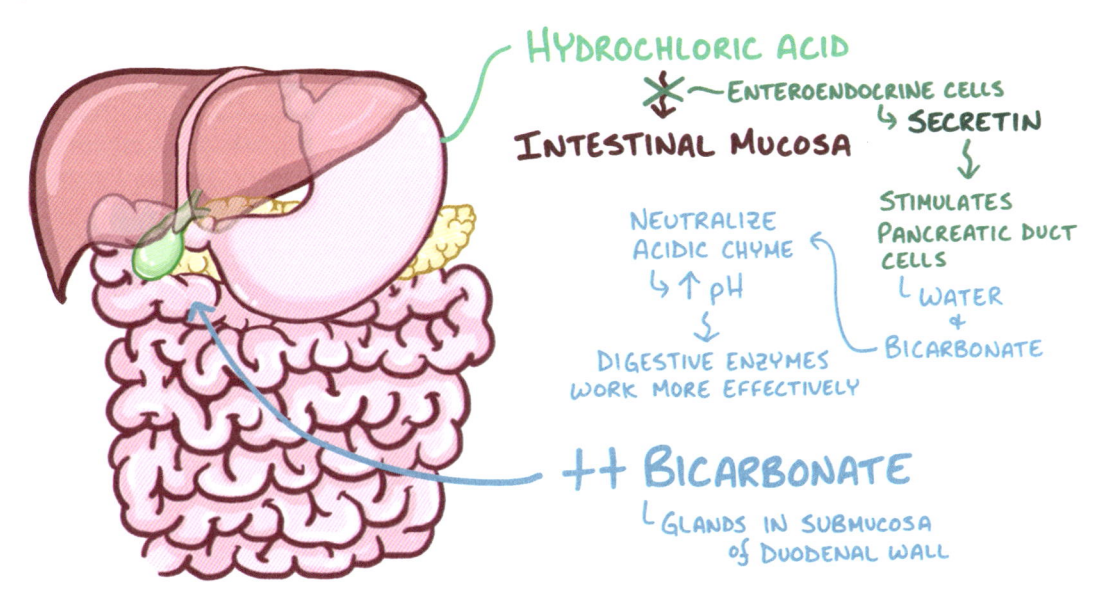

Figure 4.12

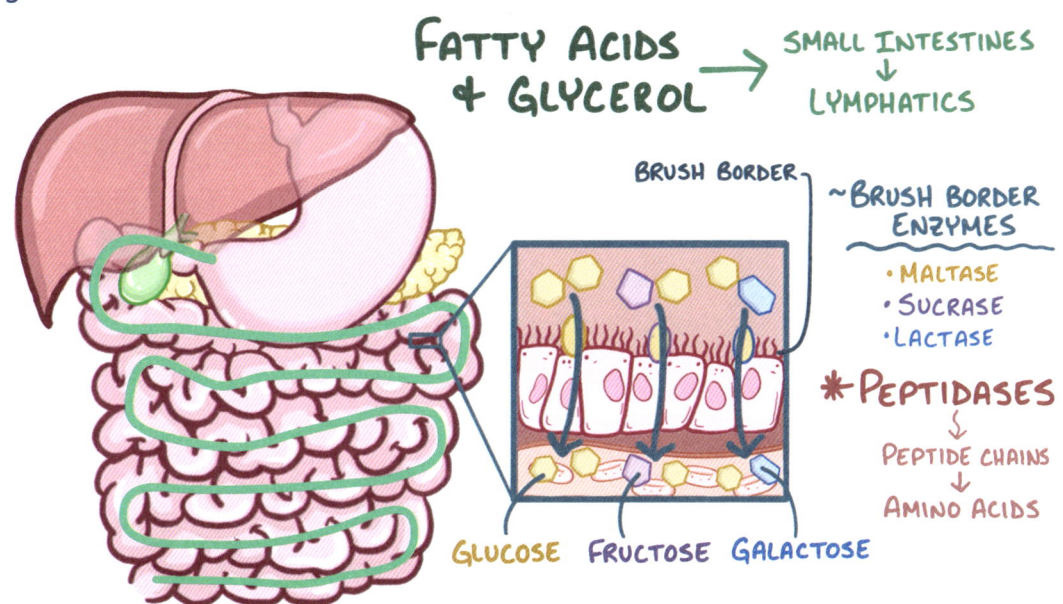

OSMOSIS.ORG 49

THE LARGE INTESTINE

Whatever isn't absorbed, like fiber, continues its journey onward through the ileocecal sphincter and into the very last part of the gastrointestinal tract: the large intestine, also known as the colon. The large intestine is basically a long loop of 1.5 meters, or about 5 feet, that frames the small intestine. It consists of six parts: the cecum, which has a tiny worm-like outpouching called the appendix; the ascending colon, climbing along the right side of the abdomen; the transverse colon, right beneath the diaphragm; the descending colon, running down the left side of the abdomen; the S-shaped sigmoid colon; and, finally, the rectum **(Figure 4.13)**.

When chyme hits the cecum, it's met by trillions of bacteria that colonize the large intestine. Collectively, these bacteria are called the gut microbiome. This microbiome is still being studied, and thus is not yet understood, but we do know that these bacteria help produce essential B and K vitamins, as well as gases like carbon dioxide, methane, and sulfurous compounds—which have been known to be released in awkward moments . . .

Figure 4.13

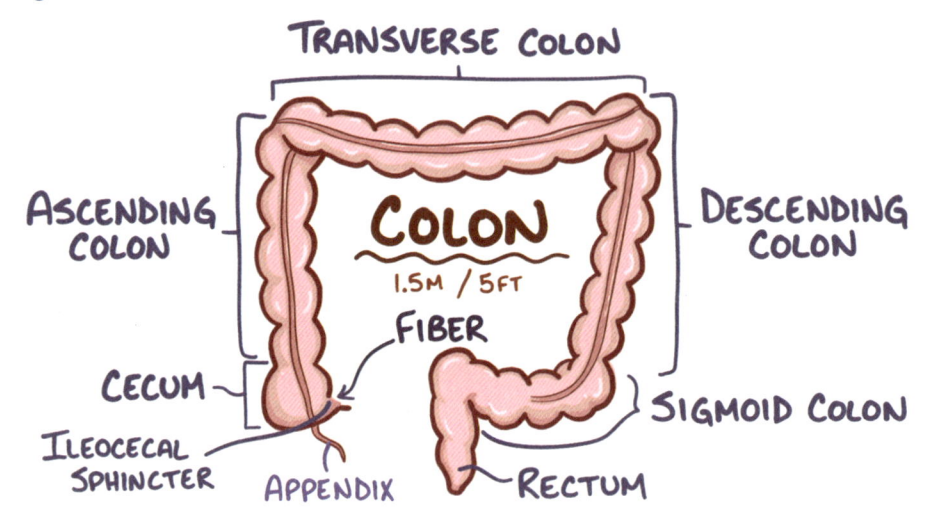

Figure 4.14

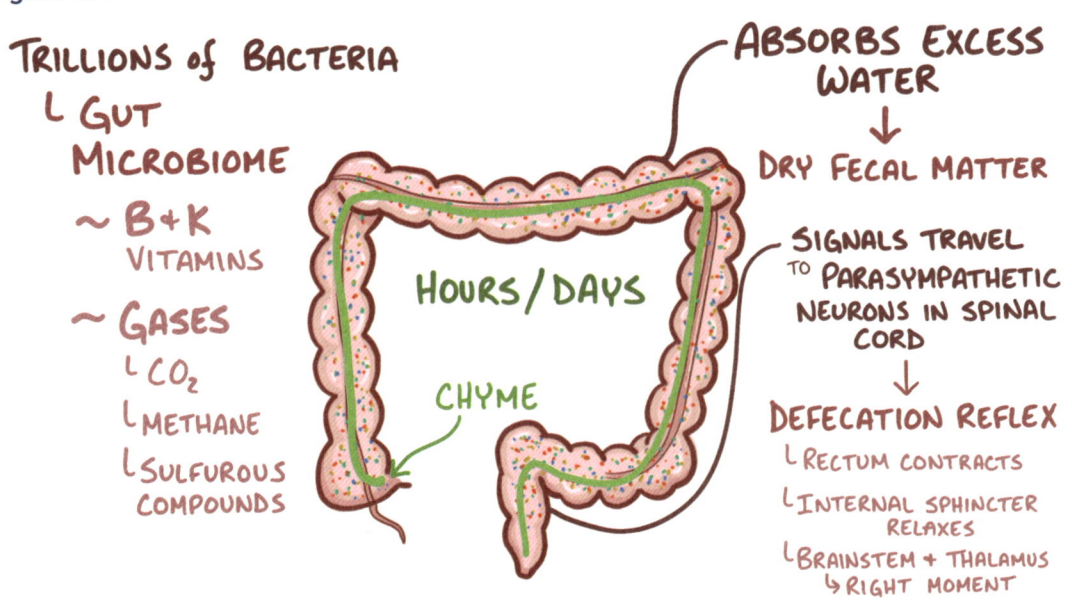

THE RECTUM

The chyme slowly moves through the large intestine through small waves of peristalsis that take place over hours or even days. The large intestine absorbs excess water from the chyme, and that helps condense it into dry fecal matter. That feces eventually ends up in the rectum.

Once the rectum is filled and stretched, signals travel to parasympathetic neurons in the spinal cord, initiating the defecation reflex. These parasympathetic neurons make the rectum contract and the internal anal sphincter relax. Meanwhile, signals are sent to the brainstem and thalamus, and when these decide the right moment has come, they allow the external anal sphincter to relax—and feces goes, hopefully, into the toilet bowl **(Figure 4.14)**.

SUMMARY

All right, as a quick recap, food is ingested through the mouth, chewed by the teeth, mixed with saliva, and turned into a bolus. The bolus is then moved by peristalsis through the esophagus and into the stomach, where hydrochloric acid is secreted and pepsin begins the digestion process. Next is the small intestine, where most of the digestion and absorption occurs, with the help of the liver's bile from the gallbladder and the pancreatic enzymes. Finally, the large intestine absorbs water and the feces forms and is excreted through the anus **(Figure 4.15)**.

Figure 4.15

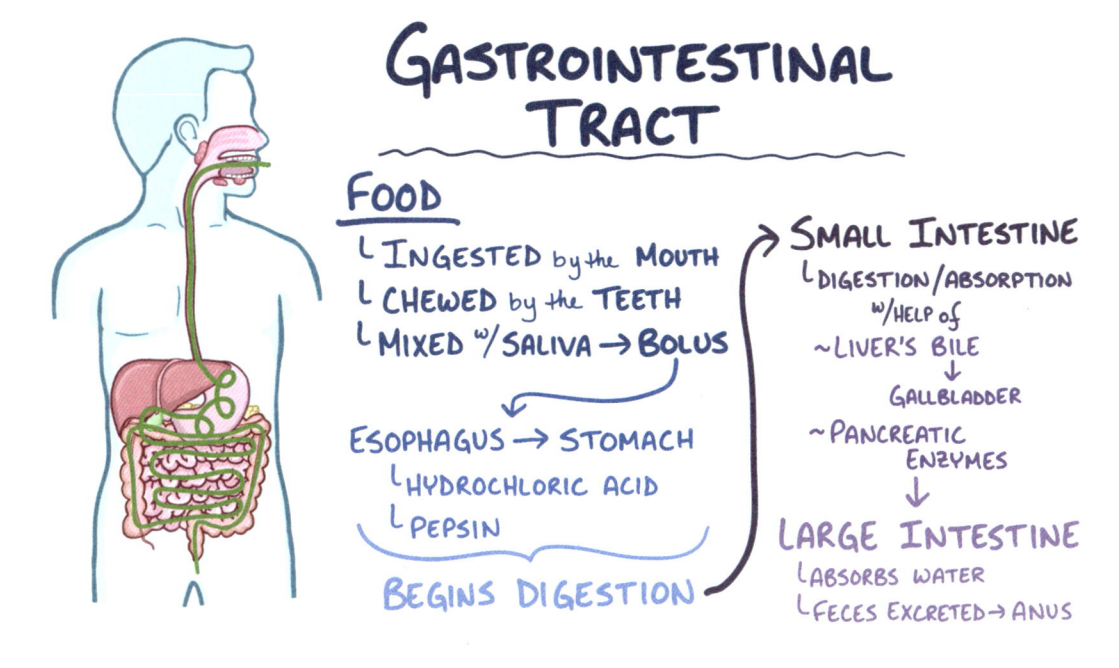

THE ENDOCRINE SYSTEM

osms.it/endocrine_system

The endocrine system is made up of various endocrine glands that each secrete hormones into the bloodstream. When hormones reach their target cell, they bind to a receptor on the cell's membrane or within that cell. In response, the target cell changes what it's doing. So, at the end of the day, the endocrine system helps establish homeostasis—a sense of balance even when there are changes in the external environment **(Figure 5.1)**.

STEROID HORMONES

Now, structurally, hormones can be either steroids or nonsteroids. Steroid hormones are made from cholesterol. They are produced by the adrenal glands, which sit above each kidney, and the gonads, either the testes or ovaries. Steroid hormones are hydrophobic or nonpolar—this means they hate watery environments. They travel through the bloodstream bound to a transport protein to reach their target cells. Because steroid hormones are relatively small and nonpolar, they can diffuse right across the phospholipid membrane of target cells. Once inside the cell, they bind to a receptor that activates certain genes in the nucleus **(Figure 5.2)**.

Figure 5.1

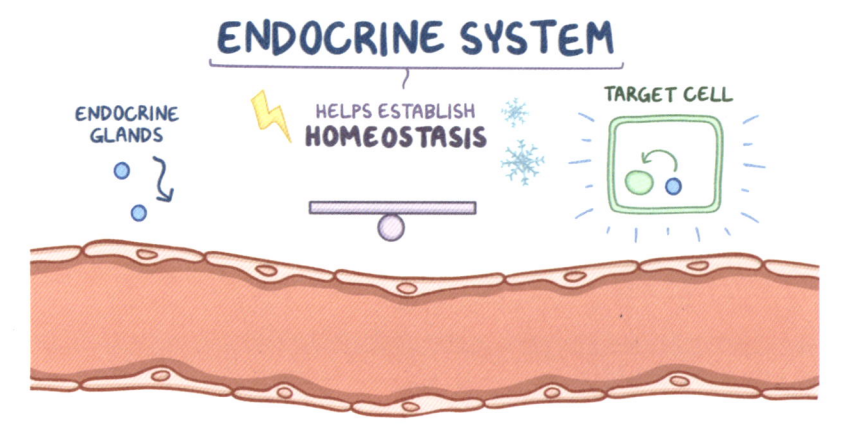

Figure 5.2

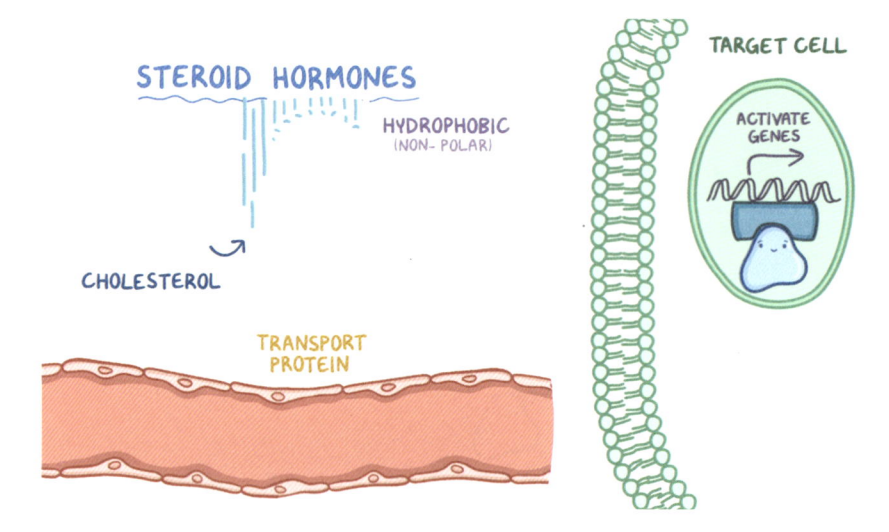

NONSTEROID HORMONES

Nonsteroid hormones, on the other hand, are either peptides or proteins. They may be chains of amino-acids, or they may derive from a single amino acid. Peptidic hormones, like insulin and glucagon, are hydrophilic—this means they love coursing through our blood. However, when they reach the cell membrane of a target cell, they can't pass through the phospholipid bilayer. Instead, they bind to cell surface receptor proteins. Once the receptors bind to a nonsteroid hormone, they change shape, and that activates various proteins and enzymes that go on to create changes in gene expression within the cell. Ultimately, once the nonsteroid hormone binds to the receptor, there's a change in the cell, even though the hormone never actually enters the cell **(Figure 5.3)**.

TYROSINE-DERIVED HORMONES

Finally, there are amino acid hormones that derive from the amino acid tyrosine, the thyroid hormone. There are also adrenaline and noradrenaline hormones, also known as epinephrine and norepinephrine. These hormones are synthesized differently **(Figure 5.4)**. Their molecular makeup makes them behave like steroids or peptides. For instance, thyroid hormones behave like steroid hormones: they travel the bloodstream bound to a transport protein, cross the cell membrane to bind to an intracellular receptor, and signal changes in gene expression in the nucleus **(Figure 5.5)**. Adrenaline and noradrenaline, on the other hand, behave like peptide hormones: they travel through the blood unbound, and bind to cell surface receptors on cells, which then set off intracellular changes **(Figure 5.6)**. This reaction is partly responsible for the increased blood flow to the heart and muscles that occurs during a fight-or-flight response (for example, when you're fighting with an airline so you can catch a flight) **(Figure 5.7)**.

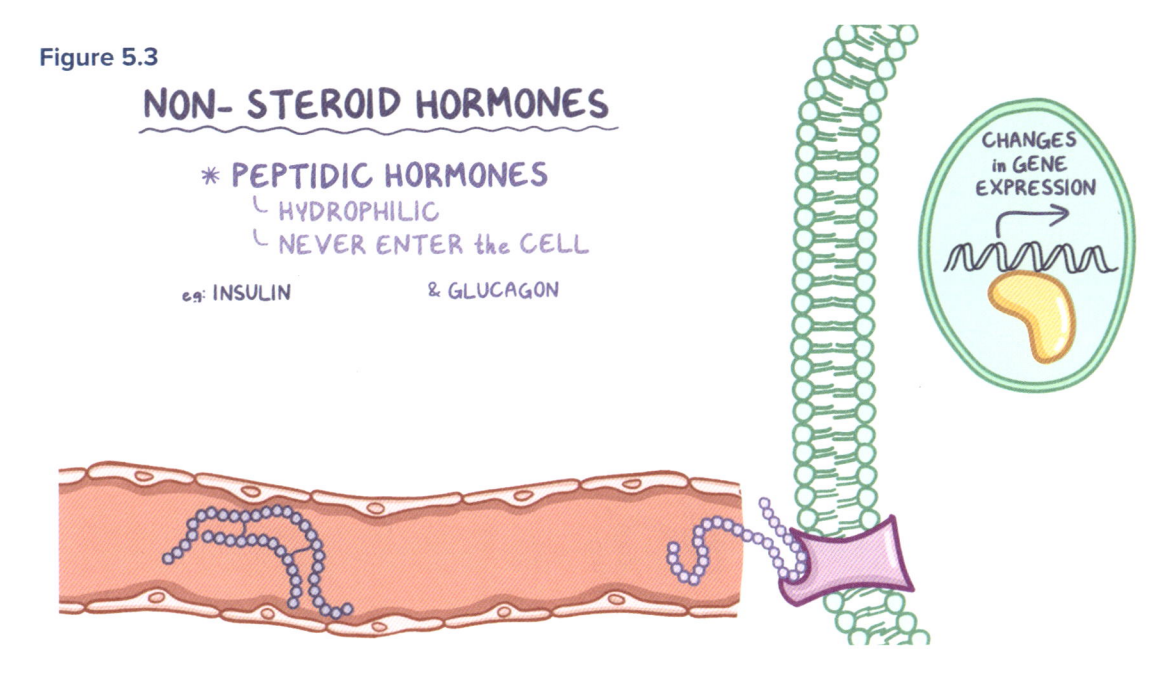

Figure 5.3

Figure 5.4

NON-STEROID HORMONES

* AMINO-ACID HORMONES ← TYROSINE
  - THYROID HORMONES
  - ADRENALINE (EPINEPHRINE)
  - NORADRENALINE (NOREPINEPHRINE)

} SYNTHESIZED DIFFERENTLY → BEHAVE DIFFERENTLY

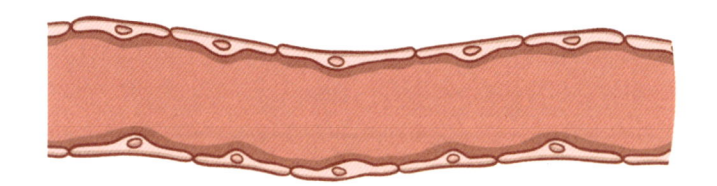

Figure 5.5

NON-STEROID HORMONES

* AMINO-ACID HORMONES
  - THYROID HORMONES → BEHAVE like STEROIDS

TARGET CELL
CHANGES in GENE EXPRESSION

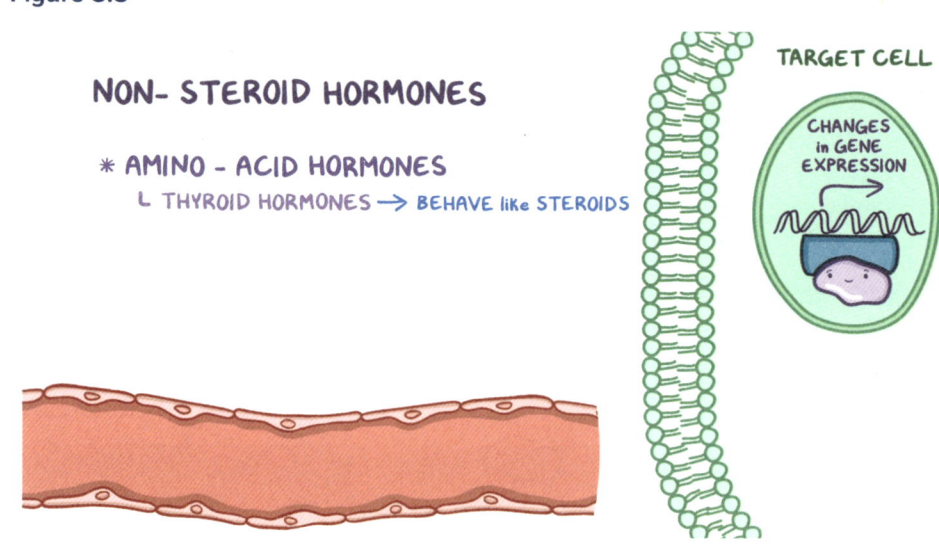

Figure 5.6

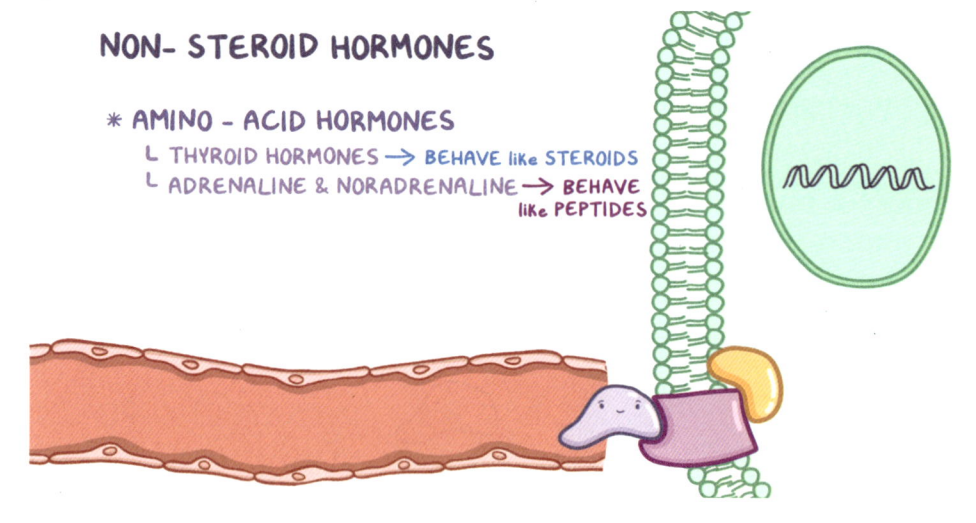

NON-STEROID HORMONES

* AMINO-ACID HORMONES
  - THYROID HORMONES → BEHAVE like STEROIDS
  - ADRENALINE & NORADRENALINE → BEHAVE like PEPTIDES

Figure 5.7

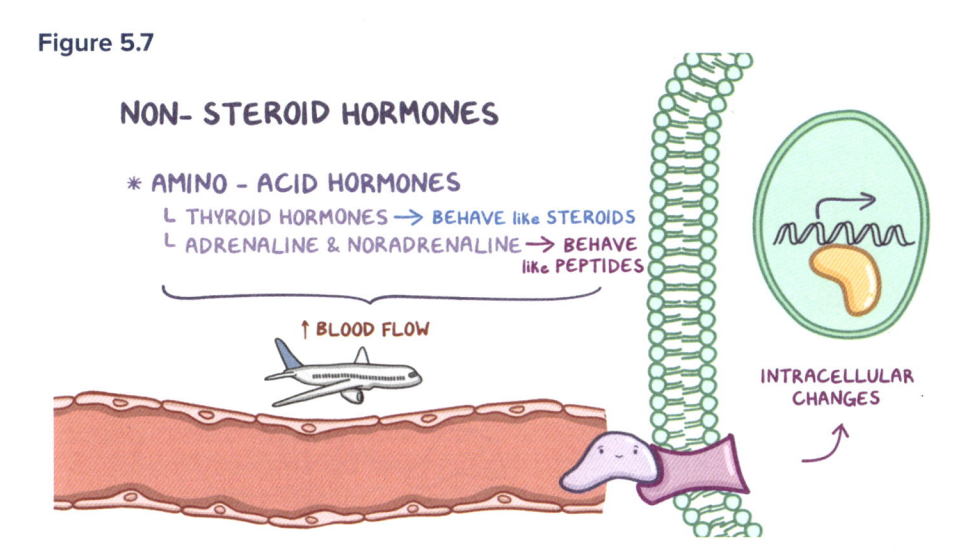

NON- STEROID HORMONES

* AMINO - ACID HORMONES
  - THYROID HORMONES → BEHAVE like STEROIDS
  - ADRENALINE & NORADRENALINE → BEHAVE like PEPTIDES

↑ BLOOD FLOW

INTRACELLULAR CHANGES

THE HYPOTHALAMUS & PITUITARY GLAND

Now, the endocrine glands are scattered throughout the body, much like a remote work environment. Let's get acquainted with our work crew! All the way up into the brain, there's the hypothalamus, the CEO. Right below it is the pituitary gland, the first officer. The hypothalamus and pituitary are physically connected by a thin stalk and they work closely together to make hormones that help control the production of other endocrine glands, like the thyroid, the adrenal glands, and the gonads **(Figure 5.8)**. The hypothalamus is made up of several nuclei: clusters of neurons with various roles, including secretion of hormones. The pituitary gland is made up of two lobes: the anterior lobe, which is made up of glandular tissue, and the posterior lobe, which is made up of the axons of neurons coming down from the supraoptic and paraventricular nucleus in the hypothalamus.

Now, the hypothalamus is the link between the nervous and the endocrine system. It receives information from the entire body regarding all sorts of things, such as body temperature, blood osmolarity, or even the presence of danger. It responds to this information by producing hormones that are stored in the posterior pituitary, to be released later, or hormones that act on the anterior pituitary, making it secrete hormones of its own. So, in effect, the hypothalamus gives the order, and the pituitary enforces it **(Figure 5.9)**.

This is possible because there are anatomical connections between the hypothalamus and both the anterior and posterior pituitary. Between the hypothalamus and the anterior lobe of the pituitary, there's the hypothalamo-hypophyseal-portal system. This is a system of tiny capillaries that moves hormones quickly from the hypothalamus to the anterior pituitary. These hypothalamic hormones can be stimulatory or inhibitory.

STIMULATORY HYPOTHALAMIC HORMONES

Let's start with the stimulatory hormones, also known as releasing hormones. These include thyrotropin-releasing hormone, or TRH; corticotropin-releasing hormone, or CRH; gonadotropin-releasing hormone, or GnRH; and, growth hormone-releasing hormone, or GHRH **(Figure 5.10)**.

These stimulatory hormones make the anterior pituitary synthesize its own hormones in response. TRH leads to the production of thyroid-stimulating hormone, or TSH, which reaches the thyroid and tells it to make more thyroid hormone. When plasma thyroid hormone levels increase, this sends a negative feedback signal to the pituitary to make less TSH, keeping thyroid hormone levels in an optimal range.

Figure 5.8

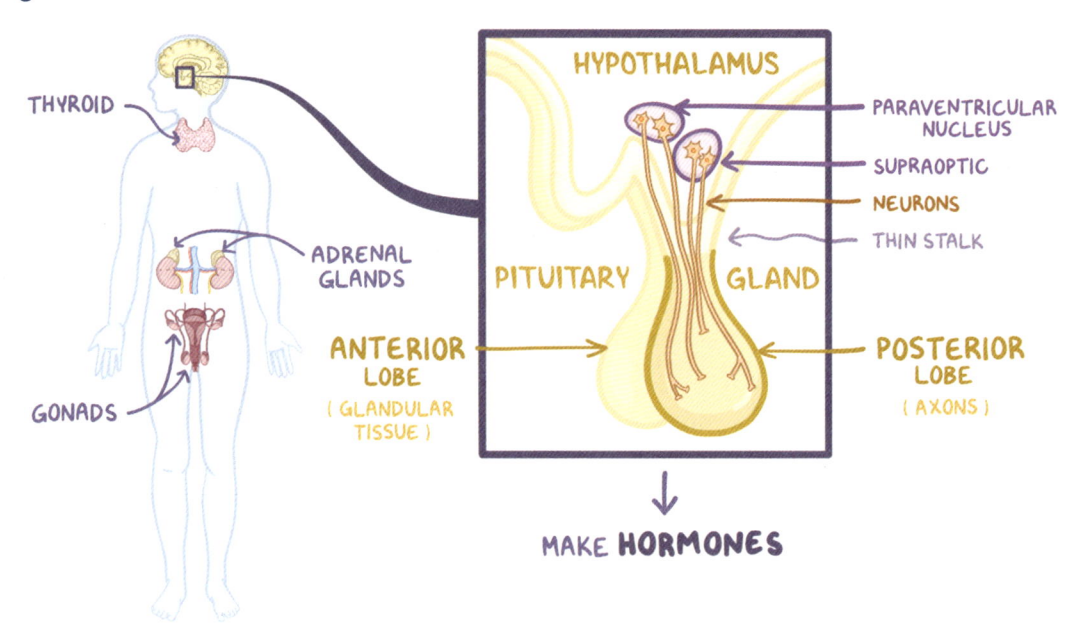

Figure 5.9

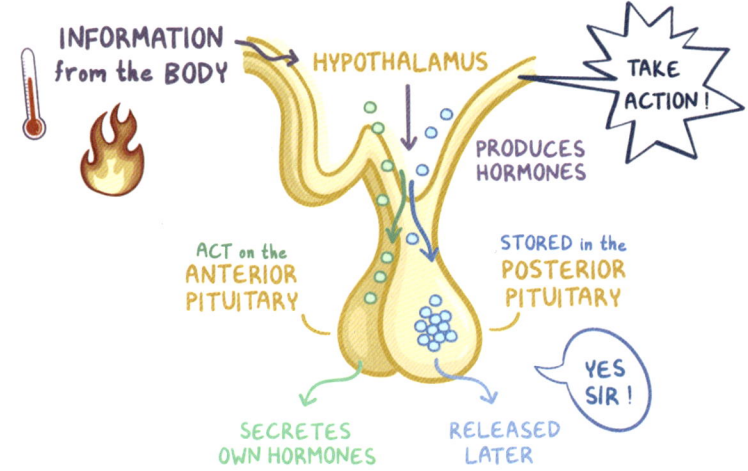

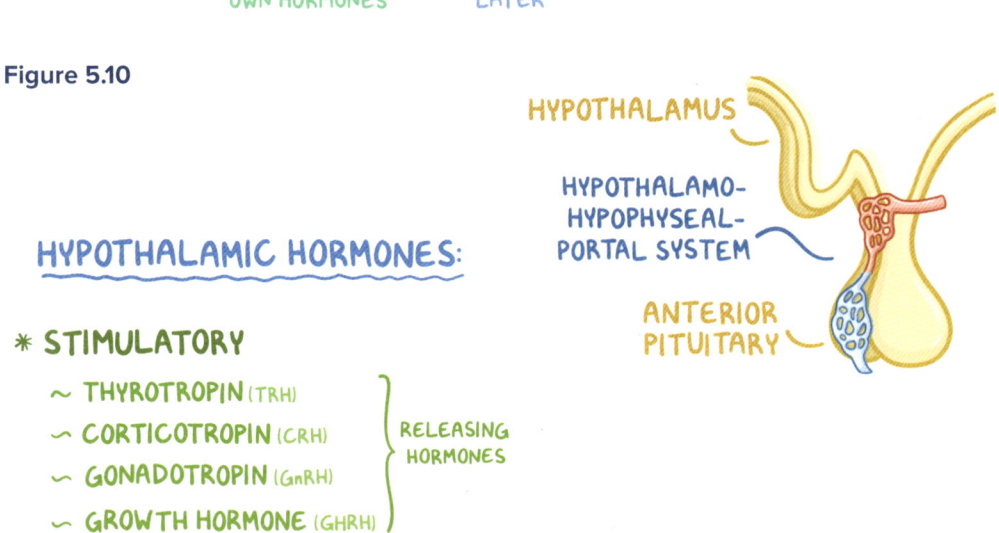

Figure 5.10

HYPOTHALAMIC HORMONES:

* **STIMULATORY**
  - THYROTROPIN (TRH)
  - CORTICOTROPIN (CRH) ⎫ RELEASING
  - GONADOTROPIN (GnRH) ⎬ HORMONES
  - GROWTH HORMONE (GHRH) ⎭

Next, there's CRH, which makes the pituitary produce adrenocorticotropic hormone, or ACTH, which goes to the adrenal glands and makes them secrete more of a hormone called cortisol. As before, high levels of cortisol inhibit the production of ACTH through a negative feedback mechanism **(Figure 5.11)**.

Following this, there's GnRH, which makes the pituitary secrete gonadotropins: follicle-stimulating hormone, or FSH, and luteinizing hormone, or LH **(Figure 5.12)**. Gonadotropins act on the gonads and regulate the production and maturation of gametes: sperm for the testes and oocytes for the ovaries. They also regulate the production of sex hormones: testosterone, estrogen, and progesterone. As a general rule, sex hormones also operate by a negative feedback mechanism via the pituitary **(Figure 5.13)**. There is an exception with individuals who are biologically female: right before ovulation, estrogen levels increase, and the pituitary becomes even more sensitive to hypothalamic GnRH. This acts as a positive feedback signal, leading to a massive surge of FSH and LH that leads to ovulation **(Figure 5.14)**.

Finally, GHRH makes the anterior pituitary secrete more growth hormone, or GH, which helps the long bones and other bodily tissues grow **(Figure 5.15)**.

INHIBITORY HYPOTHALAMIC HORMONES

So, those were the stimulatory hypothalamic hormones. The inhibitory hypothalamic hormones are much easier to remember. There are only two: growth hormone-inhibiting hormone, or GHIH, also known as somatostatin, and prolactin-inhibiting factor, also known as dopamine **(Figure 5.16)**. GHIH is also synthesized by other organs in our body, like our digestive tract, and it tells the pituitary to secrete less growth hormone **(Figure 5.17)**. Things are a bit trickier when it comes to the prolactin-inhibiting factor. Because prolactin increases milk production in the breasts, it's only needed during breastfeeding. So, outside breastfeeding, the hypothalamus continually secretes prolactin-inhibiting factor, which goes to the anterior pituitary and inhibits prolactin production so that no milk is produced. However, during breastfeeding, when the baby starts suckling, a signal is sent to the hypothalamus to halt production of prolactin-inhibiting factor. This inhibits the inhibitor, allowing the anterior pituitary to make prolactin **(Figure 5.18)**.

The hypothalamus is connected to the posterior pituitary through the pituitary stalk, which is made up of the axons of hypothalamic neurons coming specifically from the paraventricular and supraoptic nuclei. Both these nuclei secrete antidiuretic hormone—also known as ADH, or vasopressin—and oxytocin, which travel down the axons of these neurons and reach the posterior lobe of the pituitary gland. Down the length of these axons, there are small dilations called Herring bodies, which store the hormones until they get a signal to release them **(Figure 5.19)**.

When the time is right, the axons release ADH or oxytocin into the posterior pituitary capillaries and, from there, into the systemic circulation. The axons release ADH when there is either a high blood osmolarity or a low blood volume. ADH helps retain water from the urine and also causes vasoconstriction of blood vessels, which helps decrease osmolarity and increase blood pressure **(Figure 5.20)**. The other hormone, oxytocin, dilates the cervix and stimulates uterine contractions during childbirth, and makes the muscle cells in the breasts contract to eject milk during breastfeeding **(Figure 5.21)**. So, outside motherhood, its levels are generally low, but they do increase a little during pleasant social interactions, such as hugs and physical contact, or even after an orgasm—hence that lovely "afterglow."

Figure 5.11

HYPOTHALAMUS
CRH
ANTERIOR PITUITARY
⊖
ADRENAL GLANDS
↓ CORTISOL
⊕
↓ ADRENOCORTICOTROPIC HORMONE (ACTH)

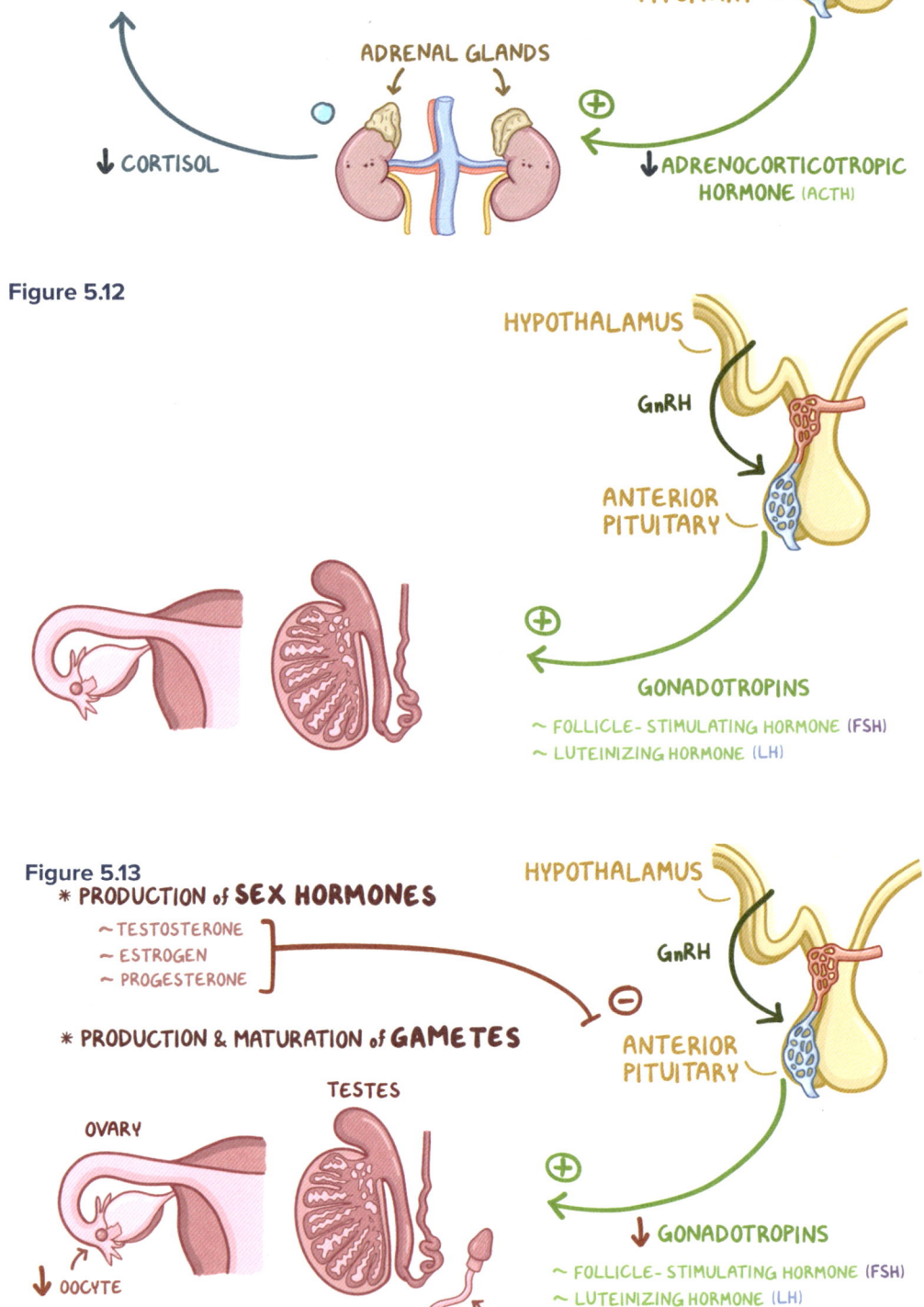

Figure 5.12

HYPOTHALAMUS
GnRH
ANTERIOR PITUITARY
⊕
GONADOTROPINS
~ FOLLICLE- STIMULATING HORMONE (FSH)
~ LUTEINIZING HORMONE (LH)

Figure 5.13

* PRODUCTION of **SEX HORMONES**
  ~ TESTOSTERONE
  ~ ESTROGEN
  ~ PROGESTERONE

* PRODUCTION & MATURATION of **GAMETES**

OVARY
TESTES
↓ OOCYTE
↓ SPERM

HYPOTHALAMUS
GnRH
⊖
ANTERIOR PITUITARY
⊕
↓ GONADOTROPINS
~ FOLLICLE- STIMULATING HORMONE (FSH)
~ LUTEINIZING HORMONE (LH)

Chapter 5 The Endocrine System

Figure 5.14

EXCEPTION: in FEMALES

OVULATION

ESTROGEN, LH, FSH

HYPOTHALAMUS
GnRH
ANTERIOR PITUITARY
⊕
↑↑ GONADOTROPINS
~ FOLLICLE-STIMULATING HORMONE (FSH)
~ LUTEINIZING HORMONE (LH)

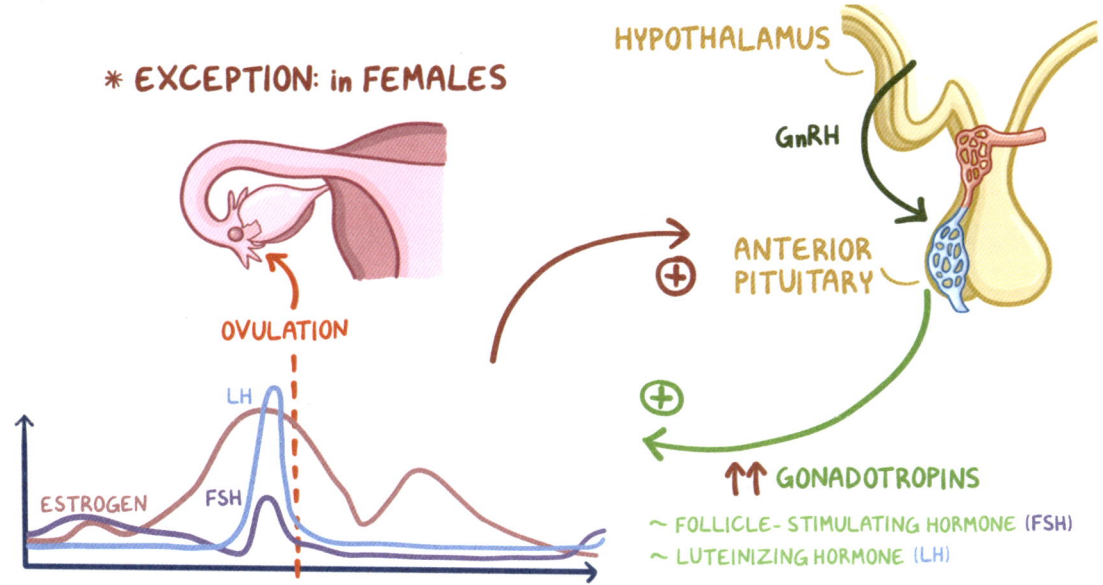

Figure 5.15

HYPOTHALAMUS
GHRH
ANTERIOR PITUITARY
⊕
GROWTH HORMONE (GH)
LONG BONES & OTHER TISSUES

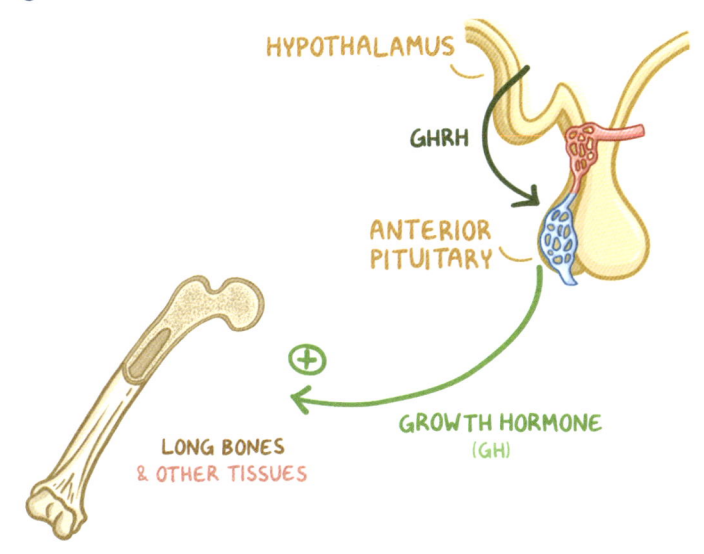

Figure 5.16

HYPOTHALAMIC HORMONES:

* **STIMULATORY**
* **INHIBITORY**
  ~ GROWTH HORMONE INHIBITING HORMONE (GHIH, or SOMATOSTATIN)
  ~ PROLACTIN INHIBITING FACTOR (DOPAMINE)

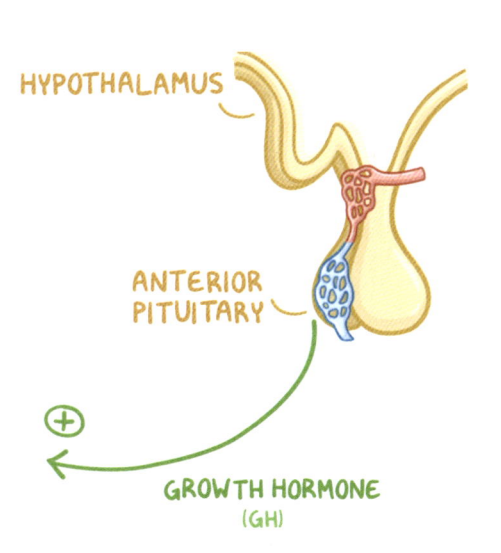

HYPOTHALAMUS
ANTERIOR PITUITARY
⊕
GROWTH HORMONE (GH)

OSMOSIS.ORG 59

Figure 5.17

HYPOTHALAMUS

GHIH ⊖

ANTERIOR PITUITARY

DIGESTIVE TRACT

⊕ ↓ GROWTH HORMONE (GH)

Figure 5.18

⊖ HYPOTHALAMUS

CONTINUOUSLY SECRETED → PROLACTIN INHIBITING FACTOR ✗

ANTERIOR PITUITARY

⊕ PROLACTIN

DURING BREASTFEEDING

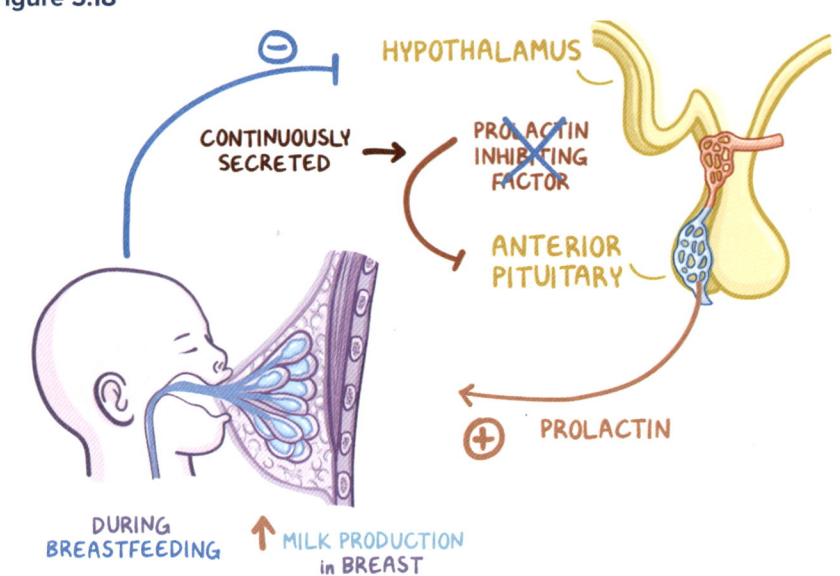

↑ MILK PRODUCTION in BREAST

Figure 5.19

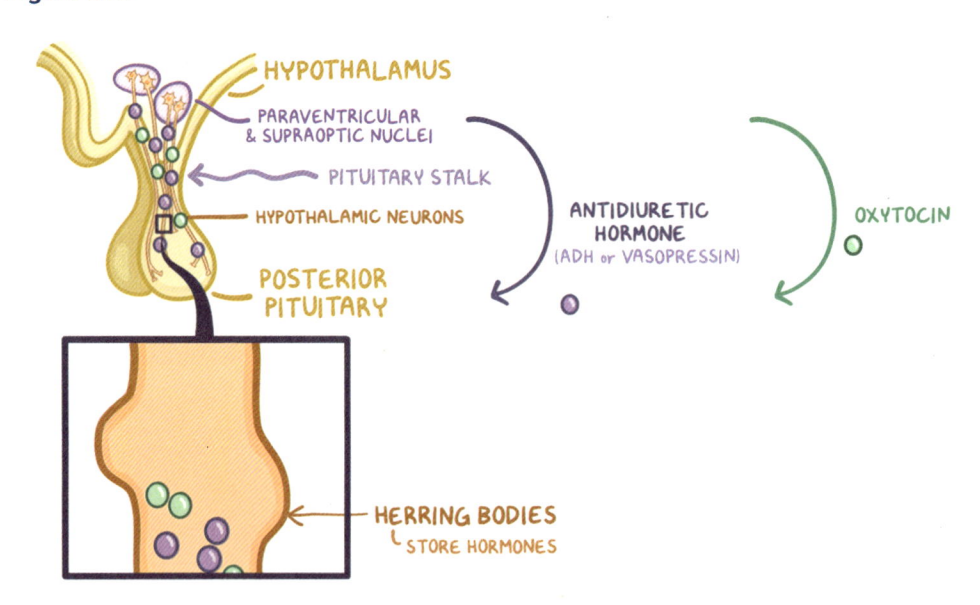

HYPOTHALAMUS
PARAVENTRICULAR & SUPRAOPTIC NUCLEI
PITUITARY STALK
HYPOTHALAMIC NEURONS
POSTERIOR PITUITARY

ANTIDIURETIC HORMONE (ADH or VASOPRESSIN)

OXYTOCIN

HERRING BODIES
store hormones

60 OSMOSIS.ORG

Figure 5.20

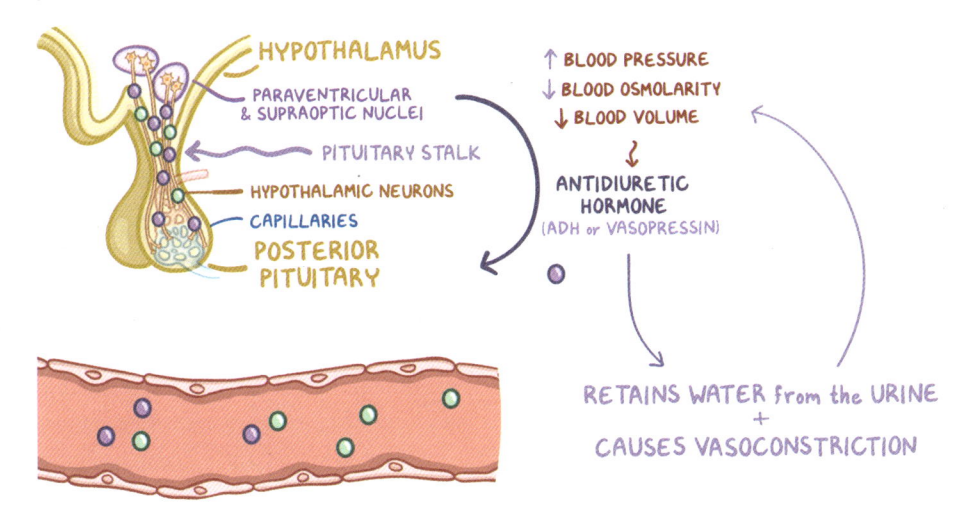

Figure 5.21

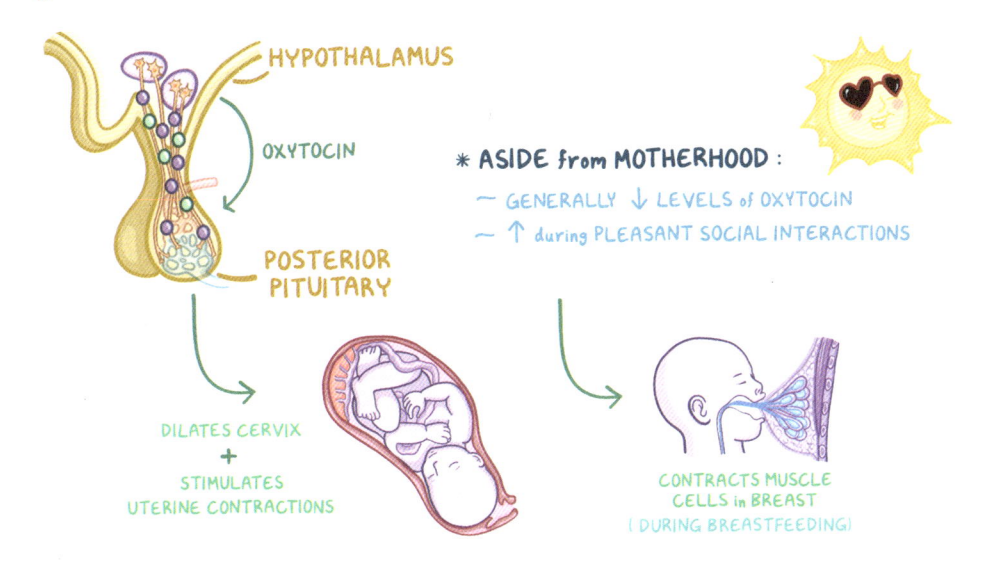

THE OTHER ENDOCRINE GLANDS

Let's look at the other glands in our work crew! Also in our head, behind the hypothalamus and the pituitary, there is the tiny pineal gland. The pineal gland is made up of cells called pinealocytes, which synthesize and release melatonin. Melatonin is mostly secreted during the night, and it regulates our body's circadian rhythm—or the "inner clock" that tells us when we should be sleeping and when we should be awake **(Figure 5.22)**.

Next, there's the thyroid gland at the front of the neck. It's made up of a left and a right lobe, like two wings of a butterfly. The thyroid gland is made up of thousands of follicles that make triiodothyronine, or T_3, and thyroxine, or T_4. Once inside the cell, T_4 is mostly converted into T_3, and it can begin to exert its effect. T_3 speeds up the basal metabolic rate **(Figure 5.23)**. In this way, the thyroid gland is like the operations manager: helping to boost productivity. In between the thyroid follicles, there are also parafollicular cells, or C cells, which secrete a hormone called calcitonin. On the back of each thyroid lobe, there are also two parathyroid glands—one above, and one below—so that there are four in total. They make parathyroid hormone. Both calcitonin and parathyroid hormone are involved in calcium, phosphate, and bone metabolism and are regulated by calcium levels in the blood **(Figure 5.24)**.

Figure 5.22

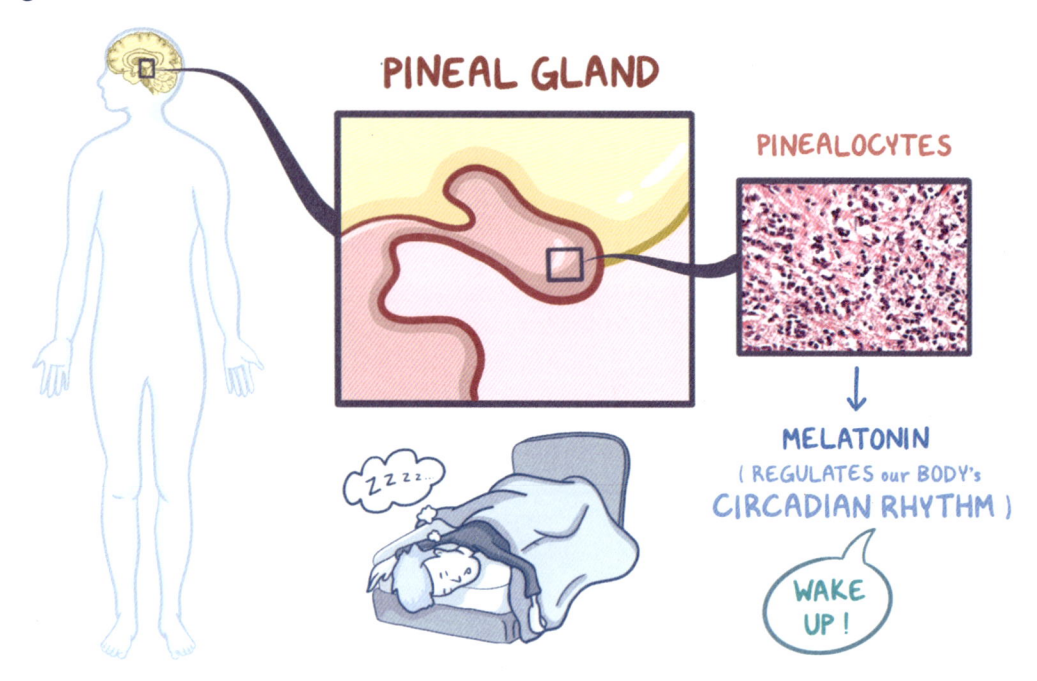

PINEAL GLAND

PINEALOCYTES

↓

MELATONIN
(REGULATES our BODY's CIRCADIAN RHYTHM)

WAKE UP!

Zzzz...

Figure 5.23

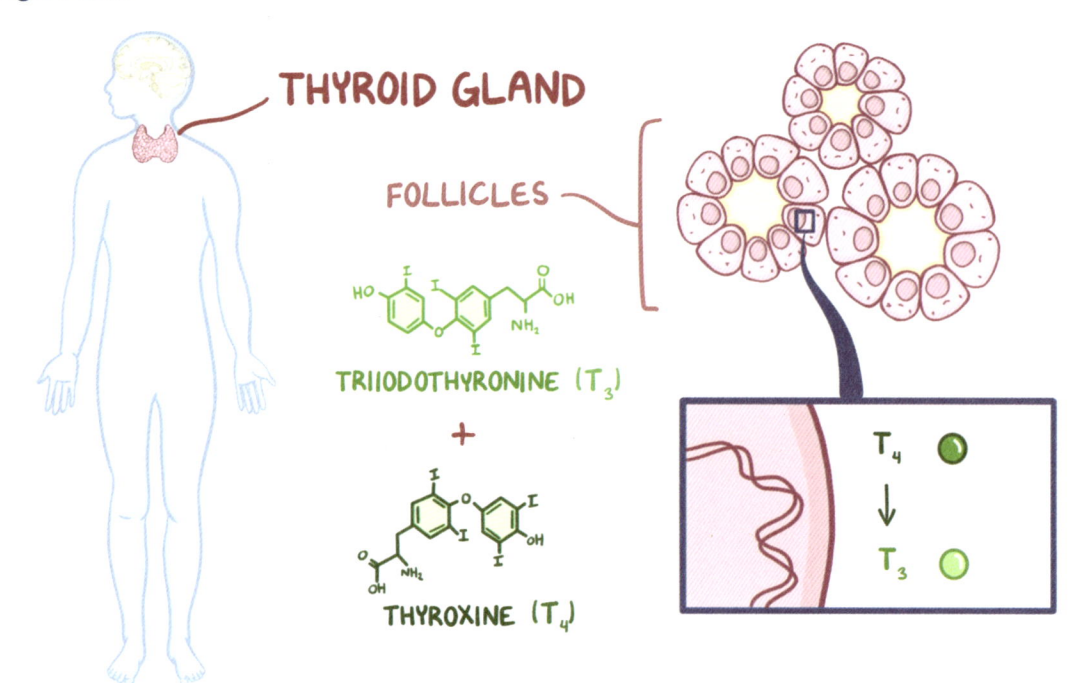

THYROID GLAND

FOLLICLES

TRIIODOTHYRONINE (T_3)

+

THYROXINE (T_4)

T_4 → T_3

62   OSMOSIS.ORG

Chapter 5 The Endocrine System

Next up, we have the adrenal glands, which are just above each of the kidneys. Each adrenal gland is made up of an outer layer, called the cortex, surrounding a core called the medulla. The cortex of the adrenal gland can further be divided into three zones that produce steroid hormones: the zona glomerulosa, which produces aldosterone; the zona fasciculata, which produces cortisol; and the zona reticularis, which produces small amounts of sex hormone precursors **(Figure 5.25)**. Aldosterone is secreted when there is low pressure or too much potassium in the blood. Upon release, aldosterone prevents loss of water and sodium in the urine and increases the elimination of potassium. Cortisol is also known as the "stress hormone," and it's secreted during fight-or-flight situations, along with adrenaline and noradrenaline, which are secreted nearby in the adrenal medulla **(Figure 5.26)**.

Finally, there's the pancreas, which has an exocrine part, that helps with digestion, and an endocrine part, that secretes insulin and glucagon. In this way, the pancreas is like the person on the team who's working two full-time jobs **(Figure 5.27)**!

The exocrine part of the pancreas secretes digestive enzymes directly into the duodenum, which help break down food into nutrients the small intestine can absorb. The endocrine part is made up of beta and alpha cells that, respectively, secrete insulin and glucagon in response to blood sugar levels. When there's high blood sugar, like right after a meal, beta cells secrete insulin into the blood, which binds to specific receptors on all the cells in our body, helping them take in glucose and use it for energy. This lowers our blood sugar levels after meals.

When there's low blood sugar, the alpha cells take charge and secrete glucagon. Glucagon knows the liver has a glucose "stash" called glycogen, so it binds to a receptor on liver cells, which respond by activating enzymes that break down glycogen and release glucose into the bloodstream. That helps us maintain our blood sugar levels between meals **(Figure 5.28)**.

Figure 5.24

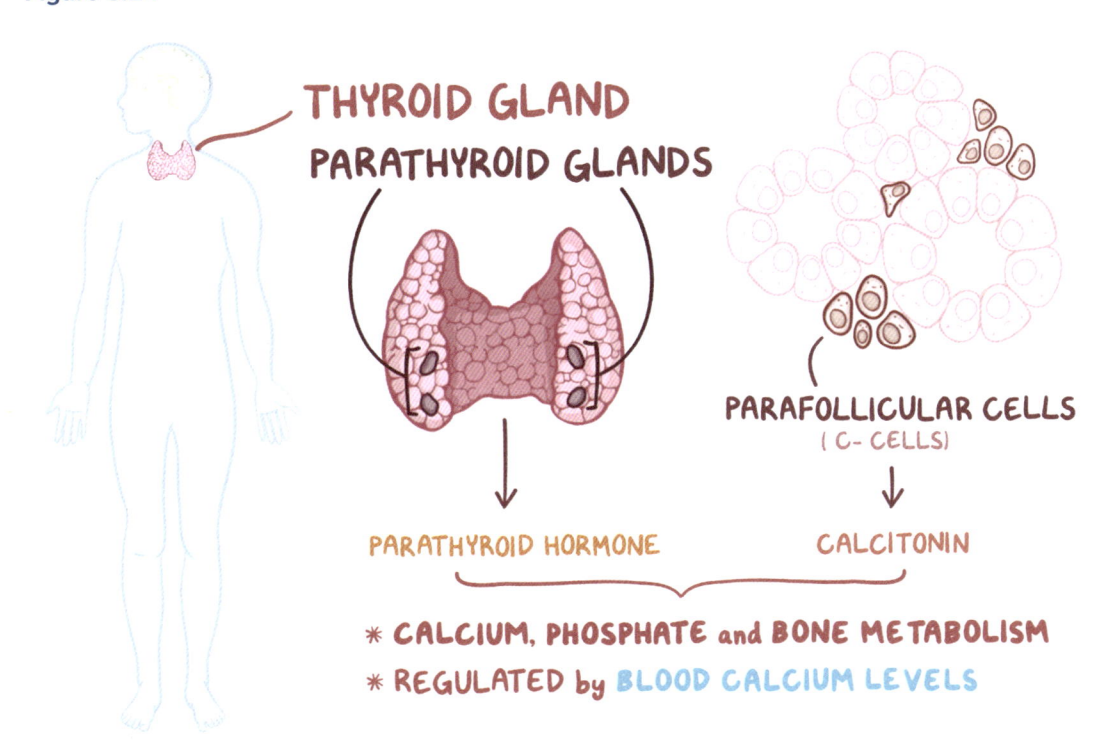

Figure 5.25

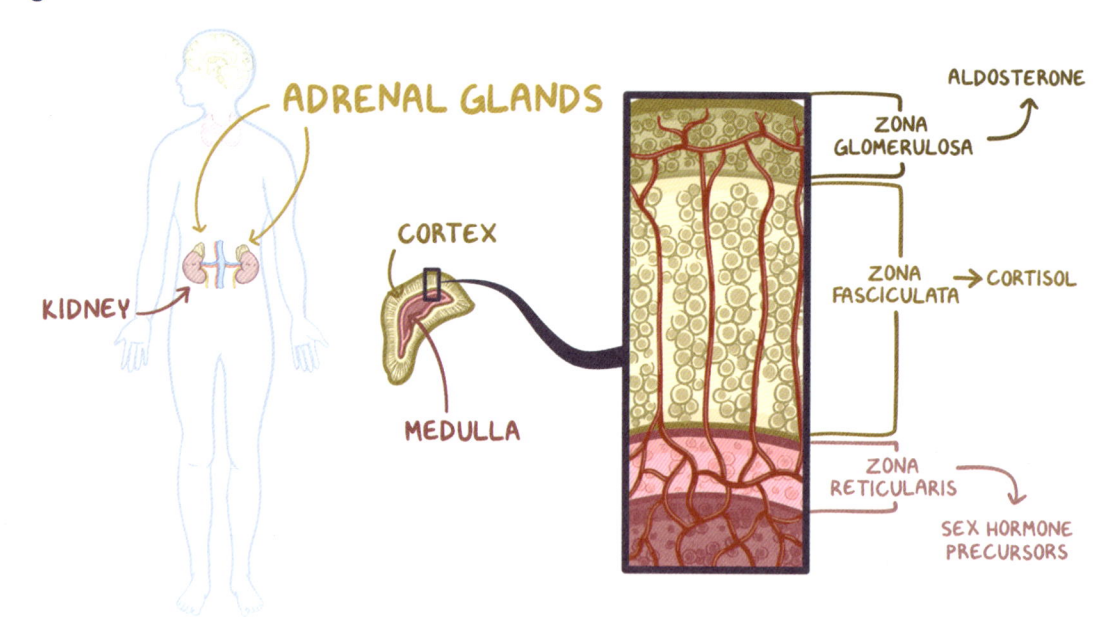

Figure 5.26

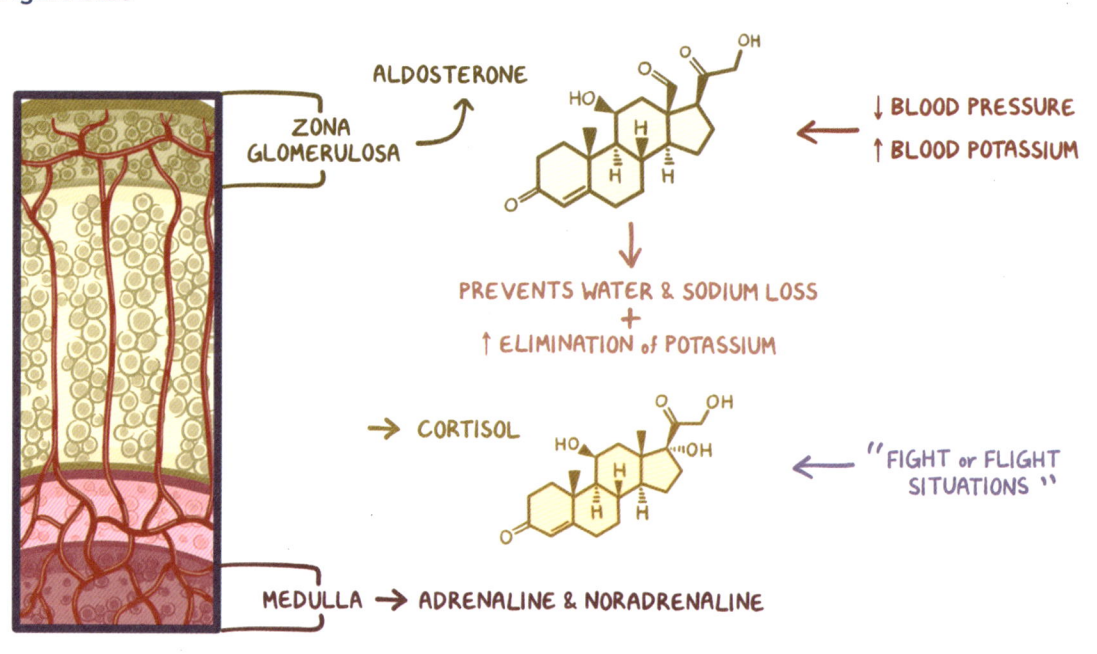

Chapter 5 The Endocrine System

Figure 5.27

PANCREAS
* **ENDOCRINE**
  └ SECRETES INSULIN & GLUCAGON
  ↑
  BLOOD SUGAR LEVELS

* **EXOCRINE**
  └ HELPS with DIGESTION

ALPHA CELLS (GLUCAGON)   BETA CELLS (INSULIN)

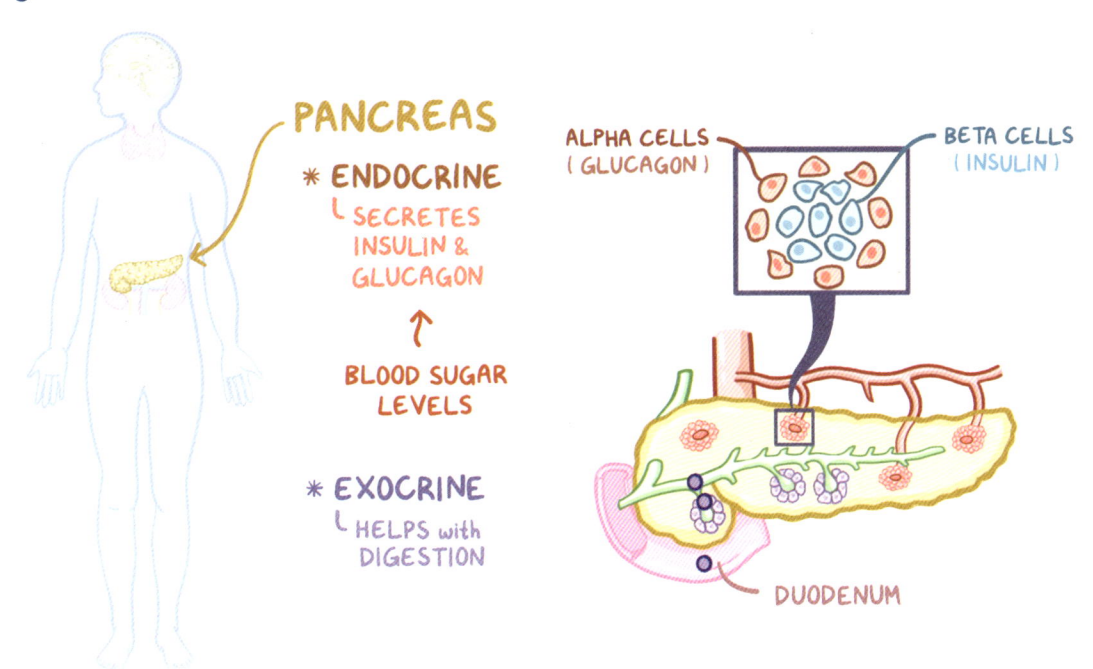

DUODENUM

Figure 5.28

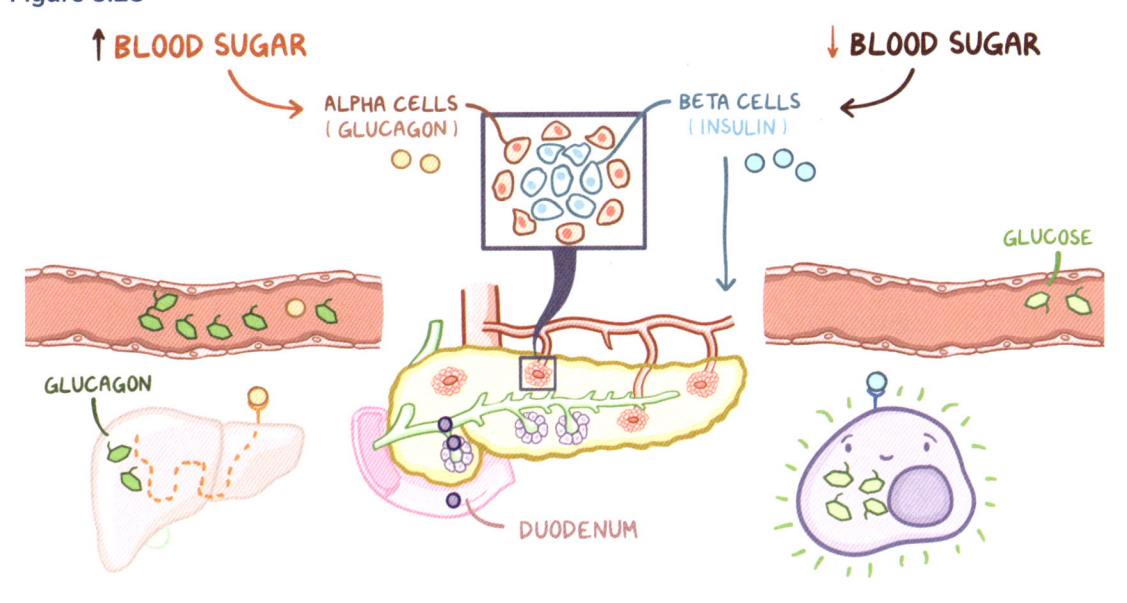

↑ BLOOD SUGAR   ↓ BLOOD SUGAR

ALPHA CELLS (GLUCAGON)   BETA CELLS (INSULIN)

GLUCOSE

GLUCAGON

DUODENUM

OSMOSIS.ORG 65

SUMMARY

All right, as a quick recap, in the endocrine system there are: steroid hormones, which are hydrophobic and diffuse across cell membranes and bind intracellular receptors; peptide hormones, which are hydrophilic and bind to cell surface receptors; and tyrosine-derived hormones that behave either like steroid hormones or like peptide hormones. Homeostasis begins with the hypothalamus, which secretes stimulatory and inhibitory hormones that affect the anterior pituitary, as well as hormones that diffuse directly into the blood at the posterior pituitary. Ultimately, these hormones affect other endocrine glands, like the thyroid, the adrenal glands, and the gonads. Other endocrine glands that are not under direct control of the hypothalamus are the parathyroids, which make parathyroid hormone, and the pancreas, which secretes insulin and glucagon **(Figure 5.29)**.

Figure 5.29

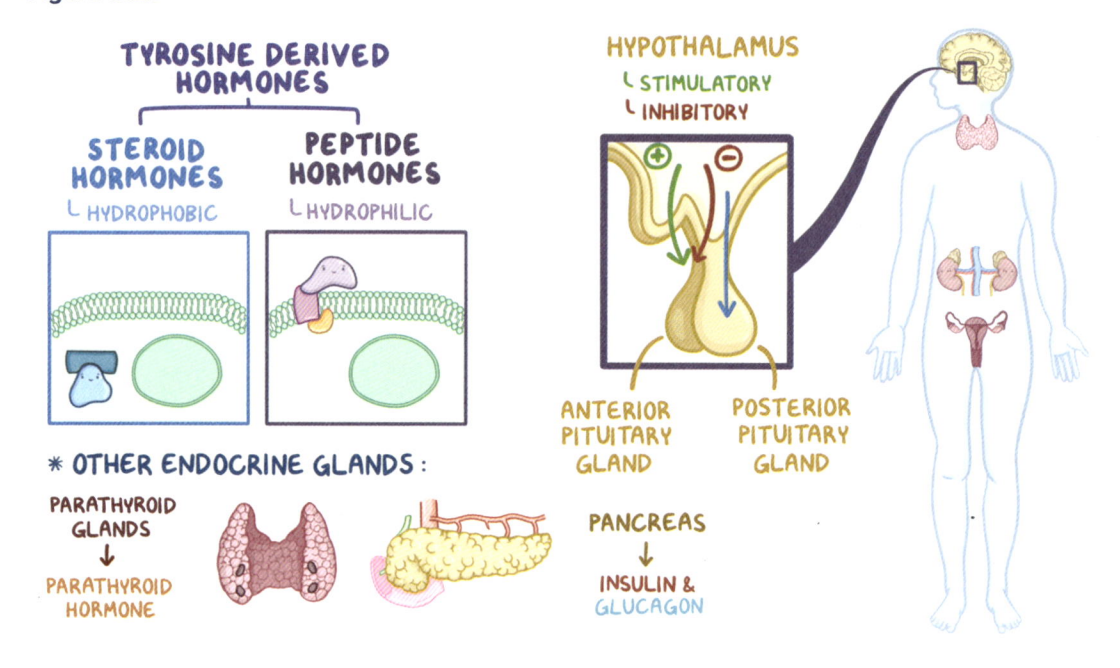

THE IMMUNE SYSTEM

osms.it/immune_system

It is thanks to our immune system that we, as humans, survive—despite the many dangers, such as the harmful microorganisms and toxins in our surrounding environments and the threat of our own cells developing into tumor cells.

The immune system is made up of organs, tissues, cells, and molecules that, together, generate an immune response that protects us from harmful microorganisms, removes toxins, and destroys tumor cells. These immune responses can identify a threat, mount an attack, eliminate a pathogen, and develop mechanisms to remember the offender in case we encounter it again—all within 10 days! In some cases, as with a particularly stubborn pathogen or an immune attack on our own tissue, the response can last much longer—from months to even years—and this leads to chronic inflammation **(Figure 6.1)**.

THE FIRST BRANCH: INNATE IMMUNE RESPONSE

Your immune system is like a military with two main branches: the innate immune response and the adaptive immune response. The first of these branches, the innate immune response, includes cells that are nonspecific. This means that although they can distinguish an invader from a human cell, they can't distinguish one invader from another invader. The innate response is feverishly fast—working within minutes or hours. It's also responsible for causing fevers. (Get it? Feverishly fast.)

The tradeoff for that speed is that there's no memory associated with innate responses. In other words, the innate response will respond to the same pathogen in the exact same way no matter how many times it has encountered the pathogen before. The innate immune response includes things that you may not even known belong to the immune system: chemical barriers, like lysozymes in the tears and a low pH in the stomach, and physical barriers, like the epithelium in the skin and gut and the cilia that line the airways to keep invaders out **(Figure 6.2)**.

Figure 6.1

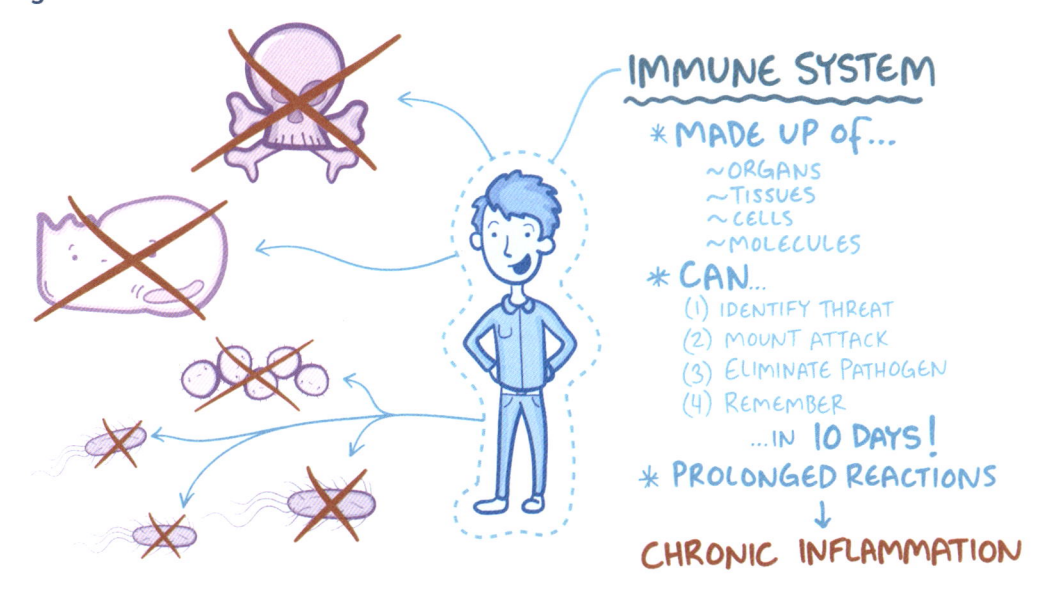

THE SECOND BRANCH: ADAPTIVE IMMUNE RESPONSE

In contrast, the adaptive immune response is highly specific to each invader. The cells of the adaptive immune response have receptors that differentiate one pathogen from another by their unique parts, which are called antigens. The receptors can distinguish between friendly bacteria and potentially deadly bacteria. The trade off for that recognition is that the adaptive response relies on cells being primed or activated, so they can fully differentiate into the right kind of fighter to kill the pathogen, and this process takes time—up to a few weeks!

The great advantage of the adaptive immune response is immunologic memory. The cells that are activated in the adaptive immune response undergo clonal expansion, which means they massively proliferate. And each time the adaptive cells see the same pathogen, they massively proliferate again, resulting in a stronger, faster response each time that pathogen comes around. Once the pathogen is destroyed, most of the clonally expanded cells die off, which is called clonal deletion. But some of the clonally expanded cells live on as memory cells, and they're ready to expand once more if that pathogen ever resurfaces **(Figure 6.3)**.

Figure 6.2

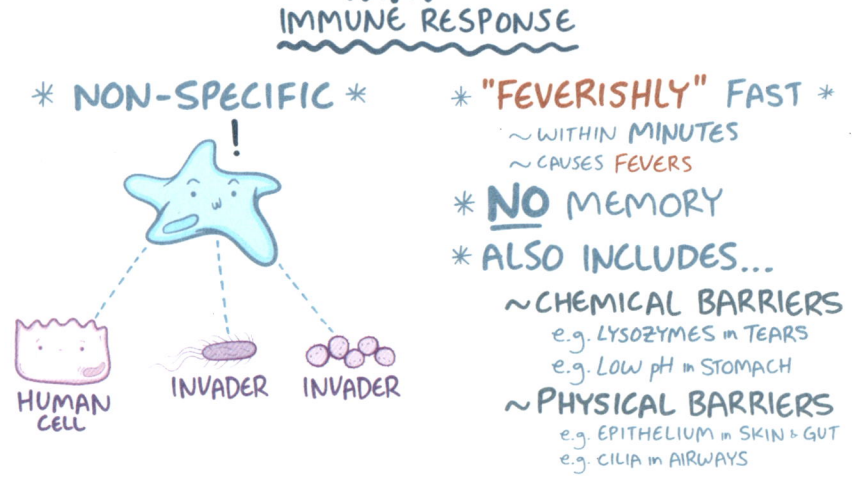

Figure 6.3

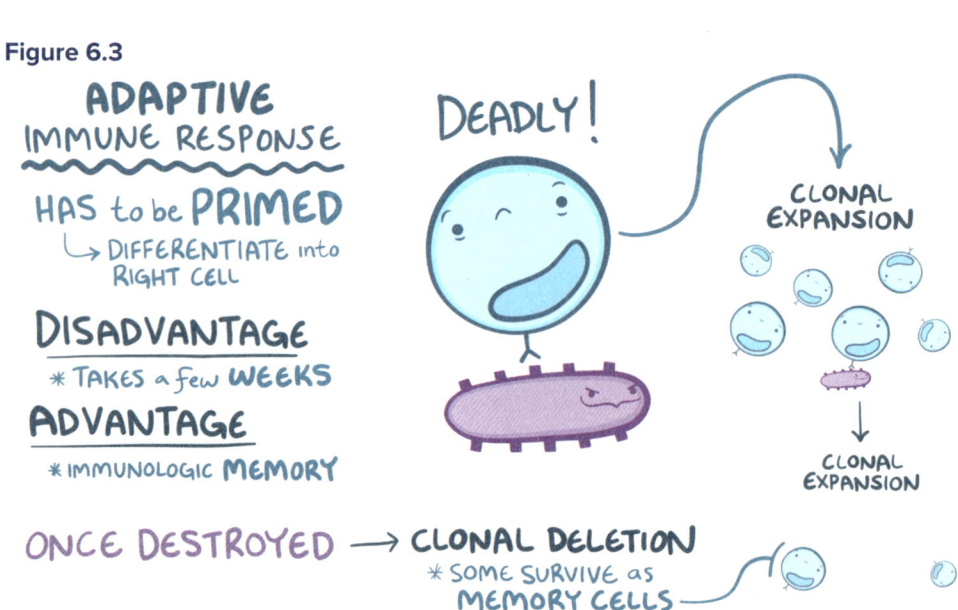

Chapter 6 The Immune System

THE SOLDIERS: WHITE BLOOD CELLS (AKA LEUKOCYTES)

Now, it's time to meet the soldiers: the white blood cells, or leukocytes. Hematopoiesis is the process of forming white blood cells, as well as red blood cells and platelets, and it takes place in the bone marrow. Hematopoiesis starts with a multipotent hematopoietic stem cell, which can develop into various cell types—thus, its future is undecided. Some become myeloid progenitor cells, whereas others become lymphoid progenitor cells **(Figure 6.4)**.

MYELOID PROGENITOR CELLS

Our first group of soldiers are the myeloid progenitor cells. These cells develop into myeloid cells, which include neutrophils, eosinophils, basophils, mast cells, dendritic cells, macrophages, and monocytes. All of these cells are part of the innate immune response and can be found in the blood, as well as in the tissues. The neutrophils, eosinophils, basophils, and mast cells are considered granulocytes because they contain granules in their cytoplasm. The trio of neutrophils, eosinophils, and basophils are also known as polymorphonuclear cells, or PMNs, because their nuclei, instead of being round in shape like that of the mast cells, contain multiple lobes **(Figure 6.5)**.

Figure 6.4

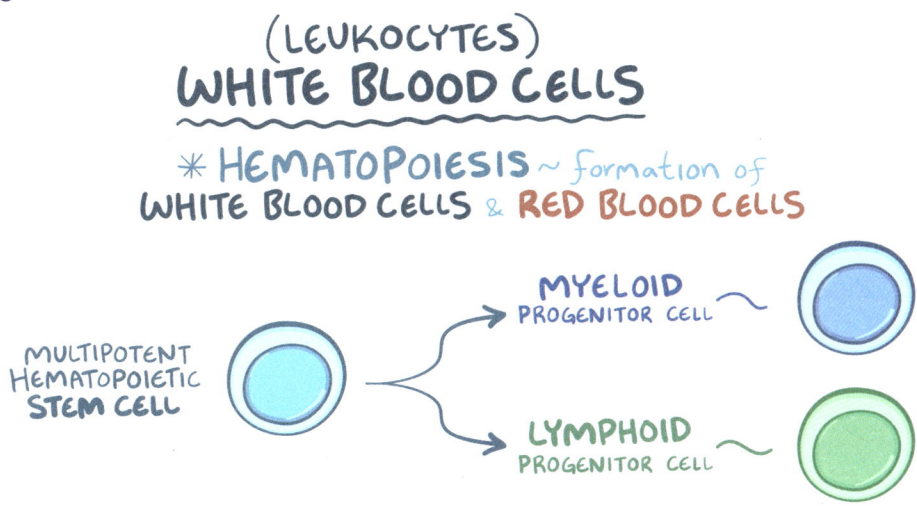

Figure 6.5

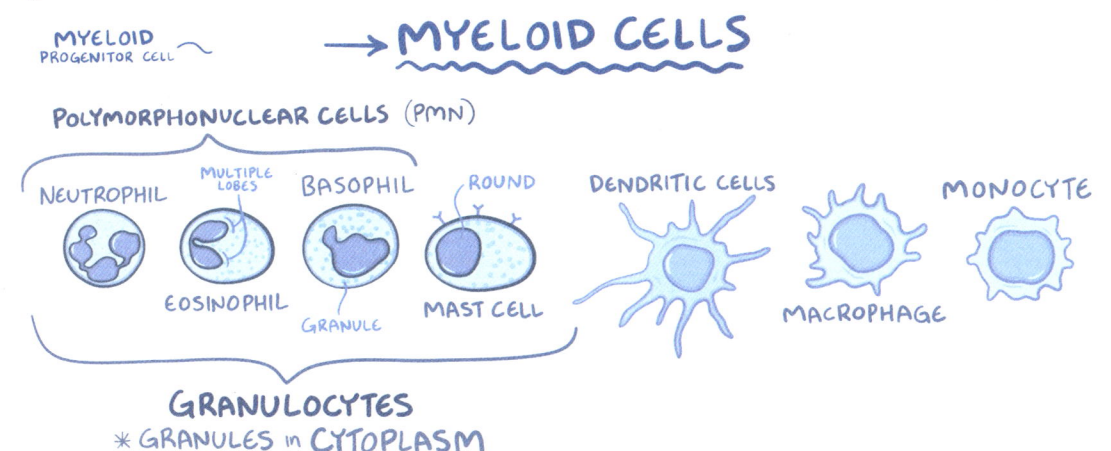

During an immune response, the bone marrow produces many PMNs, most of which are neutrophils **(Figure 6.6)**. Neutrophils use a process called phagocytosis: they approach a pathogen and reach around it with their cytoplasm to "swallow" it whole, so that it ends up in a phagosome. From there, the neutrophils destroy the pathogen in two steps: using their cytoplasmic granules and creating an oxidative burst. First, the cytoplasmic granules fuse with the phagosome to form the phagolysosome. The granules contain molecules that lower the pH of the phagolysosome, making it very acidic, and this kills about 2% of the pathogens **(Figure 6.7)**. Meanwhile, the neutrophil continues swallowing more and more pathogens until it's full, and it is at this point that it unleashes the oxidative burst. During an oxidative burst, the neutrophil produces a large amount of highly reactive oxygen molecules, like hydrogen peroxide. These molecules destroy nearby proteins and nucleic acids. This process kills the neutrophil, but each sacrificed neutrophil is able to wipe out many pathogens **(Figure 6.8)**.

In comparison to neutrophils, the remaining PMNs, eosinophils and basophils, are far less common. They both contain granules with histamine and other proinflammatory molecules. Eosinophils stain pink with the dye eosin, which is where they get their name. Eosinophils are also phagocytic, and they're best known for fighting large and unwieldy parasites because they are much larger than neutrophils and have receptors that are specific to parasites. Basophils stain blue with the dye hematoxylin and, unlike neutrophils and eosinophils, they are non-phagocytic. Like eosinophils, they can be helpful in combating large parasites, but they also cause inflammation in asthma and allergy responses. Finally, mast cells, like basophils, are also non-phagocytic. They, too, are involved in asthma and allergic responses **(Figure 6.9)**.

Figure 6.6

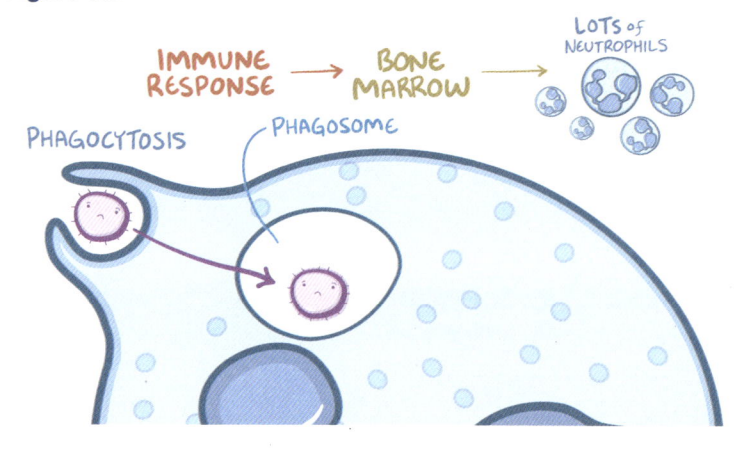

Figure 6.7

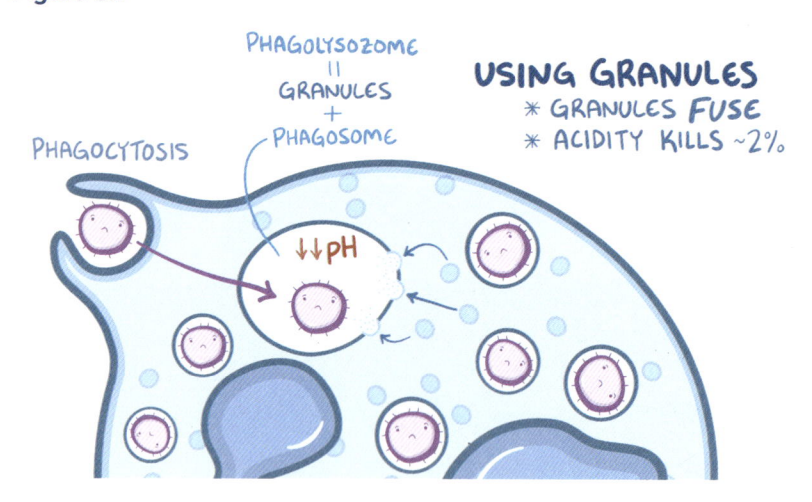

Chapter 6 The Immune System

Figure 6.8

OXIDATIVE BURST
* PRODUCES HIGHLY REACTIVE O_2 SPECIES
  - e.g. H_2O_2
* DESTROYS PROTEINS & NUCLEIC ACIDS

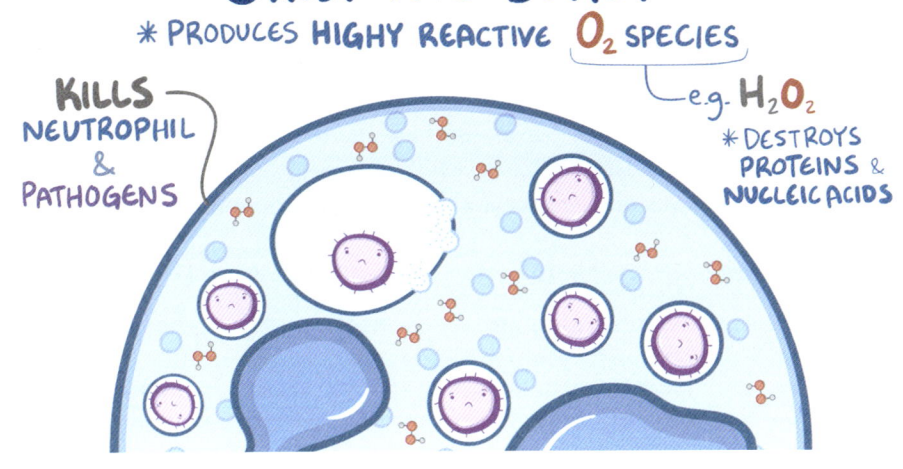

KILLS NEUTROPHIL & PATHOGENS

Figure 6.9

LESS COMMON
* CONTAIN HISTAMINE & OTHER PROINFLAMMATORY MOLECULES

EOSINOPHIL
* STAIN PINK with EOSIN
* PHAGOCYTIC
* KNOWN for FIGHTING PARASITES
* LARGER than NEUTROPHILS

BASOPHIL
* STAIN BLUE with HEMATOXYLIN
* NON-PHAGOCYTIC
* HELPFUL for FIGHTING PARASITES
* CAUSE INFLAMMATION in ASTHMA & ALLERGIC RESPONSES

MAST CELL
* NON-PHAGOCYTIC
* CAUSE INFLAMMATION in ASTHMA & ALLERGIC RESPONSES

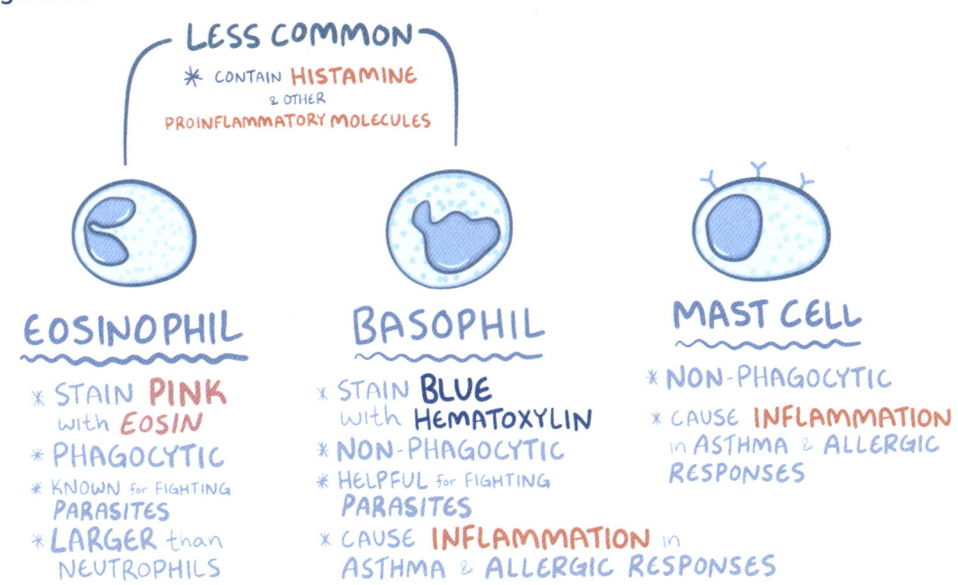

Figure 6.10

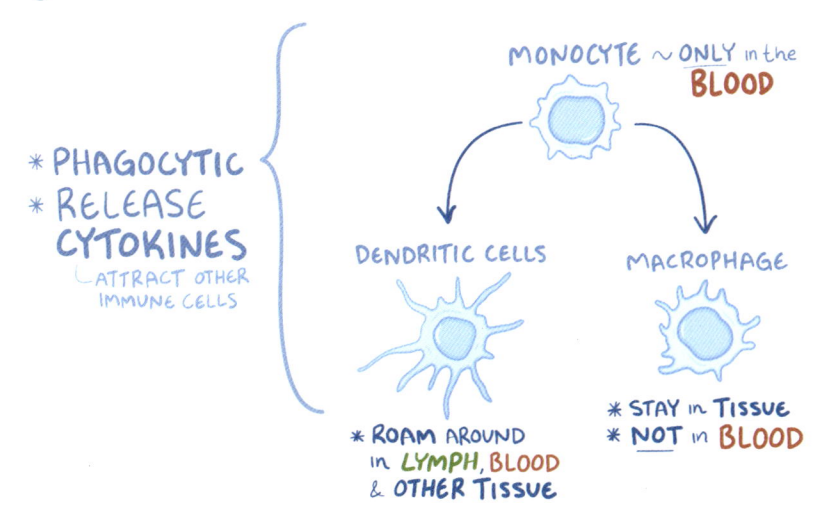

* PHAGOCYTIC
* RELEASE CYTOKINES
  - ATTRACT OTHER IMMUNE CELLS

MONOCYTE ~ ONLY in the BLOOD
→ DENDRITIC CELLS
→ MACROPHAGE

DENDRITIC CELLS
* ROAM AROUND in LYMPH, BLOOD & OTHER TISSUE

MACROPHAGE
* STAY in TISSUE
* NOT in BLOOD

OSMOSIS.ORG 71

Next up are the monocytes, macrophages, and dendritic cells. These are phagocytic cells. They gobble up pathogens and release cytokines, which are tiny molecules that help attract other immune cells to the area. Monocytes only circulate in the blood. Some monocytes migrate into tissues and differentiate into macrophages, which remain in the tissue and aren't found in the blood. Other monocytes differentiate into dendritic cells, which roam around in the lymph, blood, and tissue.

When dendritic cells are young and immature, they're excellent at phagocytosis. They are constantly eating large amounts of protein found in the interstitial fluid. When a dendritic cell phagocytoses a pathogen for the first time, it's a life-changing, coming-of-age moment. Mature dendritic cells will destroy the pathogen and break up its proteins into short amino acid chains. They then move through the lymph to the nearest lymph node **(Figure 6.11)**.

Once there, the dendritic cells perform antigen presentation. They present those amino acid chains, which are antigens, to T cells. Antigen presentation is something that can be done by dendritic cells, macrophages residing in the lymph node, and monocytes which travel to a lymph node after phagocytosing a bloodborne pathogen. All of these cells (dendritic cells, macrophages, and monocytes) are referred to as antigen-presenting cells.

Only T cells with a receptor that can bind to the specific shape of the antigen will get activated. This is called priming. It's similar to how a lock will only snap open for a key with a very specific shape. However, T cells can only see their antigen if it is presented to them on a silver platter. On a molecular level, that platter is the major histocompatibility complex, or MHC. So, the antigen-presenting cell will load the antigen onto an MHC molecule and display it to T cells, and when the right T cell comes along, it binds **(Figure 6.12)**!

Figure 6.11

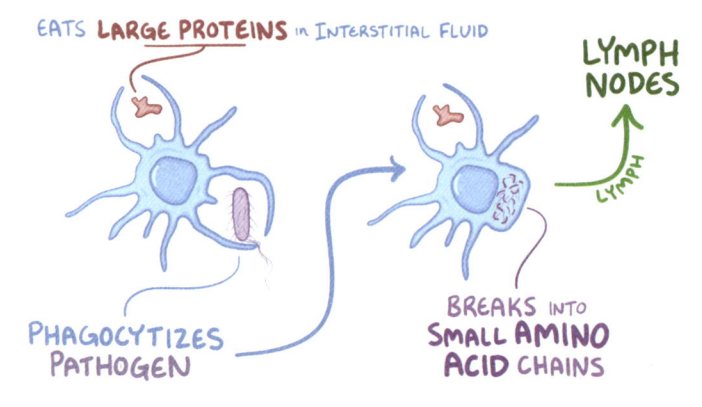

Figure 6.12

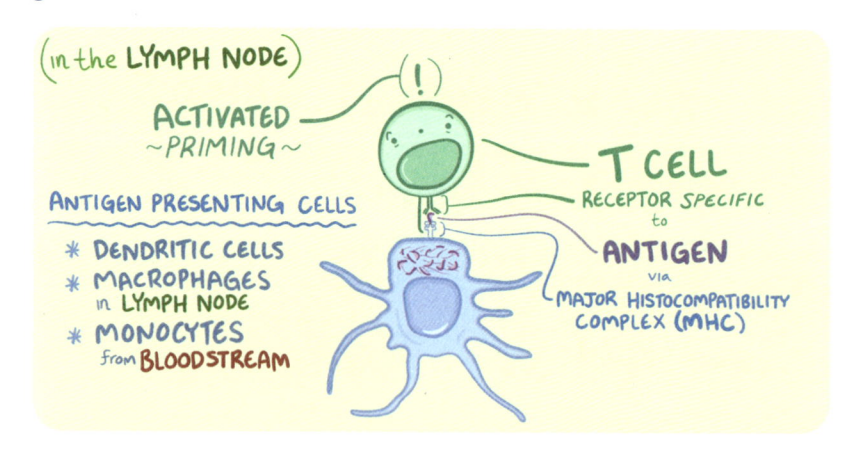

Chapter 6 The Immune System

LYMPHOID PROGENITOR CELLS

Our first group of soldiers are the lymphoid progenitor cells. These cells develop into lymphoid cells, of which there are three types: the B cells; NK cells (natural killer cells); and the T cells. B cells and NK cells complete their development where they started: in the bone marrow. Some lymphoid progenitor cells, however, migrate to the thymus, where they develop into T cells. All of the lymphocytes are able to travel in and out of both tissue and the bloodstream **(Figure 6.13)**.

NK cells are large lymphocytes with granules. They target cells infected with intracellular organisms, like viruses, as well as cells that pose a threat, like cancer cells. NK cells kill their target cells by releasing cytotoxic granules. These granules contain some molecules that punch holes in the target cell's membrane by binding directly to the phospholipids and creating pores. These granules also contain some molecules that get inside the cell and cause target cells to undergo apoptosis, which is a programmed cell death **(Figure 6.14)**.

Figure 6.13

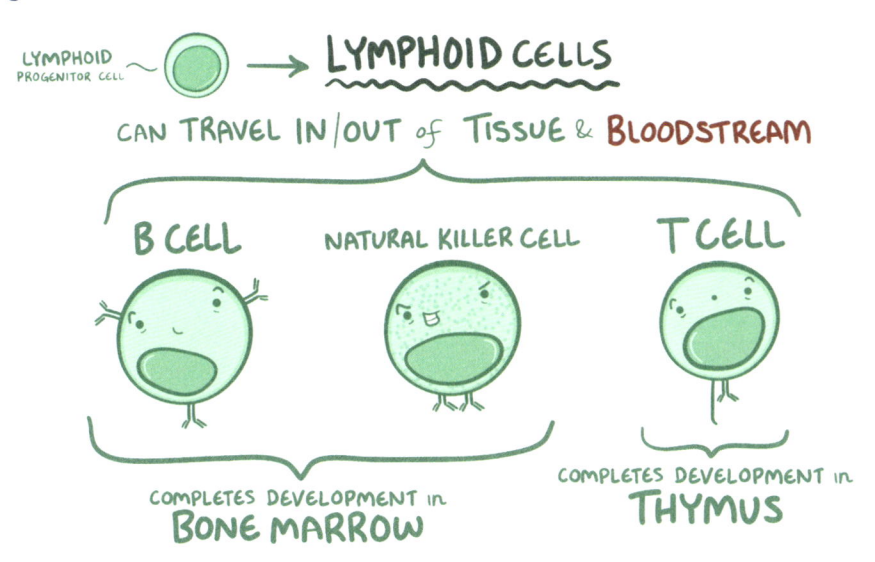

Figure 6.14

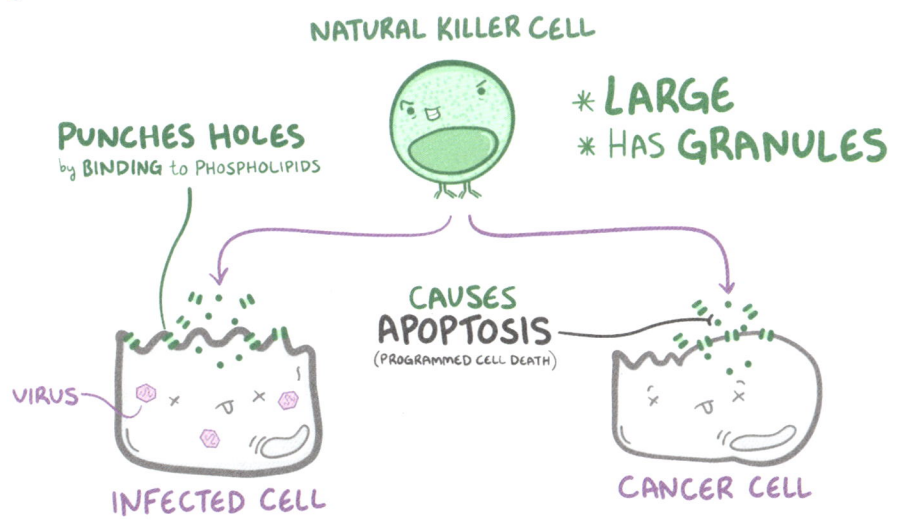

B cells, like T cells, have a receptor on their surface that allows them to only bind to an antigen that has a very specific shape. The main difference is that B cells don't need the antigen to be presented to them on an MHC molecule. They can simply bind to an antigen directly. When a B cell binds to an antigen that's on the surface of a pathogen, it is capable of phagocytosis and antigen presentation. So, technically, B cells are also antigen-presenting cells. Like other antigen-presenting cells, B cells load the antigen onto an MHC molecule, called MHC II, and display it to the T cells **(Figure 6.15)**.

When a T cell is activated, it helps the B cell mature into a plasma cell, and a plasma cell can secrete lots and lots of antibodies. Typically, it takes a few weeks for antibody levels to peak. The antibodies, or immunoglobulins, have the exact same antigen specificity as the B cell they come from. Antibodies are just the B cell receptor in a secreted form, so they can circulate in serum, which is the noncellular part of blood, attaching to pathogens and tagging them for destruction. Because antibodies aren't bound to cells and float freely in the blood, this is considered humoral immunity: a throwback to the ancient and medieval term "humors," which refers to the bodily fluids **(Figure 6.16)**.

The T cell is in charge of cell-mediated immunity. T cells are antigen specific, but they can't secrete their antigen receptor. A naive T cell can be activated or primed to turn into a mature T cell by any of the antigen-presenting cells. Most often, this activation is completed by a dendritic cell. Now, there are two main types of T cells: CD4 T cells and CD8 T cells. In both cases, the "CD" stands for cluster of differentiation. There are hundreds of CD markers in the immune system, and these markers can be used to distinguish between the different types of cells.

For example, all T cells are CD3+, because CD3 is part of the T cell receptor. Subsequently, CD4+ T cells are actually CD3+CD4+ T cells. These cells are called helper cells. They're like generals on the battlefield: they secrete cytokines that help coordinate the efforts of macrophages, B cells, and NK cells. Helper T cells can only see their antigen if it is presented on an MHC II molecule.

Here's another example. CD8+ T cells are actually CD3+CD8+ T cells. These cells are called cytotoxic T cells. They kill target cells, in a way similar to NK cells. There is, however, one major difference. CD8+ T cells only kill cells that present a specific antigen on an MHC I molecule, which is structurally similar to the MHC II molecule, whereas NK cells aren't nearly as specific in which pathogens they kill **(Figure 6.17)**.

Figure 6.15

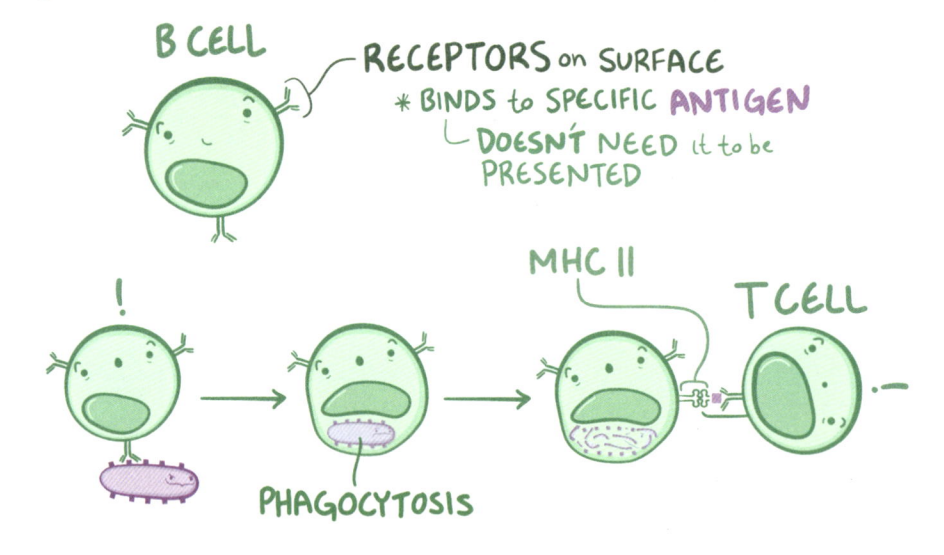

Chapter 6 The Immune System

Figure 6.16

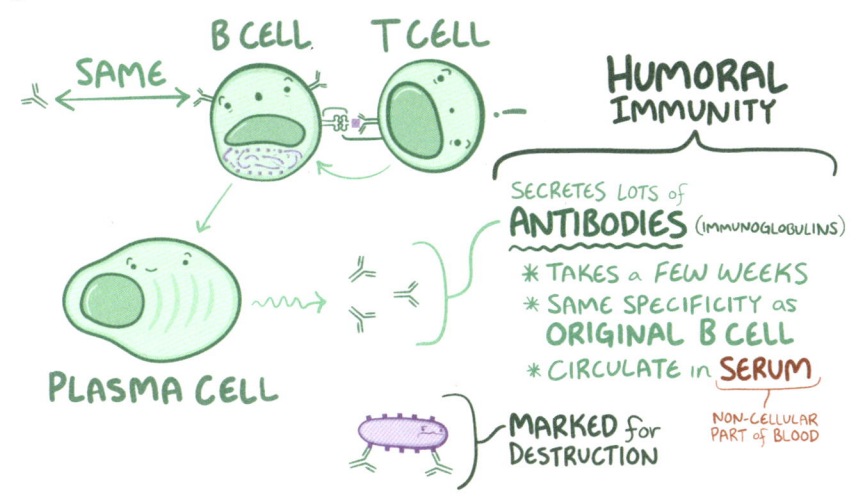

B CELL — SAME — T CELL

HUMORAL IMMUNITY
- SECRETES LOTS of ANTIBODIES (IMMUNOGLOBULINS)
- * TAKES a FEW WEEKS
- * SAME SPECIFICITY as ORIGINAL B CELL
- * CIRCULATE in SERUM (NON-CELLULAR PART of BLOOD)
- MARKED for DESTRUCTION

PLASMA CELL

Figure 6.17

T CELL
- * CELL-MEDIATED IMMUNITY
- * ANTIGEN-SPECIFIC (CAN'T SECRETE)

NAIVE T CELL → PRIMED

CLUSTER of DIFFERENTIATION (HUNDREDS in IMMUNE SYSTEM)

CD4+ T CELL (CD3+CD4+)
- * HELPER T CELL
- * SECRETE CYTOKINES THAT COORDINATE
- * CAN ONLY SEE ANTIGEN on MHC II

CD8+ T CELL (CD3+CD8+)
- * CYTOTOXIC T CELL — KILLS TARGET CELL
- * KILLS CELLS with ANTIGEN on MHC I

ANTIGEN-PRESENTING CELL (USUALLY DENDRITIC CELLS)

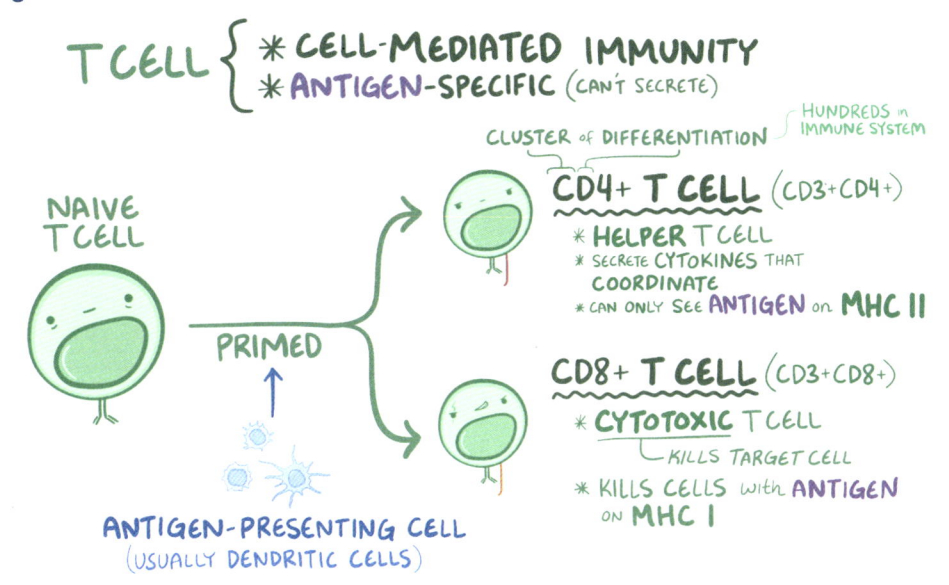

Figure 6.18

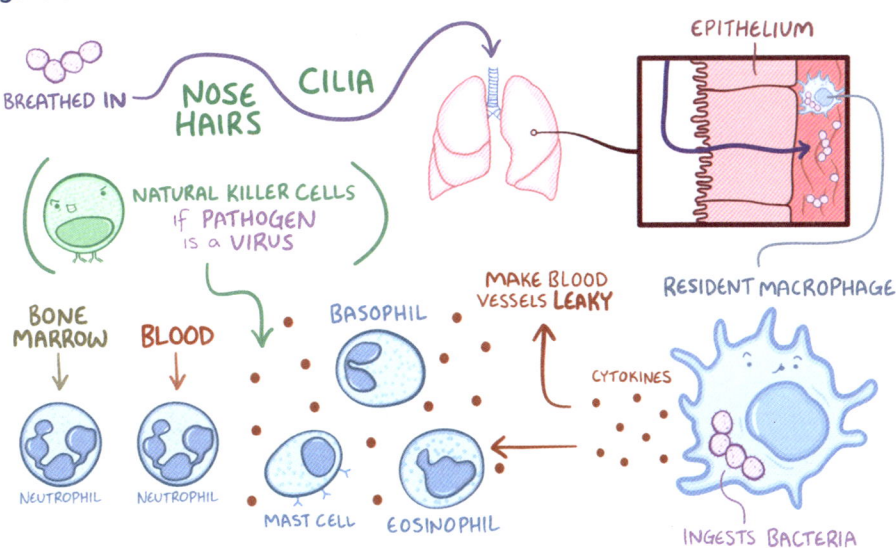

BREATHED IN → NOSE HAIRS, CILIA → EPITHELIUM

NATURAL KILLER CELLS if PATHOGEN is a VIRUS

BONE MARROW → NEUTROPHIL
BLOOD → NEUTROPHIL

BASOPHIL, MAST CELL, EOSINOPHIL

MAKE BLOOD VESSELS LEAKY ← CYTOKINES

RESIDENT MACROPHAGE — INGESTS BACTERIA

OSMOSIS.ORG 75

Figure 6.19

LUNG TISSUE → DENDRITIC CELL → LYMPH NODE { dendritic cell presenting to T cell via MHC II }

LUNG TISSUE → PATHOGEN → LYMPH NODE { CD4+ }

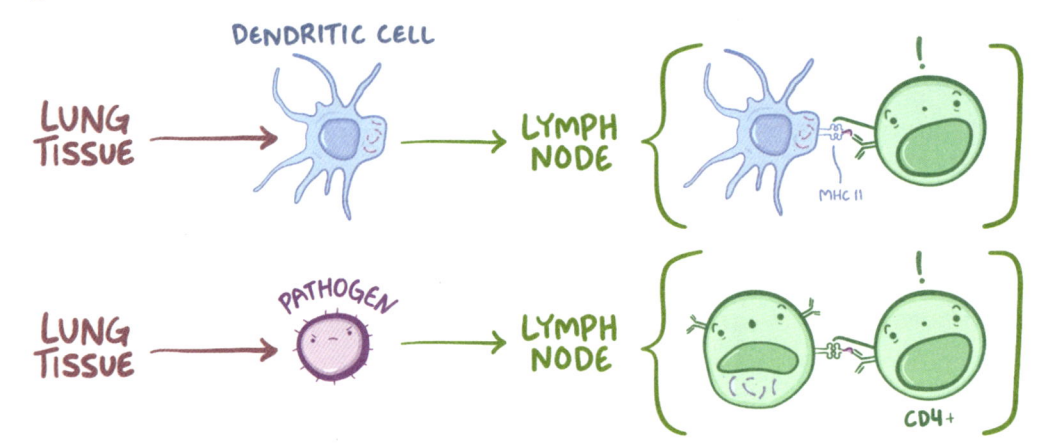

Figure 6.20

NEGLECTED CELLS **DIE**

CLONAL EXPANSION

CD4+

if VIRUS — CD8+, MHC I, VIRUS

CYTOKINES

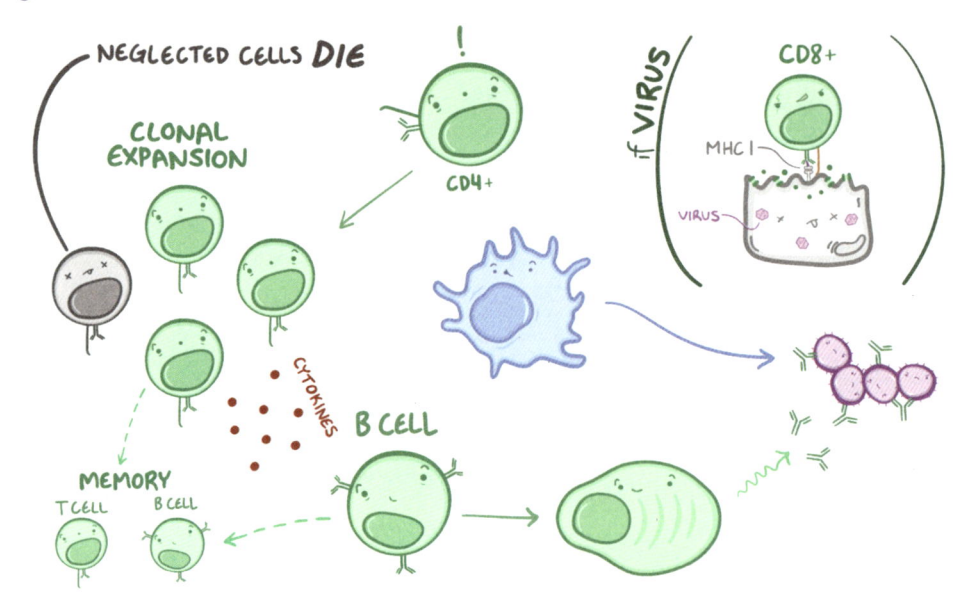

B CELL

MEMORY T CELL, B CELL

Figure 6.21

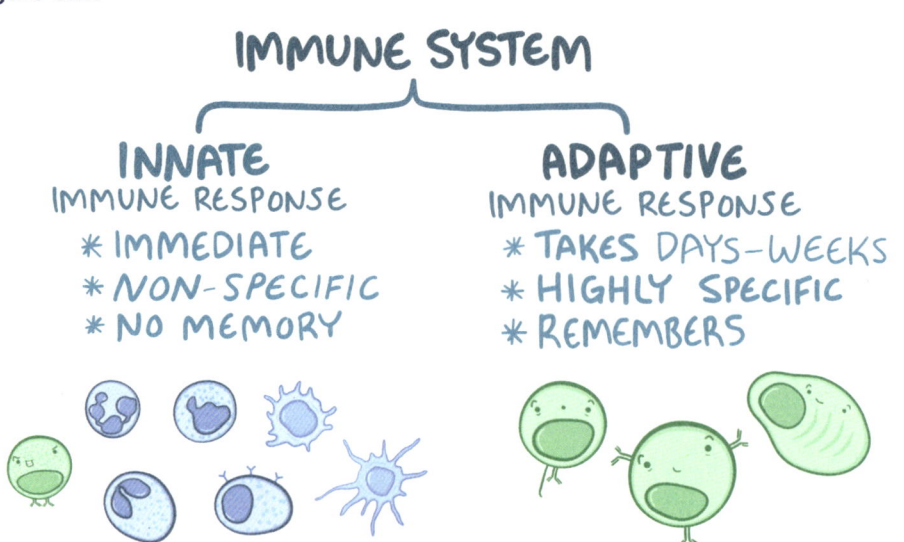

IMMUNE SYSTEM

INNATE IMMUNE RESPONSE
* IMMEDIATE
* NON-SPECIFIC
* NO MEMORY

ADAPTIVE IMMUNE RESPONSE
* TAKES DAYS–WEEKS
* HIGHLY SPECIFIC
* REMEMBERS

COMPLETE IMMUNE RESPONSE

Let's follow a complete immune response to a bacterial pathogen in the lungs. To start, the bacteria will need to be breathed in, allowed to slip by your nose hairs, sneak past the cilia in the airways, and penetrate the epithelium layer of the lungs. Once the bacterial pathogen is in the lung tissue, it will start to divide. In the lung tissue, it might encounter a resident macrophage, which will ingest the bacteria and begin releasing cytokines. These cytokines start the inflammatory process. The blood vessels become leaky and attract nearby eosinophils, basophils, and mast cells, which release their own cytokines and granules and thereby amplify the inflammation. Neutrophils from the blood, as well as fresh ones from the bone marrow, dive into the tissue and join the battle. If the pathogen is a virus, NK cells will also join in to help destroy the infected cells **(Figure 6.18)**.

At this point in the infection, dendritic cells that have digested the pathogens move to a nearby lymph node, where they present the processed antigen on an MHC II protein to a naive T cell. Sometimes, if the infection is spreading, bacteria might find its own way to a lymph node without the help of the dendritic cell. In this case, B cells might directly phagocytose the bacteria and present it to a naive CD4+ T cell **(Figure 6.19)**.

Either way, if the antigen is the right "fit" for the T cell, it will begin to differentiate and undergo clonal expansion. Differentiated CD4+ T cells will release cytokines, and these cytokines will induce B cells to differentiate into plasma cells, and these plasma cells will secrete antibodies into the lymph and then the bloodstream. These antibodies will tag pathogens, making it easier for phagocytes to eat them. At this point, if the pathogen is a virus, the CD8+ T cells will kill any infected cells that express the viral antigen on an MHC I. Over time, as the invading pathogen dies off, most of the B and T cells die of neglect. However, a few will turn into memory B cells and memory T cells, and they will linger for years to come in case they are needed for a future battle **(Figure 6.20)**.

SUMMARY

All right, as a quick recap, the immune system has two types of response: innate and adaptive. The innate immune response is immediate, but nonspecific, and lacks memory. In contrast, the adaptive immune response is highly specific and remembers everything, but it takes several days to get started and almost two weeks to peak **(Figure 6.21)**.

THE LYMPHATIC SYSTEM

osms.it/lymph_system

Lymph means "clear water" in Latin, and it describes the fluid that flows through the lymphatic vessels and lymph nodes which make up the lymphatic system. The three major roles of the lymphatic system—the reason we need it in the first place—are as follows: returning fluid from the tissues back to the heart; assisting molecules like hormones and lipids to enter the blood; and assisting immune surveillance to keep infections from running amok **(Figure 7.1)**.

RETURNING FLUID TO THE HEART

So, let's take a closer look at the lymph and where it comes from. The blood in the arteries is under a lot of pressure because it needs to reach every little nook and cranny of the body. The arteries branch out into narrower and narrower arteries, and then arterioles, and finally into capillaries, which have walls that are only one cell thick and are slightly porous. Red blood cells are too big to fit through capillary pores, but small proteins, like albumin, and fluid are able to pass through. Every day, 20 liters of protein and fluid seep out of the capillaries and become part of the interstitial fluid between cells. About 17 of those liters is quickly reabsorbed right back into the capillaries **(Figure 7.2)**.

Figure 7.1

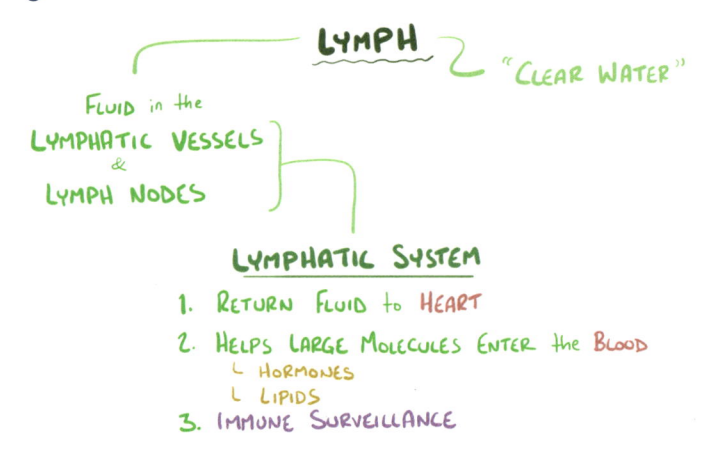

Figure 7.2

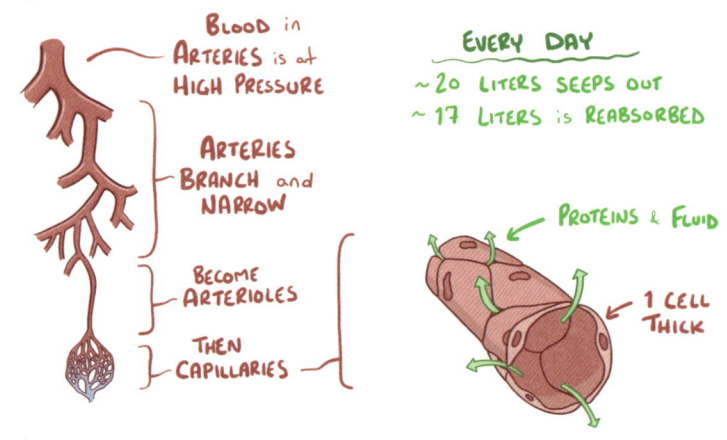

Chapter 7 The Lymphatic System

But that leaves three liters of fluid behind in the tissues each day and this three liters of fluid needs to find a way back into the blood in order for the body's interstitial fluid volume and blood volume to remain constant over time. That's where the lymphatic vessels, or lymphatics, come in: they collect excess interstitial fluid and return it to the blood. Once the interstitial fluid is in the lymphatic vessels, it's called lymph **(Figure 7.3; Figure 7.4; Figure 7.5)**.

Now, you may be wondering how 20 liters of fluid can seep out each day if the blood volume is only five liters. Just remember that those five liters are constantly in motion, so the blood gets recycled over and over again in a single day.

Unlike the circulatory system, the lymphatic system isn't a closed loop. Fluid and proteins make their way into the microscopic lymphatic capillaries and all of the collected lymph is dumped into the veins. Lymphatic capillaries are the smallest lymphatic vessels, and they're located throughout the interstitial space. Lymphatic capillaries are extremely permeable because their walls are made of endothelial cells that only loosely overlap, forming one-way minivalves. These endothelial cells are anchored to structures in the interstitial space by collagen filaments, which allow the lymphatic capillaries to remain flexible but retain their overall shape. When the pressure in the interstitial space is greater than the pressure in the lymphatic capillary, the endothelial minivalves open up, allowing fluid to enter **(Figure 7.6)**.

When the pressure in the interstitial space is less than the pressure in the lymphatic capillary, the endothelial minivalves are pushed shut, keeping the lymph inside **(Figure 7.7)**.

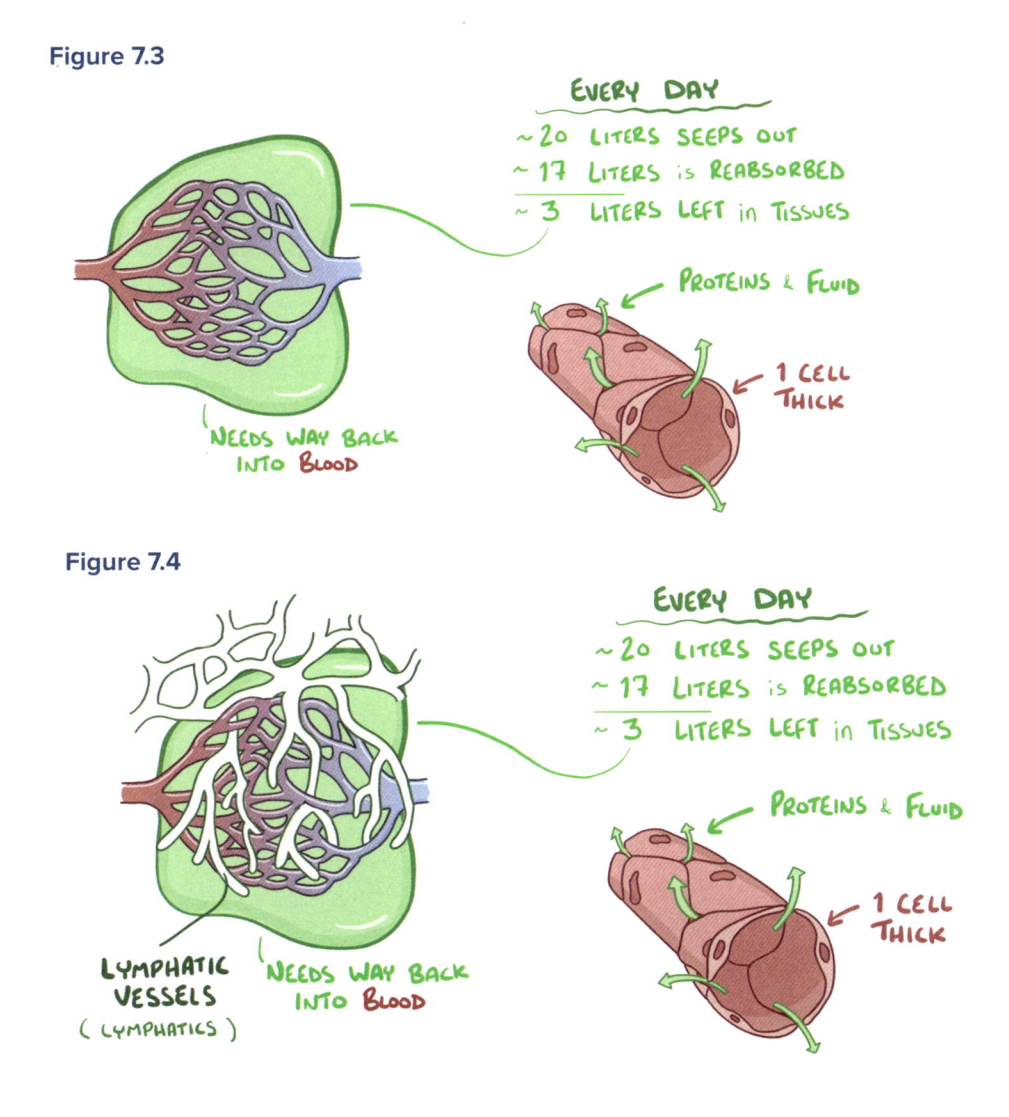

Figure 7.3

Figure 7.4

Figure 7.5

EVERY DAY
~20 LITERS SEEPS OUT
? BLOOD VOLUME is ~5L
REMEMBER BLOOD CIRCULATES
1 CELL THICK

LYMPHATIC VESSELS (LYMPHATICS) — Collect Interstitial Fluid which is then called LYMPH

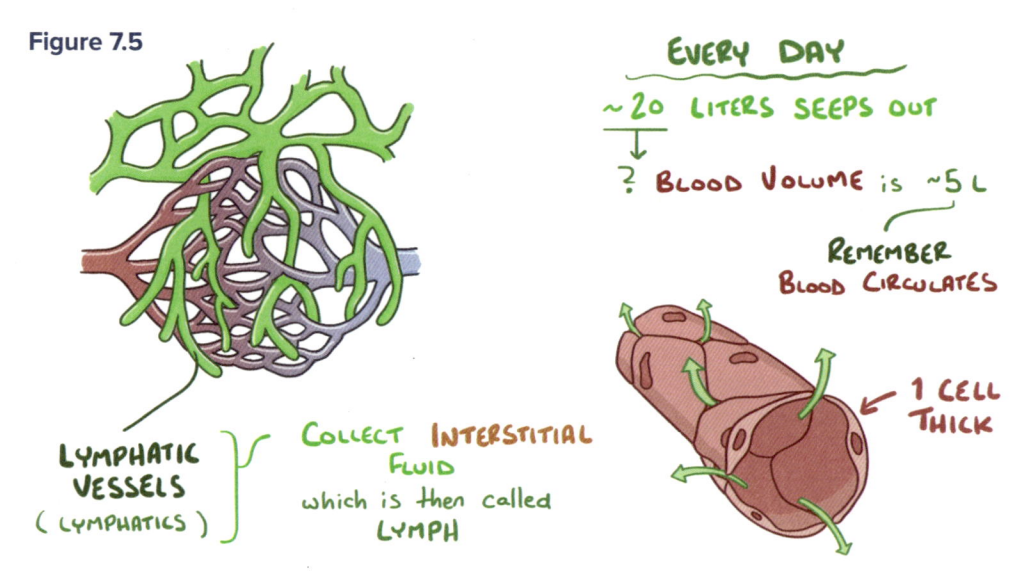

Figure 7.6

LYMPHATIC CAPILLARIES
INTERSTITIAL SPACE
COLLAGEN FILAMENTS
when PRESSURE in the INTERSTITIAL SPACE is HIGHER the ONE-WAY MINIVALVES OPEN
FLUID ENTERS

LYMPHATIC VESSELS (LYMPHATICS) — Collect Interstitial Fluid which is then called LYMPH — Dumped into VEINS

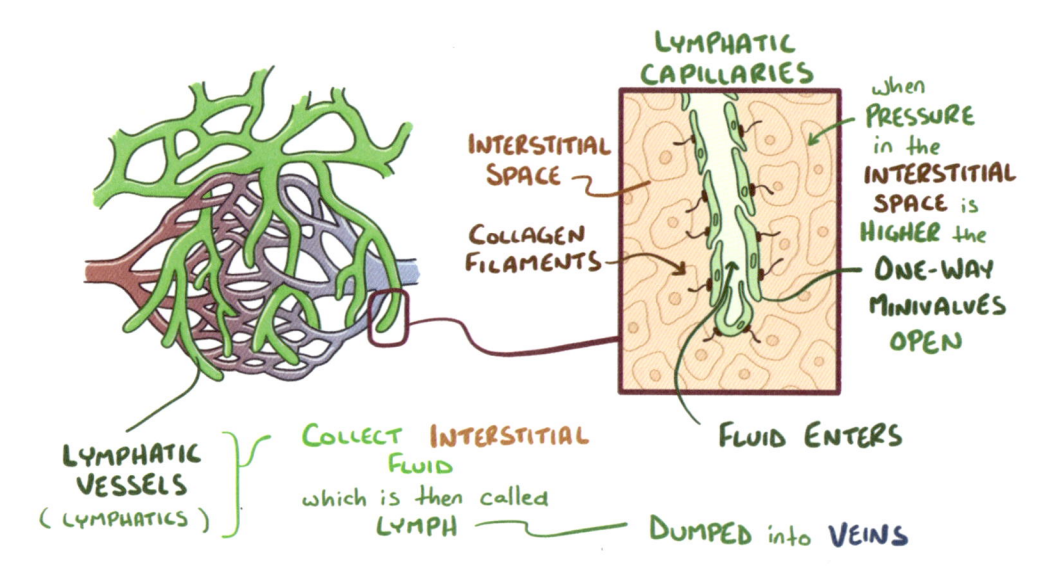

Figure 7.7

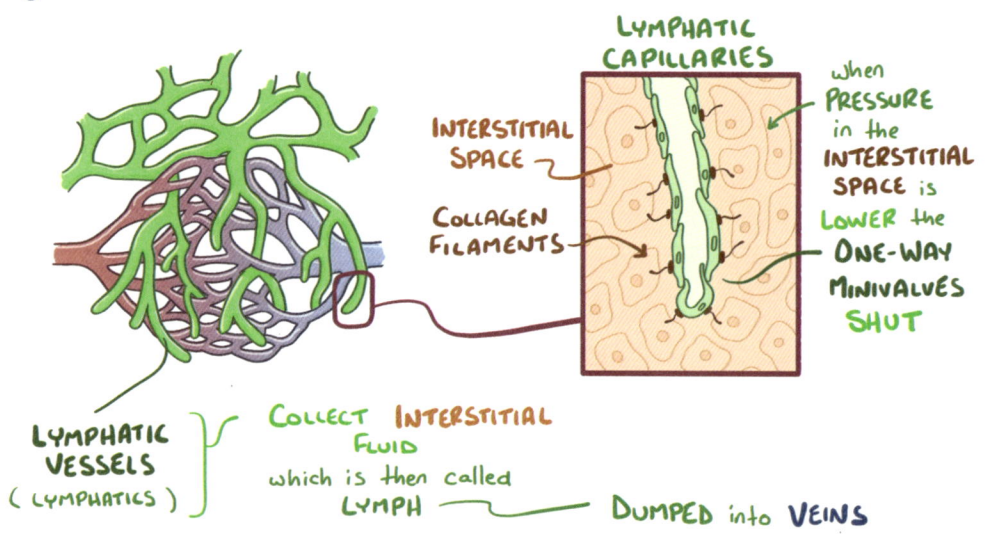

LYMPHATIC CAPILLARIES
INTERSTITIAL SPACE
COLLAGEN FILAMENTS
when PRESSURE in the INTERSTITIAL SPACE is LOWER the ONE-WAY MINIVALVES SHUT

LYMPHATIC VESSELS (LYMPHATICS) — Collect Interstitial Fluid which is then called LYMPH — Dumped into VEINS

Chapter 7 The Lymphatic System

Once the lymph is inside the lymphatic capillaries, it travels through bigger and thicker-walled vessels, then trunks, and then ducts. There's no pump pushing the lymph through the lymphatic system; instead, smooth muscle in the lymph vessels reacts to the pulsing of nearby arteries by squeezing to get things started **(Figure 7.8)**. Then, the squeezing of skeletal muscles, which contract throughout the day, exert external pressure to keep the lymph moving along, until eventually it reaches a nearby lymphatic trunk. To keep the lymph from sliding backwards, the lymphatic vessels have valves just like the veins **(Figure 7.9)**.

The lymphatic trunks are named after the regions of the body from which they drain the lymph: two lumbar trunks, two bronchomediastinal trunks, two subclavian trunks, and two jugular trunks, as well as one intestinal trunk **(Figure 7.10)**. From there, the lymph is delivered to either the right lymphatic duct or the thoracic duct. The right lymphatic duct collects lymph from the right arm and the right side of the head and chest, whereas the thoracic duct, which is much bigger, collects lymph from the rest of the body. The right lymphatic duct dumps lymph into the junction of the right jugular vein and the right subclavian vein. The thoracic duct dumps lymph into the same junction on the left side of the body. That particular spot is perfect because it's where the pressure is very low, making it much easier for the lymph to flow in.

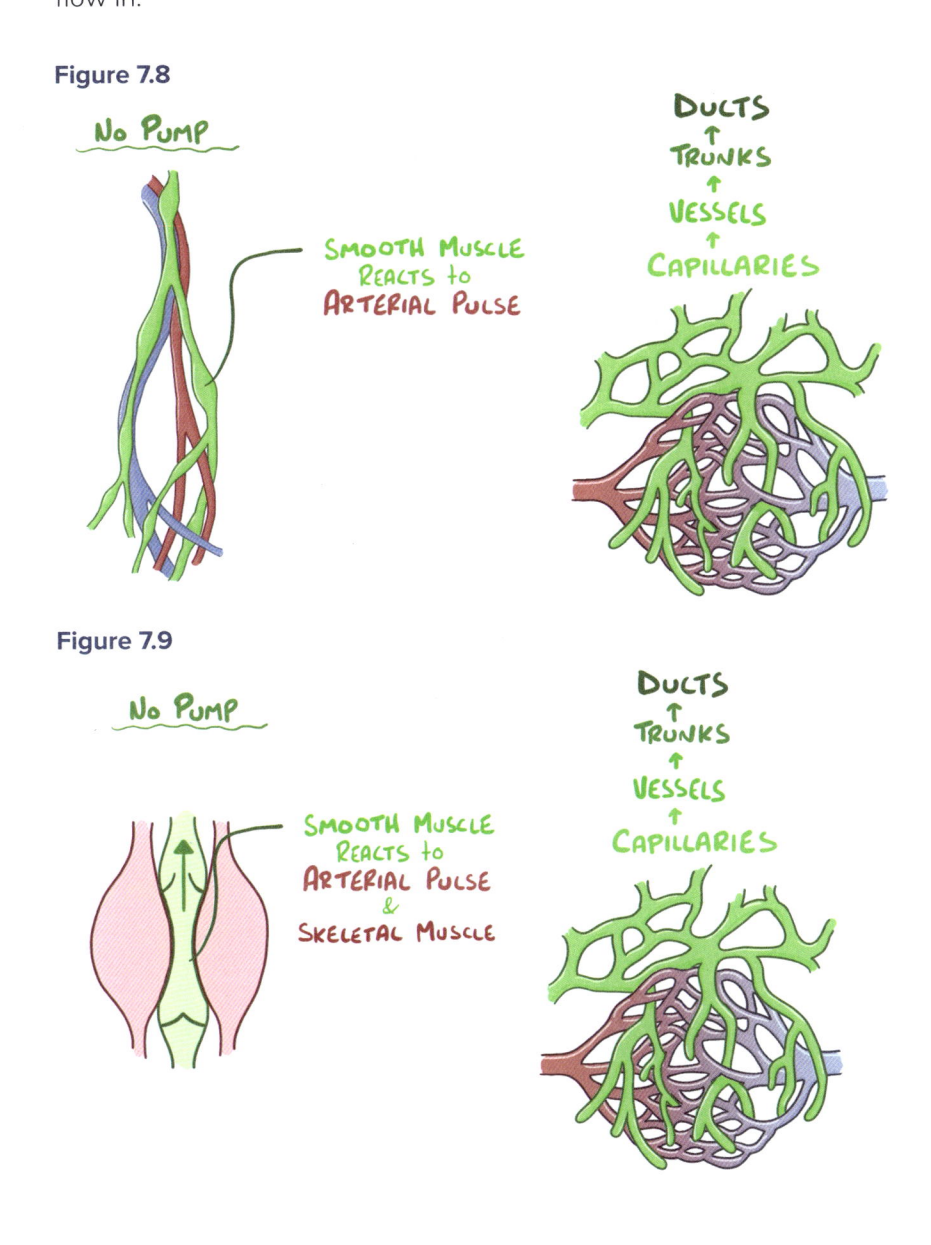

Figure 7.8

Figure 7.9

Figure 7.10

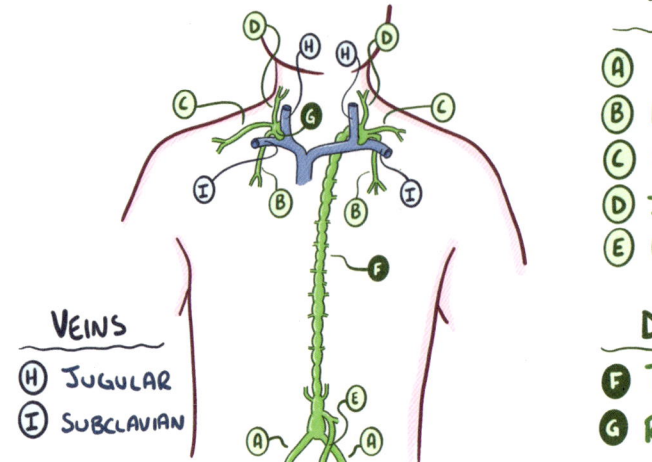

TRUNKS
- A Lumbar
- B Bronchomediastinal
- C Subclavian
- D Jugular
- E Intestinal

DUCTS
- F Thoracic
- G Right Lymphatic

VEINS
- H Jugular
- I Subclavian

Figure 7.11

Lymphatic system delivers large molecules to bloodstream

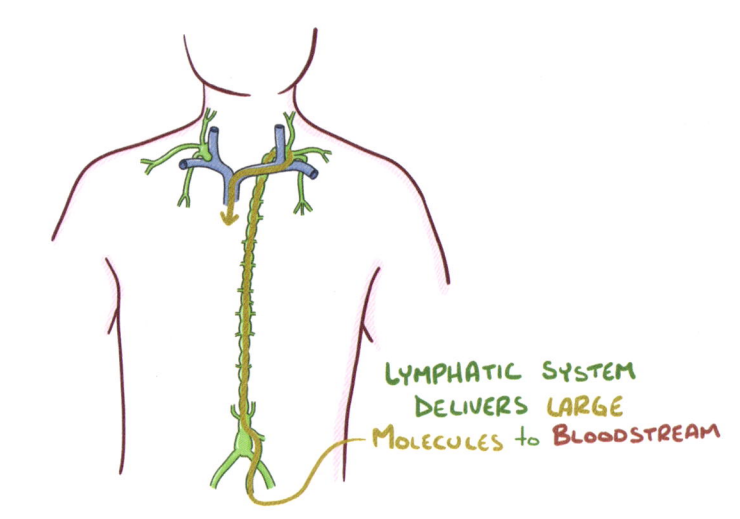

Figure 7.12

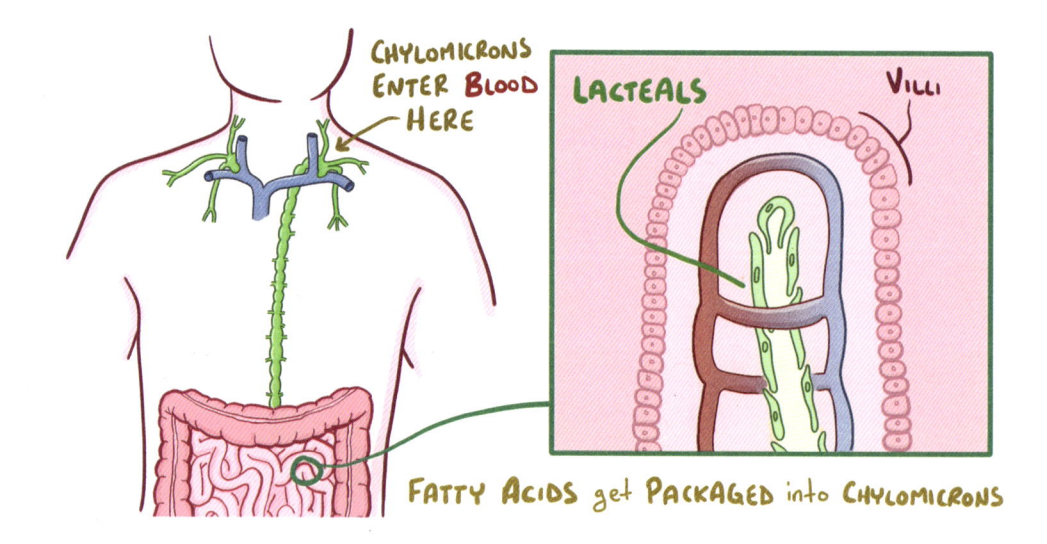

Chylomicrons enter blood here

Lacteals • Villi

Fatty acids get packaged into chylomicrons

82   OSMOSIS.ORG

Chapter 7 The Lymphatic System

ASSISTING LARGE MOLECULES ENTER THE BLOOD

The lymphatic system has several key advantages: for example, it can pick up larger molecules, like hormones, that are too large to get into the capillaries, and allow them to enter the bloodstream **(Figure 7.11)**.

The lymphatic system can also help get nutrients to the tissues. For example, during a meal, fatty acids get packaged into balls of fat called chylomicrons by the small intestine. Like the hormones, however, these are too large to move across capillaries. Instead, the chylomicrons go into special lymphatic vessels called lacteals, which get their name from the milky appearance of the lymph that flows through them. The chylomicrons slowly make their way up into the thoracic duct and get dumped into the venous blood **(Figure 7.12)**.

ASSISTING IMMUNE SURVEILLANCE

The lymphatic system also plays an important role in immune function. Lymphoid organs remove foreign material from the lymph to prevent it entering the bloodstream. These organs also act as lookout points for the body's immune defenses.

Some lymphoid organs are in the form of diffuse lymphoid tissue, meaning they are just a loose arrangement of lymphoid cells and protein. This is typical in the lining of the gastrointestinal and respiratory tract. Lymph nodes are another type of lymphoid organ. They are tightly packed balls of lymphoid cells and protein. Hundreds of lymph nodes cluster along the lymph vessels, each one a few millimeters to about 1–2 cm in size. When they're concentrated along the lymph trunks, you can feel them, especially in the neck, armpit, and groin. They can also be found in the intestinal wall, where they're called Peyer's patches **(Figure 7.13)**.

When an infection gets into the tissue, it can slip into a lymphatic capillary and move into a lymphatic vessel. Unfiltered lymph fluid drains into a nearby lymph node, and now any pathogen or piece of pathogen is quickly detected by a dendritic cell—a type of antigen-presenting cell that serves up pieces of anything it destroys to other immune cells.

In the lymph nodes, dendritic cells continuously sample the lymph and present antigens to the B cells—a type of lymphocyte that can make antibodies. B cells are designed to only react to foreign antigens, and if the dendritic cell presents something foreign, the B cell turns into a plasma cell and begins cranking out antibodies. These antibodies then flow into the lymph and exit the lymph node.

Figure 7.13

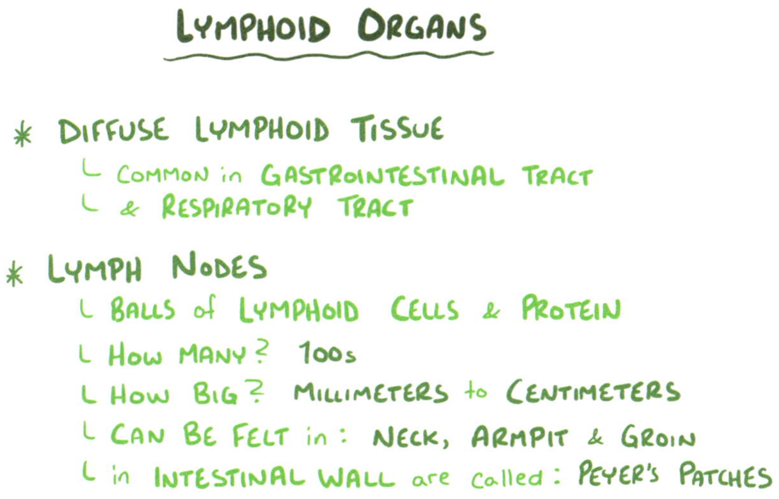

LYMPHOID ORGANS

* **DIFFUSE LYMPHOID TISSUE**
  - COMMON in GASTROINTESTINAL TRACT
  - & RESPIRATORY TRACT

* **LYMPH NODES**
  - BALLS of LYMPHOID CELLS & PROTEIN
  - HOW MANY? 100s
  - HOW BIG? MILLIMETERS to CENTIMETERS
  - CAN BE FELT in: NECK, ARMPIT & GROIN
  - in INTESTINAL WALL are called: PEYER'S PATCHES

There are also circulating T cells—another type of lymphocyte that moves between the lymph nodes, lymph, and blood, always on the lookout for pathogens and infected or abnormal cells that have been tagged by antibodies **(Figure 7.14)**.

Another lymphoid organ is the spleen, which is about the size of a fist, and sits on the left side of the body below the diaphragm and on top of the stomach **(Figure 7.15)**.

The spleen has both white pulp and red pulp. The white pulp is where antibody-coated bacteria are filtered out of circulation and antibodies are generated by B cells. In a sense, the white pulp of the spleen is like a giant lymph node. Unlike a lymph node, which receives unfiltered lymphatic fluid, the spleen receives blood. The red pulp of the spleen is where old and defective blood cells are destroyed and their parts—the hemoglobin, heme chain, and iron—are either broken down or recycled. The spleen also helps keep red blood cells and platelets available, in case they are suddenly needed by the body. It's an organ that's got your back in an emergency **(Figure 7.16)**!

Figure 7.14

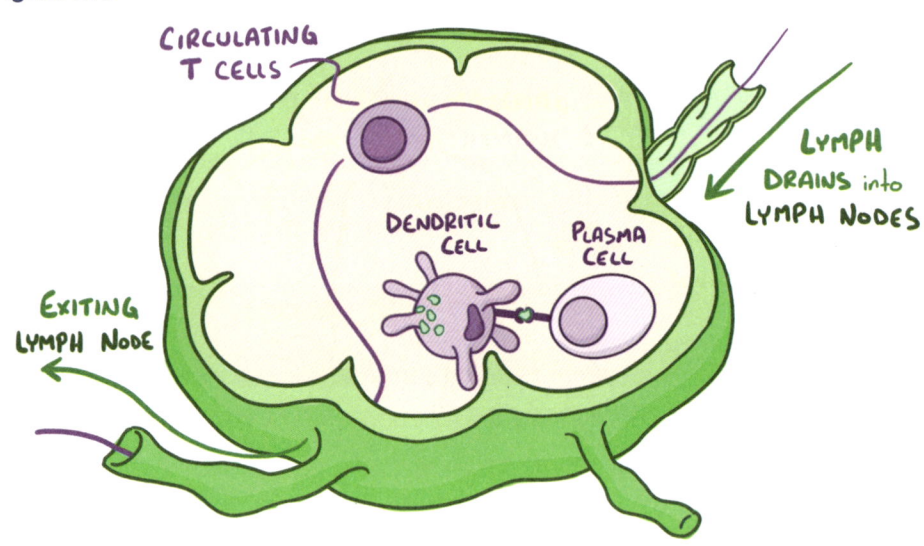

Figure 7.15

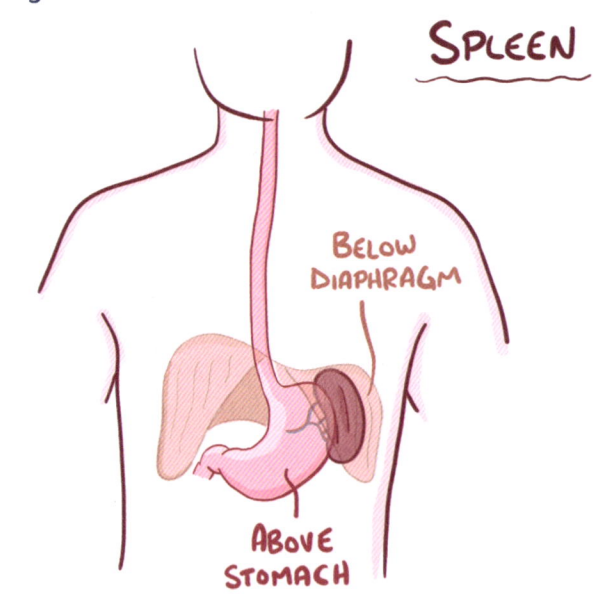

Chapter 7 The Lymphatic System

Figure 7.16

SPLEEN — KEEPS RBCs & PLATELETS AVAILABLE for EMERGENCIES

WHITE PULP
* ANTIBODY-COATED BACTERIA are FILTERED OUT
* ANTIBODIES are MADE by B CELLS
* FILTERS BLOOD

RED PULP
* OLD BLOOD CELLS are DESTROYED
  └ RECYCLES the PARTS

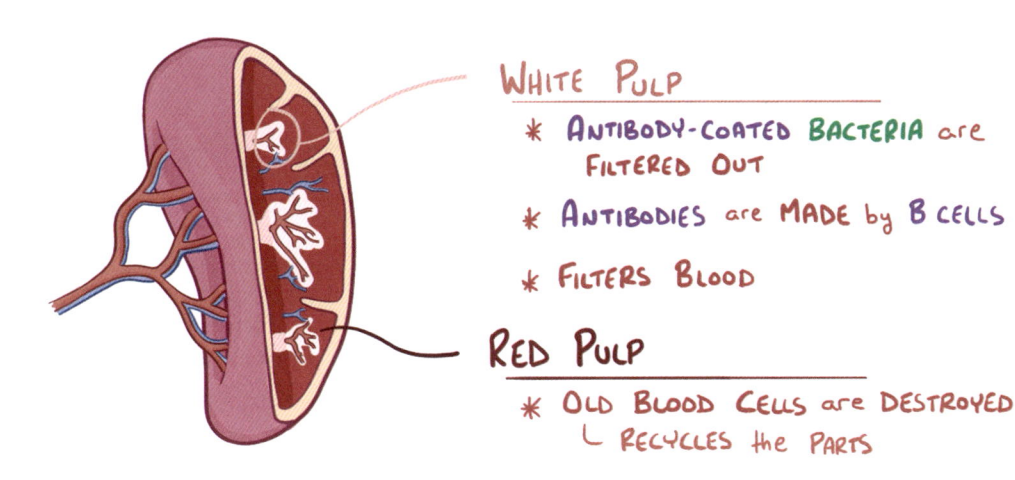

Figure 7.17

THYMUS
- MOST ACTIVE in the NEONATAL & PRE-ADOLESCENT PERIODS — ATROPHIES AFTER PUBERTY
* INVOLVED in the DEVELOPMENT of T CELLS
- DESTROYS T CELLS that REACT to SELF-ANTIGENS

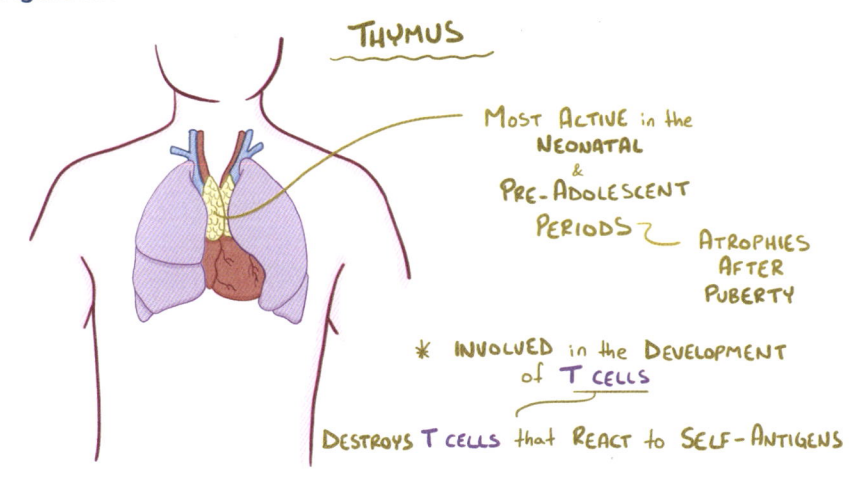

Figure 7.18

TONSILS
FORM a RING of LYMPHOID TISSUE AROUND the THROAT

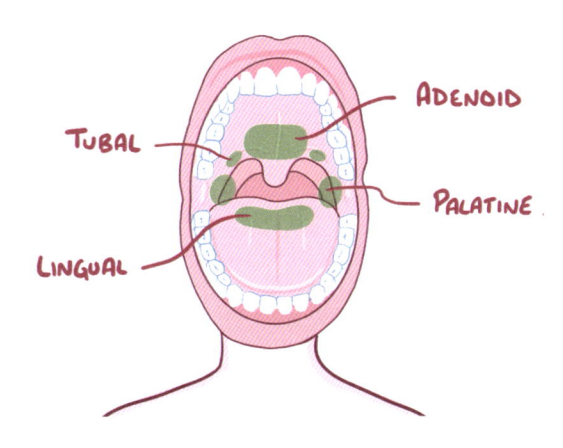

- TUBAL
- ADENOID
- PALATINE
- LINGUAL

OSMOSIS.ORG 85

Another lymphoid organ is the thymus, which is in the upper part of the chest, just below where a necklace might lie. The thymus is most active in the neonatal period and pre-adolescent years. After puberty, it slowly atrophies and is replaced by fat. The thymus is involved in the development of T cells: making sure that any T cells that react to self-antigens—antigens that are normally found in the body—are promptly destroyed **(Figure 7.17)**.

A final set of lymphoid organs worth mentioning are the tonsils, which include the adenoid tonsils, tubal tonsils, palatine tonsils, and lingual tonsils. Together, they form a ring of lymphoid tissue around the throat and their main job is to trap pathogens from the food you eat and air you inhale **(Figure 7.18)**.

SUMMARY

All right, as a quick recap, the lymphatic system refers to the one-way network of lymphatic vessels that allows lymph—a clear fluid squeezed out of the blood—to transport nutrients to the cells and act as a method of waste removal. Lymph is cleansed at lymph nodes throughout the lymphatic system, which play an important role in immune function **(Figure 7.19)**.

Figure 7.19

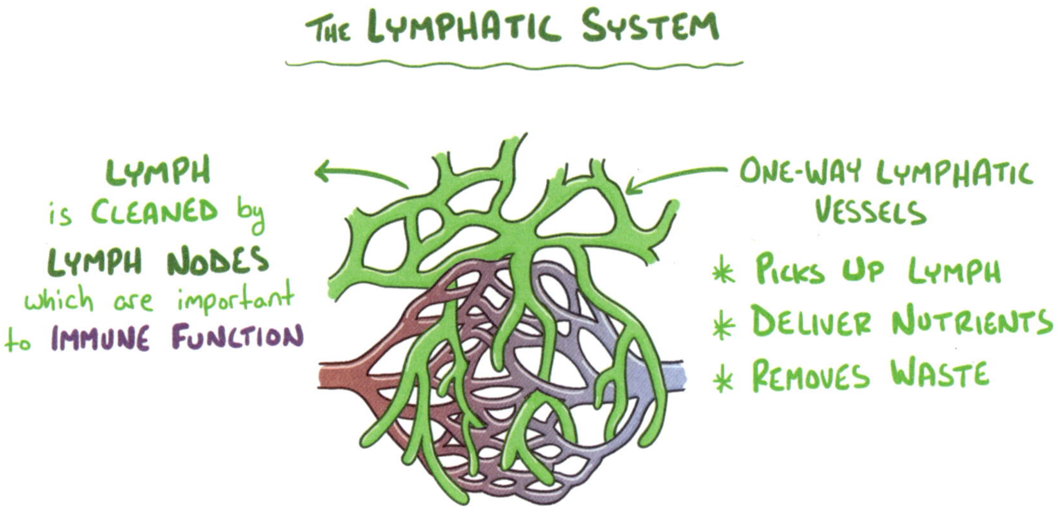

THE HEMATOLOGIC SYSTEM

osms.it/hemo_system

The word "blood" evokes many things—from tiny paper cuts to major injuries—but spilling the red liquid is almost never a good thing. That's because blood helps us move nutrients and waste around the body, regulate our pH level, and prevent infections. Some components of blood even help prevent blood loss during an injury **(Figure 8.1)**.

The components of blood can be separated out by simply spinning the blood in a centrifuge. This is a machine that whips a vial of blood in a circle over and over, really quickly—a bit like what happens to clothes in a washing machine. When blood is centrifuged, the heaviest blood components move to the bottom and the lightest components move to the top. Overall, three distinct layers form: the erythrocytes—also known as red blood cells—at the bottom; the buffy coat, which contains platelets and immune cells, in the middle; and the plasma at the top **(Figure 8.2)**.

Figure 8.1

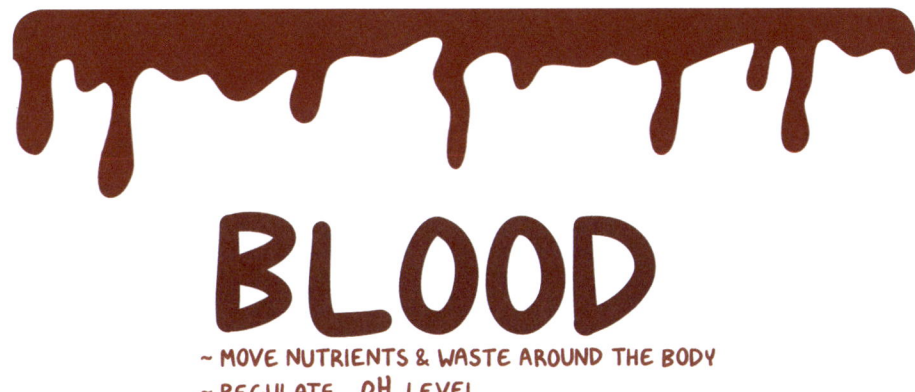

BLOOD
- MOVE NUTRIENTS & WASTE AROUND THE BODY
- REGULATE pH LEVEL
- PREVENT INFECTIONS
- COMPONENTS PREVENT LOSS OF BLOOD DURING INJURY

Figure 8.2

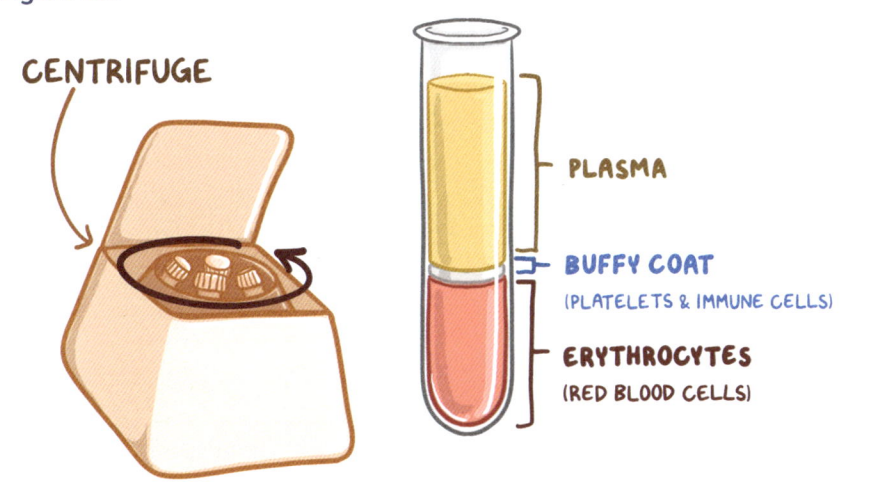

CENTRIFUGE

- PLASMA
- BUFFY COAT (PLATELETS & IMMUNE CELLS)
- ERYTHROCYTES (RED BLOOD CELLS)

ERYTHROCYTES

If we start at the bottom, there's the large layer that takes up approximately 45% of the total blood volume. This is made up of erythrocytes. This value is called the hematocrit. A decreased hematocrit means there are too few erythrocytes, either because they're not being made or because they are being destroyed. On the other hand, an increased hematocrit may be due to dehydration, because if there's less liquid in the blood the portion taken up by erythrocytes rises. Alternatively, an increased hematocrit may be due to the production of too many erythrocytes, which can occur in some diseases.

The main function of erythrocytes is to carry oxygen to tissues and bring carbon dioxide to the lungs so it can be exhaled from the body. Erythrocytes are shaped liked thin biconcave discs—meaning they have a depressed center which makes them flexible enough to fit through even the smallest blood vessels. This shape also increases their surface area which helps them conduct gas exchange efficiently. Erythrocytes lack organelles, like the nucleus, which creates even more room for hemoglobin proteins which carry oxygen. While red blood cells are fantastic for gas exchange, the fact that they don't have any organelles means that they only live for about 120 days. For this reason, red blood cells are always being regenerated in the bone marrow **(Figure 8.3)**.

THE BUFFY COAT

The thin white middle layer just above the erythrocytes is called the buffy coat. It contains platelets and leukocytes—also known as white blood cells. This layer generally accounts for less than 1% of the total blood volume. Most of this volume is taken up by the leukocytes. The platelets account for much less of this volume. They are small pieces that split from larger cells called megakaryocytes in the bone marrow. The main role of platelets is to clump together and form a plug that helps seal a damaged blood vessel and prevent blood loss **(Figure 8.4)**.

Figure 8.3

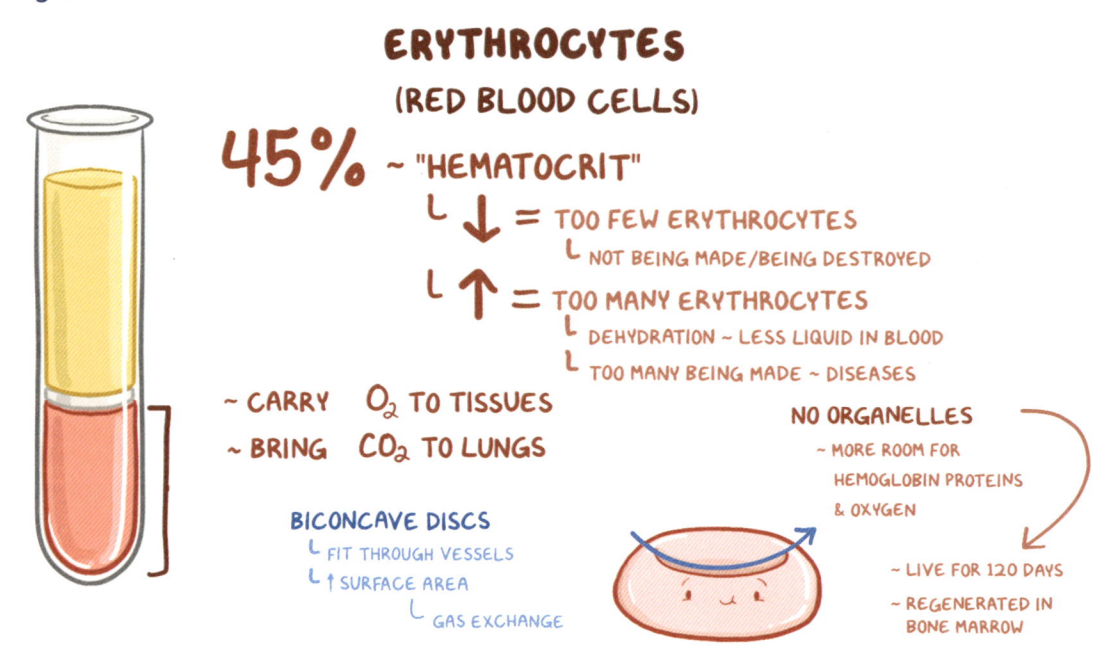

Chapter 8 The Hematologic System

The leukocytes are the only complete cells in the blood. This means they have all the usual organelles. There are many different types of leukocytes and they all help to ward off pathogens like bacteria and viruses, destroy cancerous cells, and neutralize toxins. Leukocytes that contain granules—tiny sacs filled with inflammatory molecules—are called granulocytes. Neutrophils are the most common granulocyte. They make up about 60% of the leukocytes and are usually the first to respond to an infection. Other granulocytes include eosinophils and basophils, but these only make up about 2–5% of leukocytes. Eosinophils are largely responsible for fighting off parasitic infections, while basophils are key in responding to allergic reactions **(Figure 8.5)**.

Leukocytes that don't contain granules include lymphocytes and monocytes. Lymphocytes include B cells, T cells, and natural killer cells **(Figure 8.6)**. They make up about 35% of leukocytes. They are responsible for the adaptive immune response, which includes antibody production and is what allows our immune system to have "memory." This "memory" enables us to effectively respond to pathogens that have caused infections in the past. Monocytes make up about 5% of leukocytes. These cells help gobble up bacteria or other pathogens via phagocytosis **(Figure 8.7)**.

Figure 8.4

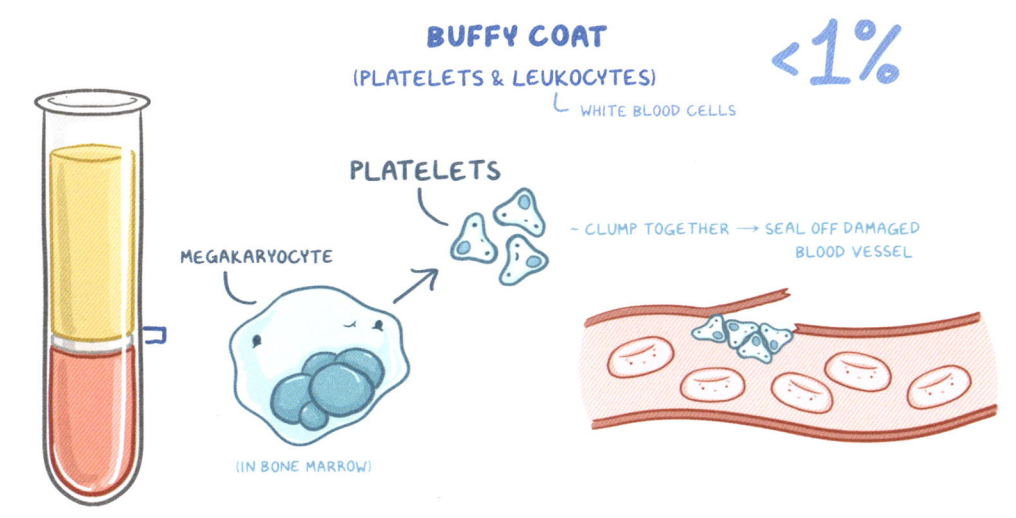

Figure 8.5

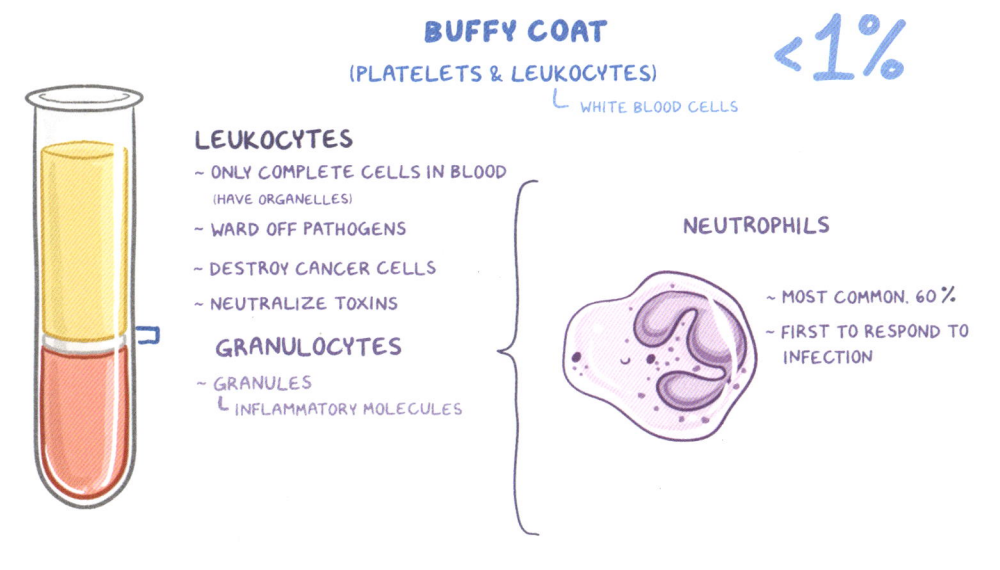

Unlike the other blood components, leukocytes have the ability to leave the blood and enter into tissues using a process called diapedesis. In diapedesis, the leukocytes slip in between endothelial cells that line the blood vessels. In a way, leukocytes are like a mobile army: utilizing the blood as a highway to get to different areas of the body.

PLASMA

Finally, the top layer contains plasma. The plasma makes up approximately 55% of the total blood volume and is acellular, meaning it has no cells. About 90% of plasma is water, and the rest is composed of proteins, electrolytes, and dissolved gases.

The most abundant protein found in the blood is albumin. Albumin is made in the liver and it helps maintain oncotic pressure, which is the force that helps keep water in the bloodstream. In addition, albumin is a transport protein. It shuttles fatty acids, calcium, lipid soluble hormones, and even some medications around the body.

Globulins are another group of plasma proteins. They include gamma globulins, which are antibodies that stick to pathogens and label them for destruction. They also include alpha and beta globulins, which transport fats, metal ions, and fat-soluble vitamins.

Fibrinogen is another abundant plasma protein. It's involved in clot formation for damaged vessels. Fibrinogen helps platelets attach to one another to form the initial platelet plug. Other clotting factor proteins in the plasma will then come along to stabilize the clot. All of these clotting factor proteins, including fibrinogen, can be removed from a sample of plasma. When these clotting factor proteins are removed, what remains is the serum **(Figure 8.8)**.

Figure 8.6

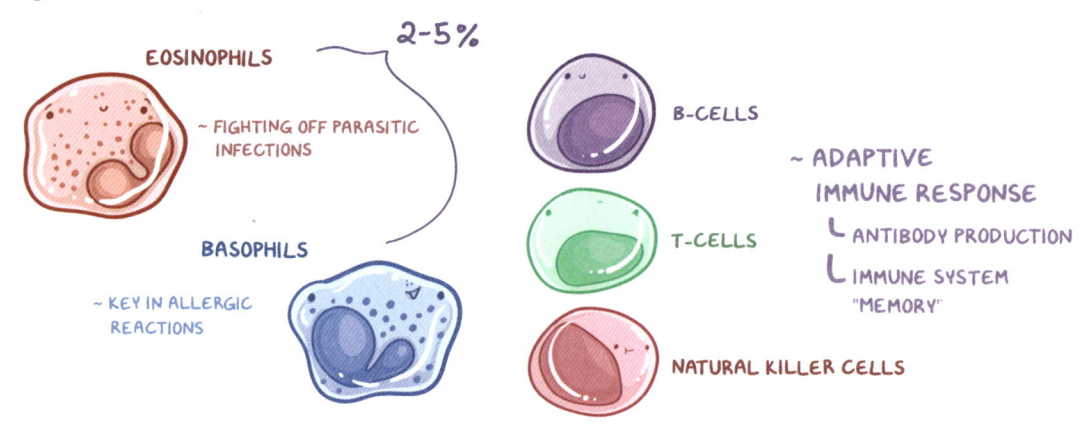

EOSINOPHILS 2-5%
~ FIGHTING OFF PARASITIC INFECTIONS

BASOPHILS
~ KEY IN ALLERGIC REACTIONS

B-CELLS
T-CELLS
~ ADAPTIVE IMMUNE RESPONSE
  └ ANTIBODY PRODUCTION
  └ IMMUNE SYSTEM "MEMORY"

NATURAL KILLER CELLS

Figure 8.7

MONOCYTES 5%
~ GOBBLE UP BACTERIA (PHAGOCYTOSIS)
~ LEAVE BLOOD → ENTER TISSUE (DIAPEDESIS)

Chapter 8 The Hematologic System

Electrolytes that are found in the plasma include: sodium, potassium, calcium, bicarbonate, and chloride. These electrolytes play vital roles in maintaining normal acid base physiology in the blood and help regulate blood osmolarity—the overall concentration of blood. Other solutes in the plasma include hormones, nutrients like glucose, and respiratory gases like oxygen and carbon dioxide that are dissolved in the blood **(Figure 8.9)**.

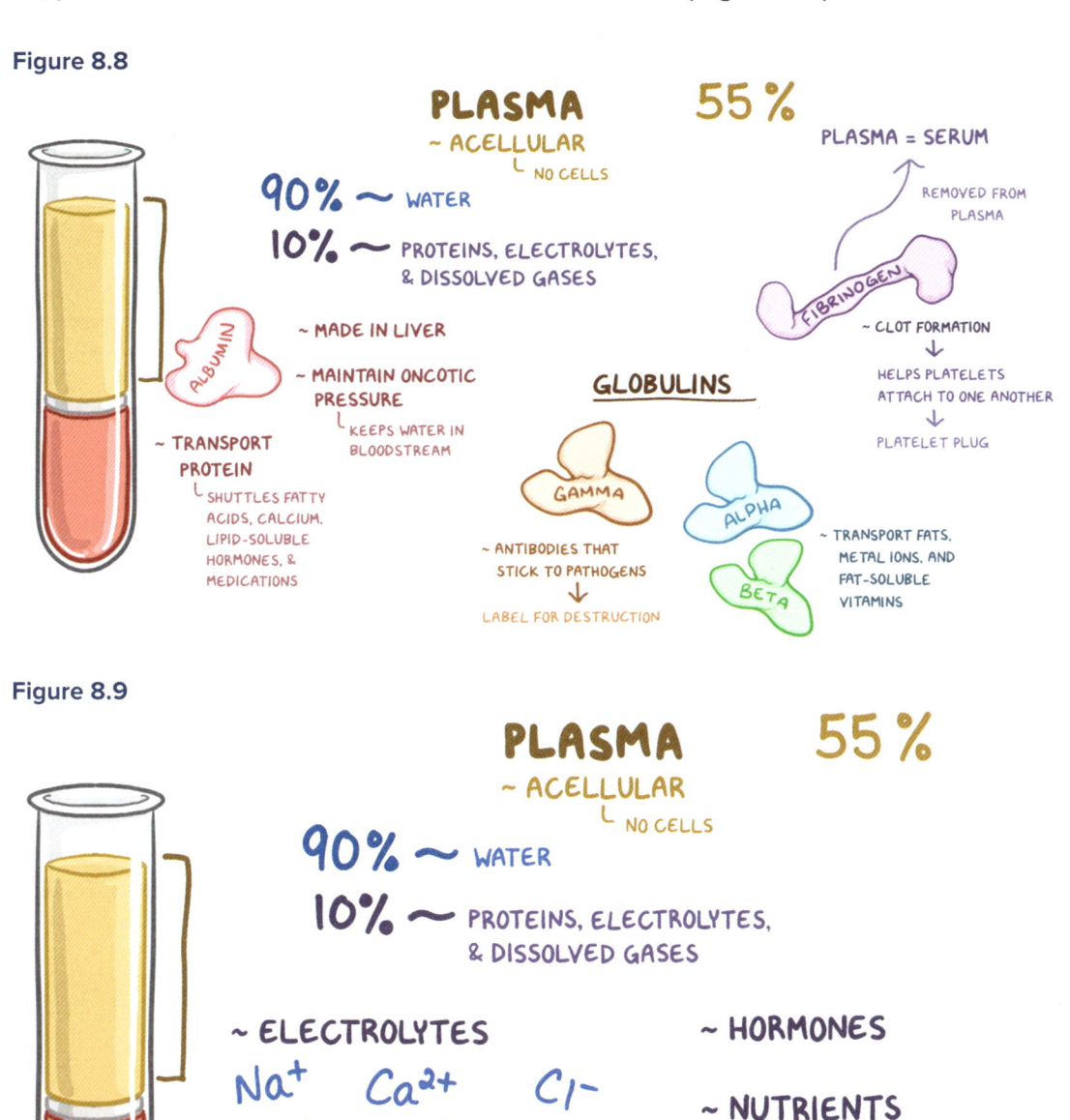

Figure 8.8

PLASMA 55%
~ ACELLULAR
    └ NO CELLS

PLASMA = SERUM
    ↑ REMOVED FROM PLASMA

90% ~ WATER
10% ~ PROTEINS, ELECTROLYTES, & DISSOLVED GASES

ALBUMIN
~ MADE IN LIVER
~ MAINTAIN ONCOTIC PRESSURE
    └ KEEPS WATER IN BLOODSTREAM
~ TRANSPORT PROTEIN
    └ SHUTTLES FATTY ACIDS, CALCIUM, LIPID-SOLUBLE HORMONES, & MEDICATIONS

FIBRINOGEN
~ CLOT FORMATION
    ↓
HELPS PLATELETS ATTACH TO ONE ANOTHER
    ↓
PLATELET PLUG

GLOBULINS
GAMMA
~ ANTIBODIES THAT STICK TO PATHOGENS
    ↓
LABEL FOR DESTRUCTION

ALPHA
BETA
~ TRANSPORT FATS, METAL IONS, AND FAT-SOLUBLE VITAMINS

Figure 8.9

PLASMA 55%
~ ACELLULAR
    └ NO CELLS

90% ~ WATER
10% ~ PROTEINS, ELECTROLYTES, & DISSOLVED GASES

~ ELECTROLYTES
Na^+ Ca^{2+} Cl^-
K^+ HCO_3^-

~ MAINTAIN NORMAL ACID BASE PHYSIOLOGY IN THE BLOOD
~ REGULATE OSMOLARITY (CONCENTRATION OF BLOOD)

~ HORMONES

~ NUTRIENTS
GLUCOSE

~ RESPIRATORY GASES
O_2 & CO_2
    └ DISSOLVED IN BLOOD

SUMMARY

All right, as a quick recap, the blood is made up of about 45% erythrocytes, 55% plasma, which is mostly water but also contains proteins like albumin, electrolytes, and dissolved gases, and, finally, less than 1% platelets and leukocytes **(Figure 8.9)**.

Figure 8.10

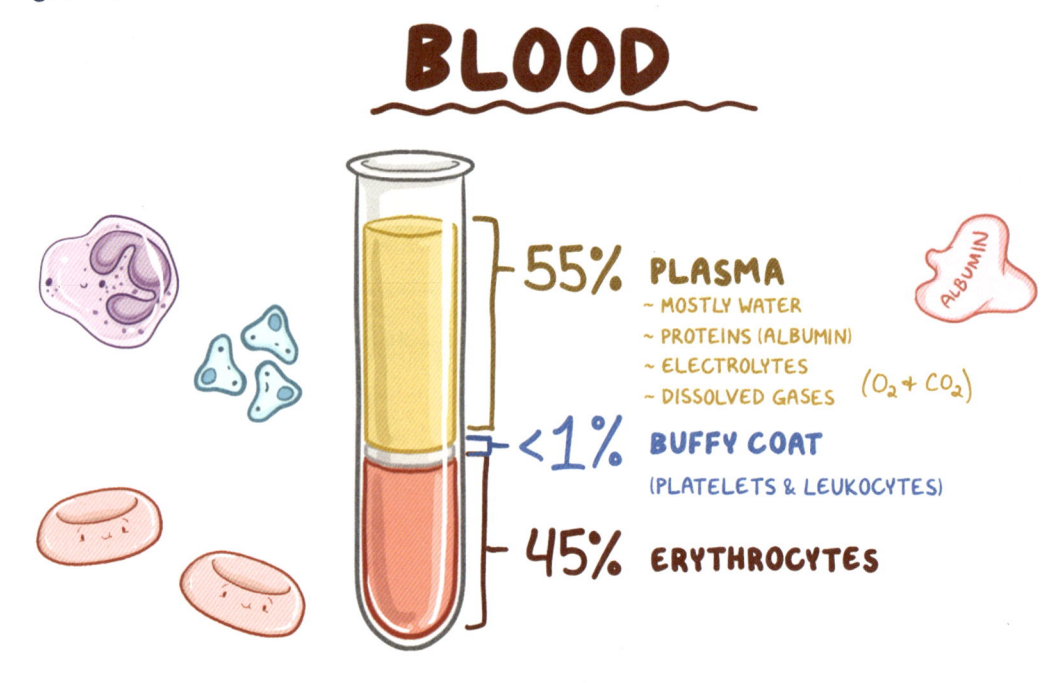

THE MUSCULAR SYSTEM

osms.it/muscle_system

The muscular system is made up of three types of muscle tissue: skeletal, cardiac, and smooth. While they differ in terms of their location, cell structure, and innervation, they do share some characteristics: each one is excitable, meaning the cells react to stimuli; each one is able to contract, meaning the cells can shorten; each one possesses extensibility, meaning the cells can stretch; and each one is elastic, meaning the tissue can recoil or bounce back to its original length **(Figure 9.1)**.

SKELETAL MUSCLE TISSUE

Let's start with the skeletal muscle tissue. Skeletal muscles usually attach to bones. In some cases, however, they attach to the skin, like the muscles in our face that control facial expression. Skeletal muscles are voluntary muscles, meaning they can be controlled consciously, but some skeletal muscles are also controlled subconsciously. Your diaphragm is an example of a muscle that can be controlled consciously and subconsciously **(Figure 9.2)**. For instance, you can consciously contract this muscle when you choose to take a big breath, but this muscle continues to contract and relax without conscious effort—when you're fast asleep or simply thinking about other things. Skeletal muscles, like the diaphragm, help you maintain your posture and stabilize joints. Because they use up a lot of energy as they contract and relax, skeletal muscles also generate a great deal of heat as a byproduct. That's why we shiver to stay warm **(Figure 9.3)**!

Now, let's take a look at the biceps brachii—a skeletal muscle in your upper arm. As with most muscles, there's the belly of the muscle and the muscle tendons. The muscle belly is the part that contracts. It's wrapped in a layer of connective tissue called the epimysium **(Figure 9.4)**.

Figure 9.1

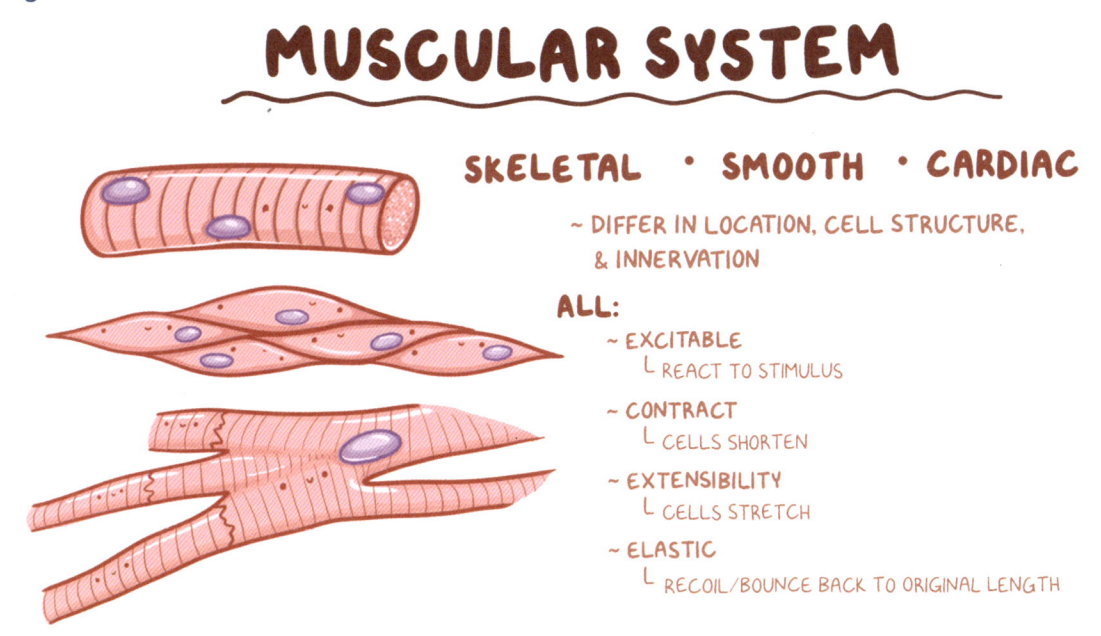

If we take a look at a cross-section of the muscle belly, we see thin layers of connective tissue called the perimysium. These separate the muscle into fascicles. Each muscle fascicle consists of a bundle of muscle fibers, and each muscle fiber is a muscle cell—or myocyte. Every myocyte is surrounded by a smaller connective tissue sheath called the endomysium. Together, the endomysium, perimysium, and epimysium form a bundle that consists of thousands of muscle fibers. This bundle is responsible for muscle structure and strength. To understand the importance of this bundle, think of how easy it may be to snap a single twig, but how difficult it is to snap a bundle of sticks. Thankfully, those thousands of muscle fibers form a mighty strong bundle **(Figure 9.5)**!

Together, these three layers of connective tissue extend beyond the muscle belly and become the tough cord-like tendon that attaches the muscle to the bone. When a tendon attaches to a bone that's not moving, it's called an origin. When a tendon attaches to a bone that's moving, it's called an insertion **(Figure 9.6)**.

Figure 9.2

SKELETAL MUSCLES

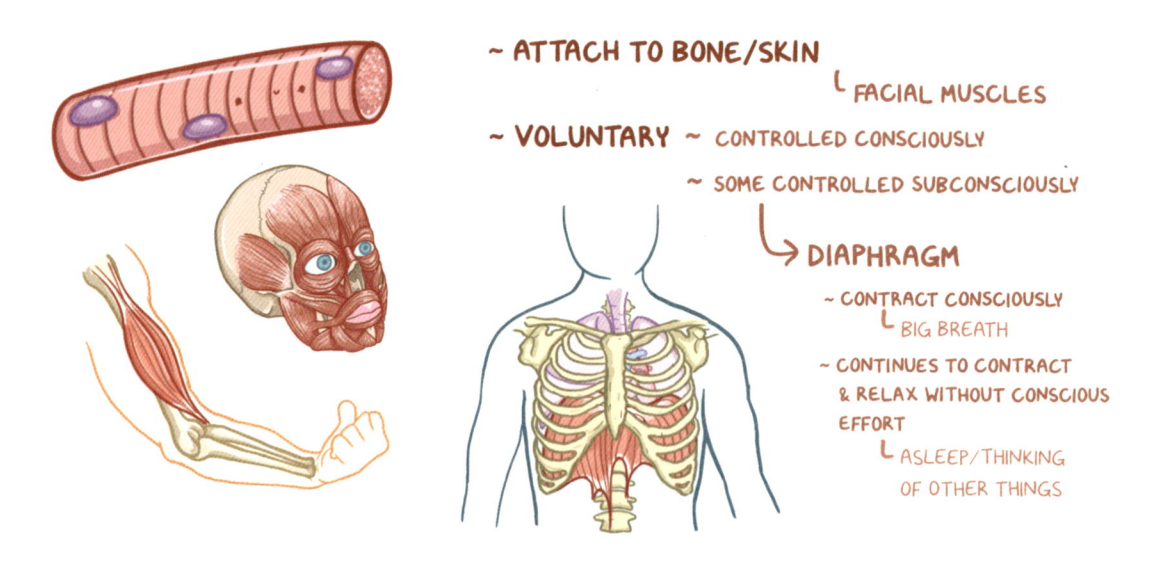

- ATTACH TO BONE/SKIN
  - FACIAL MUSCLES
- VOLUNTARY
  - CONTROLLED CONSCIOUSLY
  - SOME CONTROLLED SUBCONSCIOUSLY
    - DIAPHRAGM
      - CONTRACT CONSCIOUSLY
        - BIG BREATH
      - CONTINUES TO CONTRACT & RELAX WITHOUT CONSCIOUS EFFORT
        - ASLEEP/THINKING OF OTHER THINGS

Figure 9.3

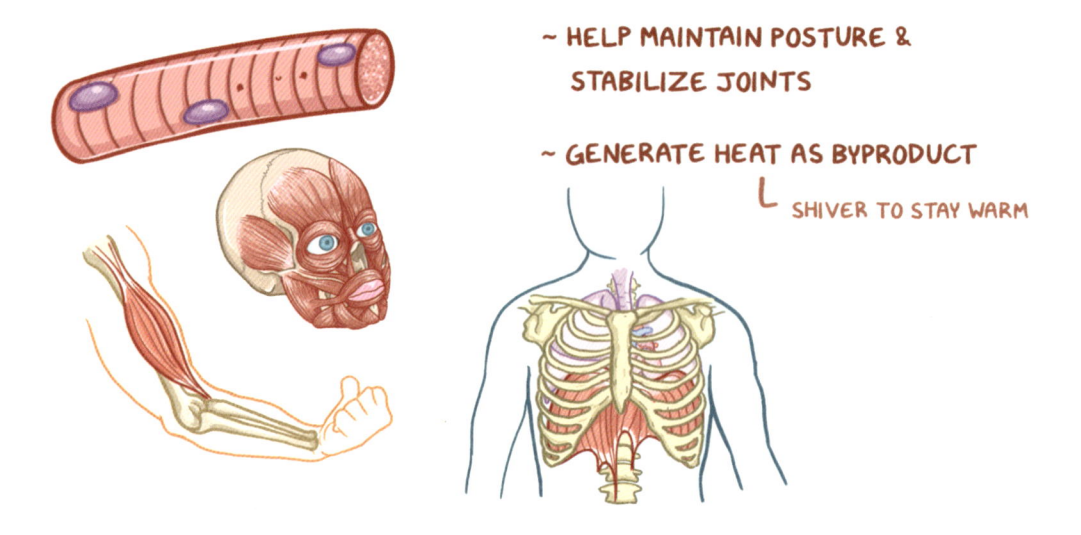

- HELP MAINTAIN POSTURE & STABILIZE JOINTS
- GENERATE HEAT AS BYPRODUCT
  - SHIVER TO STAY WARM

Chapter 9 The Muscular System

Figure 9.4

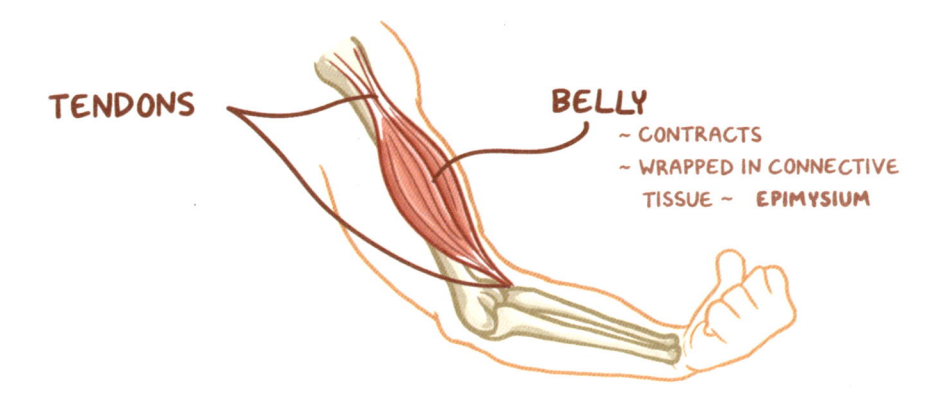

TENDONS

BELLY
~ CONTRACTS
~ WRAPPED IN CONNECTIVE TISSUE ~ EPIMYSIUM

BICEPS BRACHII

Figure 9.5

SKELETAL MUSCLES

PERIMYSIUM

FASCICLE

MUSCLE FIBER (MYOCYTE)

EPIMYSIUM

ENDOMYSIUM

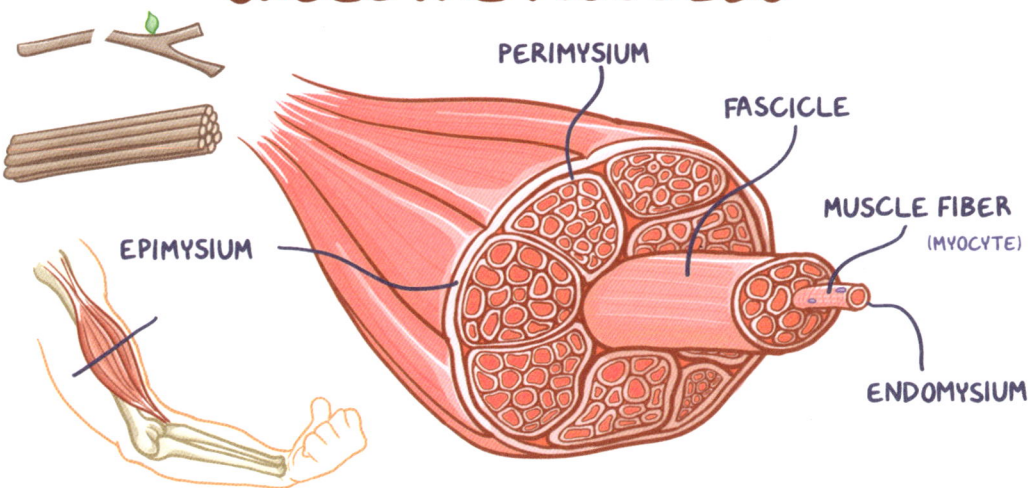

Figure 9.6

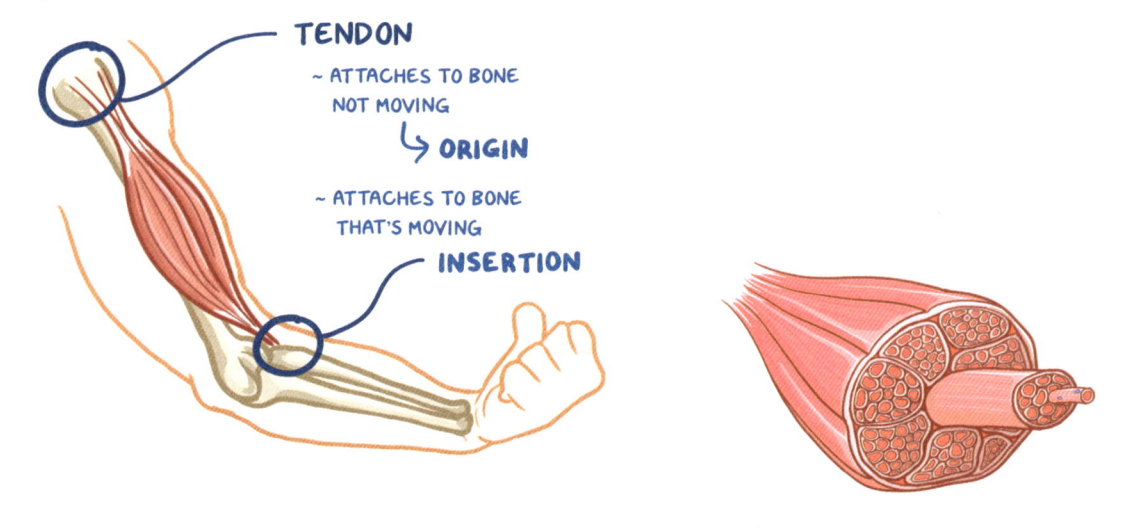

TENDON
~ ATTACHES TO BONE NOT MOVING
↳ ORIGIN

~ ATTACHES TO BONE THAT'S MOVING
INSERTION

OSMOSIS.ORG 95

Now, let's zoom in and look at a single myocyte. Myocytes are long cylindrical cells with multiple nuclei. They're located just below the cell membrane, which is called the sarcolemma. The sarcolemma is considered unique because of the tiny tunnels it creates, which project downwards from the surface into the center of the muscle fiber. These tunnels are called transverse tubules, or T tubules.

The cytoplasm of a myocyte is called sarcoplasm. It contains smooth endoplasmic reticulum, which is called sarcoplasmic reticulum. The sarcoplasmic reticulum stores a large amount of calcium and runs parallel to the T tubules. The sarcoplasm is filled with stacks of long filaments called myofibrils. Each myofibril has thin actin filaments and thick myosin filaments. These filaments don't extend through the entire length of the myocyte, but are arranged into shorter segments called sarcomeres. Each myocyte is made up of hundreds of sarcomeres, and under a microscope, the thick myosin filaments look dark, while the thin actin filaments look light. This is why skeletal muscles look striated or striped **(Figure 9.7)**!

So when we want to move, a motor signal is sent from the brain, down to the spinal cord, and then travels on a motor neuron. The motor neuron releases the neurotransmitter acetylcholine onto the sarcolemma, which has acetylcholine receptors. This causes rapid shifts in ions across the sarcolemma and down the T tubules. As a result, calcium begins to enter the myocyte. Once this happens, the sarcoplasmic reticulum releases its own calcium into the sarcoplasm. When all of this calcium flows into the myocyte, it causes the actin and myosin to bind and pull in on each other. This, in turn, causes thousands of sarcomeres within each myocyte to contract all at once—and that's how the myocyte contracts. Afterwards, the sarcoplasmic reticulum grabs most of the calcium ions and stores them again. Without calcium, the contraction ends and the muscle relaxes **(Figure 9.8)**.

CARDIAC MUSCLE TISSUE

Cardiac muscle tissue is only found in the walls of the heart. The heart is an incredible muscle that pumps blood into the lungs, where it gets oxygenated, before it's delivered to the rest of the body **(Figure 9.9)**. Similar to skeletal muscle fibers, cardiac muscle fibers are striated and organized into sarcomeres. However, they differ from skeletal muscle fibers in the following ways: cardiac muscle fibers are shorter and contain only one nucleus, which is usually in the center of the cell and is called a cardiomyocyte; these cardiomyocytes are not consciously controlled, making the cardiac muscle an involuntary muscle; and cardiomyocytes may be covered by endomysium, but they lack perimysium and epimysium.

Figure 9.7

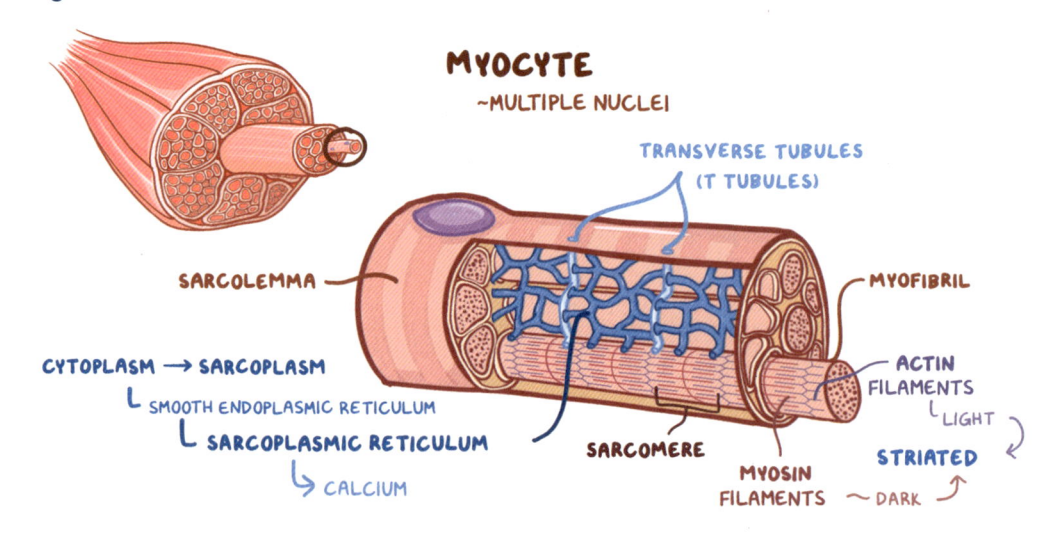

Chapter 9 The Muscular System

Figure 9.8

SKELETAL MUSCLES

- ACETYLCHOLINE
- ACETYLCHOLINE RECEPTORS
- RAPID SHIFTS IN IONS ACROSS SARCOLEMMA
- ACTIN
- MYOSIN
- Ca²⁺
- SARCOPLASMIC RETICULUM
  - RELEASES CALCIUM INTO SARCOPLASM
  - GRABS CALCIUM IONS AND STORES THEM

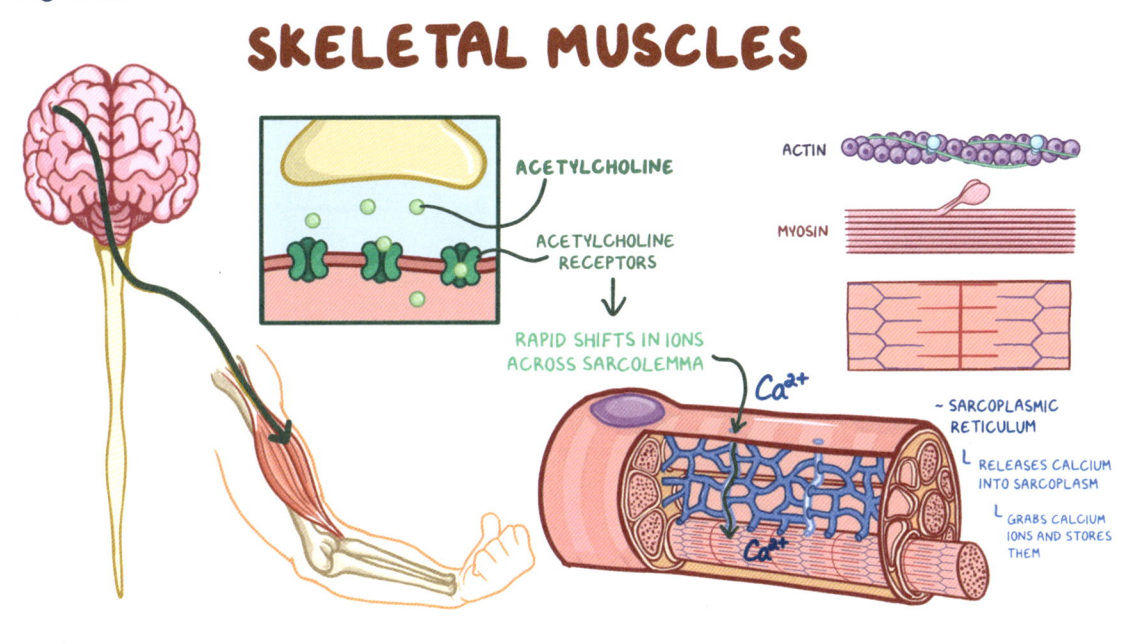

Figure 9.9

CARDIAC MUSCLE

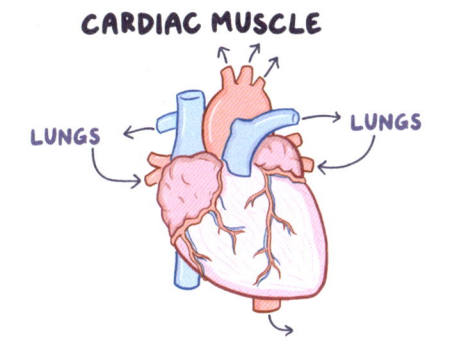

- LUNGS
- LUNGS

Figure 9.10

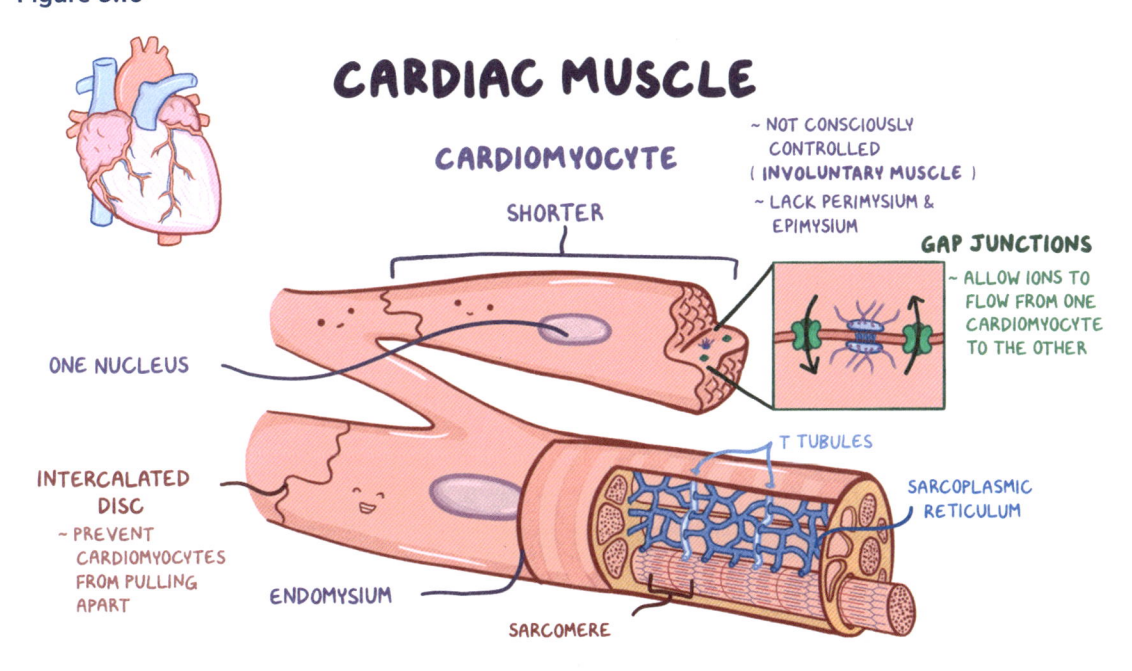

CARDIAC MUSCLE

CARDIOMYOCYTE
- NOT CONSCIOUSLY CONTROLLED (INVOLUNTARY MUSCLE)
- LACK PERIMYSIUM & EPIMYSIUM
- SHORTER

GAP JUNCTIONS
- ALLOW IONS TO FLOW FROM ONE CARDIOMYOCYTE TO THE OTHER

- ONE NUCLEUS
- INTERCALATED DISC
  - PREVENT CARDIOMYOCYTES FROM PULLING APART
- ENDOMYSIUM
- T TUBULES
- SARCOPLASMIC RETICULUM
- SARCOMERE

OSMOSIS.ORG 97

Figure 9.11

CARDIAC MUSCLE

PACEMAKER CELLS
- GENERATE AND CONDUCT ACTION POTENTIALS
  ↳ RAPID SHIFTS IN IONS

✱ **COORDINATED CONTRACTION** OF THE **HEART**

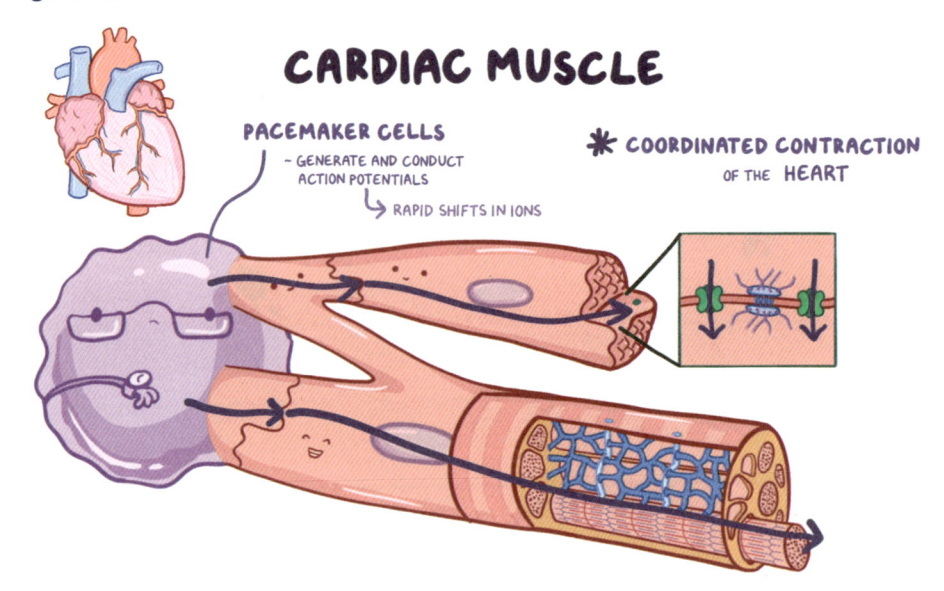

Figure 9.12

SMOOTH MUSCLE
↳ DON'T LOOK STRIATED

- THIN AND **THICK** MYOFILAMENTS
- CAVEOLAE
- ENDOMYSIUM

- ~ FUSIFORM- SPINDLE-SHAPED
- ~ ONE NUCLEUS
- ~ LACK PERIMYSIUM & EPIMYSIUM
- ~ INVOLUNTARY CONTROL

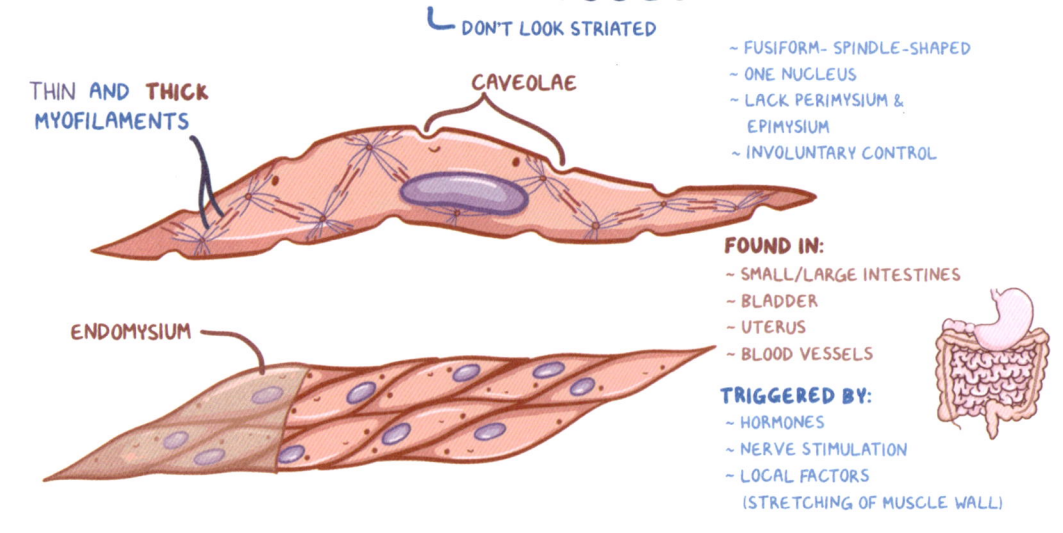

FOUND IN:
- ~ SMALL/LARGE INTESTINES
- ~ BLADDER
- ~ UTERUS
- ~ BLOOD VESSELS

TRIGGERED BY:
- ~ HORMONES
- ~ NERVE STIMULATION
- ~ LOCAL FACTORS (STRETCHING OF MUSCLE WALL)

Figure 9.13

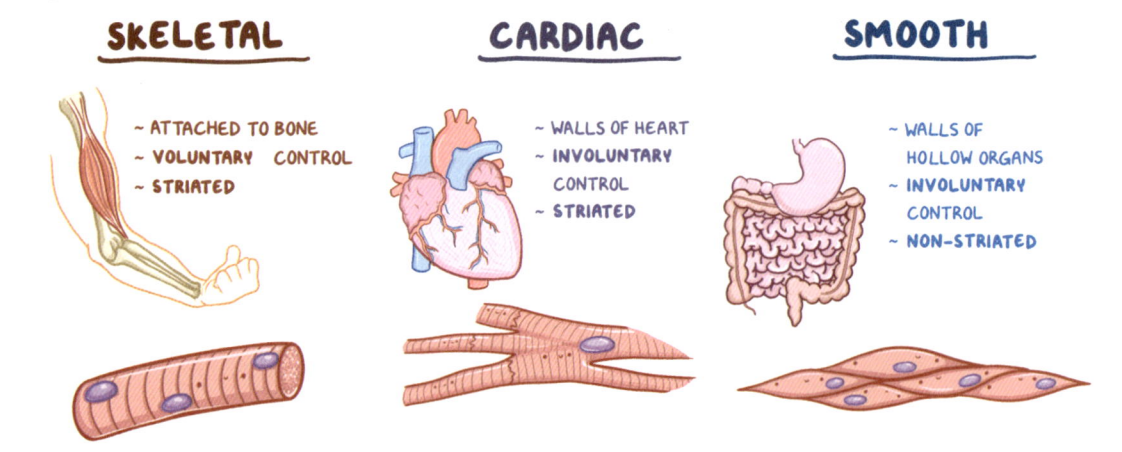

SKELETAL	CARDIAC	SMOOTH
~ ATTACHED TO BONE ~ VOLUNTARY CONTROL ~ STRIATED	~ WALLS OF HEART ~ INVOLUNTARY CONTROL ~ STRIATED	~ WALLS OF HOLLOW ORGANS ~ INVOLUNTARY CONTROL ~ NON-STRIATED

Now, just like skeletal muscle cells, the cardiomyocytes have T tubules, sarcoplasmic reticulum, and sarcomeres, but they also branch and connect to adjacent cardiomyocytes using intercalated discs. Intercalated discs are sort of like staples that prevent the cardiomyocytes from pulling apart during contraction. Intercalated discs also have gap junctions, which are like little connections that allow ions to flow from one cardiomyocyte right into another **(Figure 9.10)**.

In addition, there are specialized cardiomyocytes in the heart muscle walls called pacemaker cells. Pacemaker cells generate and conduct action potentials, which are basically rapid shifts in ions, including calcium, that enter the cell. When these ion shifts happen in one cardiomyocyte, they also start happening in the neighboring cardiomyocytes because ions can slip through intercalated discs. This results in the coordinated contraction of the entire heart **(Figure 9.11)**.

SMOOTH MUSCLE TISSUE

Finally, let's examine the smooth muscle tissue. Within the sarcoplasm of the smooth muscle cells, there are thin and thick myofilaments, but, unlike the skeletal and cardiac muscles, they're not organized into sarcomeres. In fact, that's why they're considered "smooth": they don't look striated under a microscope. Smooth muscle cells are fusiform or spindle shaped, meaning they are wide in the middle and tapered at both ends, and they have one centrally located nucleus.

They're wrapped within endomysium but, like the cardiac muscle, they lack perimysium and epimysium. In contrast to both skeletal and cardiac muscles, smooth muscle cells don't have T tubules; instead, they have smaller invaginations of the sarcolemma, called caveolae. As well, the sarcoplasmic reticulum within the smooth muscle fibers isn't as extensive as the ones in skeletal or cardiac muscles.

Smooth muscles are usually found in the walls of hollow organs, like the small intestine, large intestine, bladder, and uterus. They are also found in the blood vessels. Like cardiac muscles, smooth muscles are under involuntary control. Contractions are triggered by hormones, nerve stimulation, and local factors, such as the stretching of the muscle wall **(Figure 9.12)**.

SUMMARY

All right, as a quick recap, the muscular system is made up of skeletal, cardiac, and smooth muscle tissue. Skeletal muscles are attached to the bones, are under voluntary control, and have a striated appearance. Cardiac muscles are found within the walls of the heart, are under involuntary control, and also have a striated appearance. Finally, smooth muscles are mostly found within the walls of hollow organs, are under involuntary control, and do not have a striated appearance **(Figure 9.13)**.

THE SKELETAL SYSTEM

osms.it/skeletal_system

The human body has approximately 206 bones and together they make up the skeleton. The skeleton, in turn, is responsible for maintaining body structure, protecting important organs, like the brain and heart, and facilitating movement. Without bones, you'd be a shapeless, immobile blob **(Figure 10.1)**!

The skeleton can be broken down into the axial and the appendicular skeleton. The axial skeleton consists of bones located along the vertical axis of your body. It contains about 80 bones in total: 22 of these make up the skull, 33 the vertebrae, 24 the ribs, and, finally, the sternum. The appendicular skeleton consists of bones in your limbs, as well as the bones that attach these limb bones to the axial skeleton, like the pelvis and the scapulae. It contains about 126 bones in total: 4 of these are in the shoulders, 6 in the arms, 54 in the hands, 2 in the hips that form the pelvic girdle, 8 in the legs, and, finally, 52 in the feet **(Figure 10.2)**.

Figure 10.1

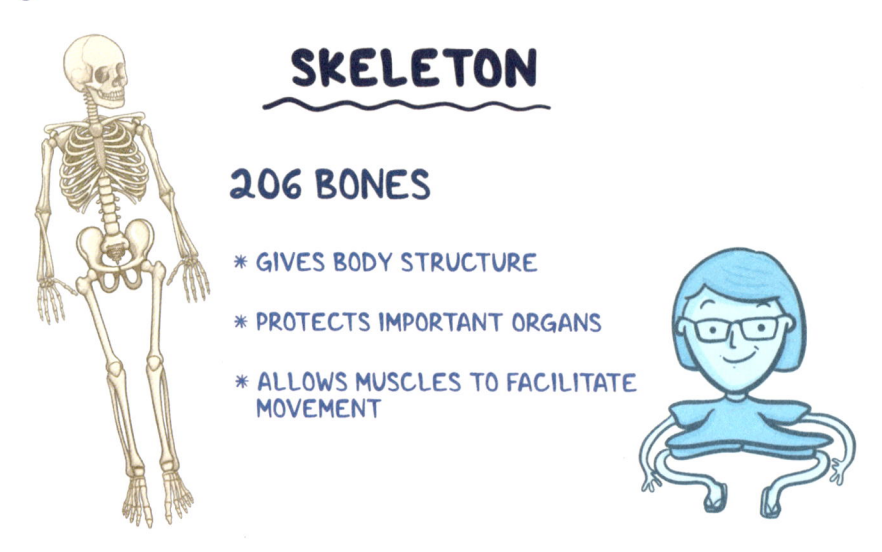

SKELETON

206 BONES

* GIVES BODY STRUCTURE
* PROTECTS IMPORTANT ORGANS
* ALLOWS MUSCLES TO FACILITATE MOVEMENT

Figure 10.2

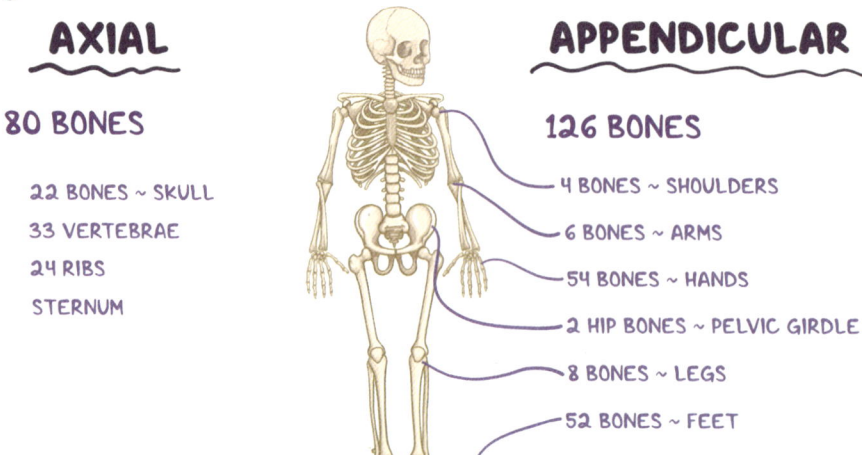

AXIAL

80 BONES

22 BONES ~ SKULL
33 VERTEBRAE
24 RIBS
STERNUM

APPENDICULAR

126 BONES

4 BONES ~ SHOULDERS
6 BONES ~ ARMS
54 BONES ~ HANDS
2 HIP BONES ~ PELVIC GIRDLE
8 BONES ~ LEGS
52 BONES ~ FEET

Chapter 10 The Skeletal System

BONE TYPES: LONG, SHORT, FLAT, SESAMOID, & IRREGULAR

Now, there are five types of bones. These types are based on shape: long, short, flat, sesamoid, and irregular. Long bones are longer than they are wide, and they are found in the limbs. Long bones include the humerus, radius, and ulna in the arms, as well as the metacarpals and phalanges in the hands and fingers. Long bones also include the femur, tibia, and fibula in the legs, as well as the metatarsals and phalanges in the feet and toes. During childhood and adolescence, long bones continue to grow. They are the bones responsible for your height **(Figure 10.3)**.

Unlike long bones, short bones have a similar length and width. This gives them a round or cube-like appearance. They include the carpal bones of the wrist and tarsal bones of the ankle. Their main job is to support the hand and foot **(Figure 10.4)**.

Figure 10.3

* LONG BONES
~ LONGER THAN WIDE

- HUMERUS
- RADIUS
- ULNA
- METACARPALS
- PHALANGES

* CHILDHOOD & ADOLESCENCE
  - LONG BONES CONTINUE TO GROW
  - HEIGHT

- FEMUR
- TIBIA
- FIBULA
- METATARSALS
- PHALANGES

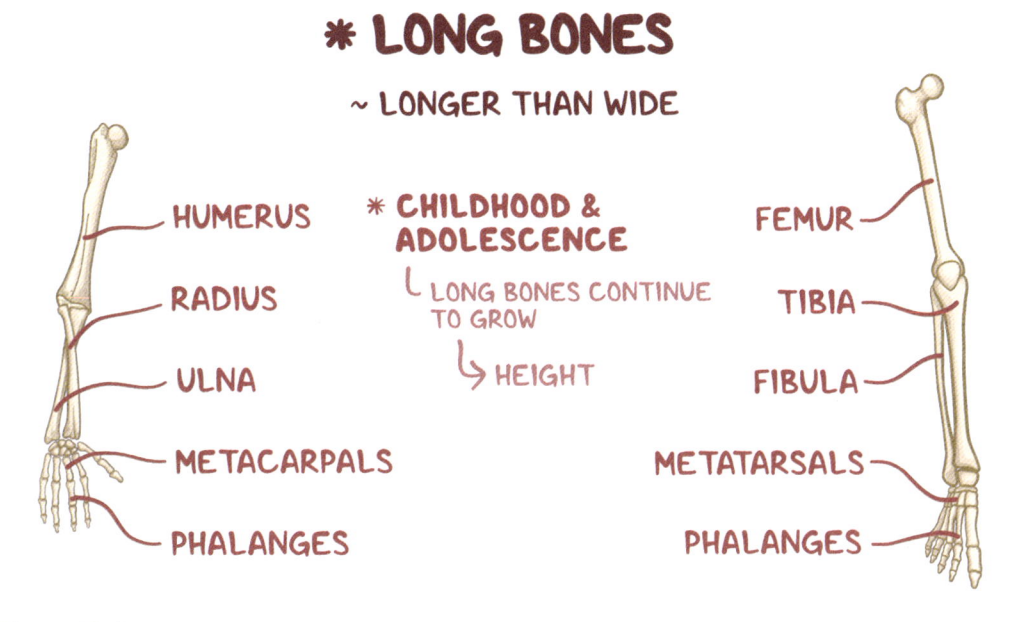

Figure 10.4

* SHORT BONES
~ SIMILAR LENGTH & WIDTH

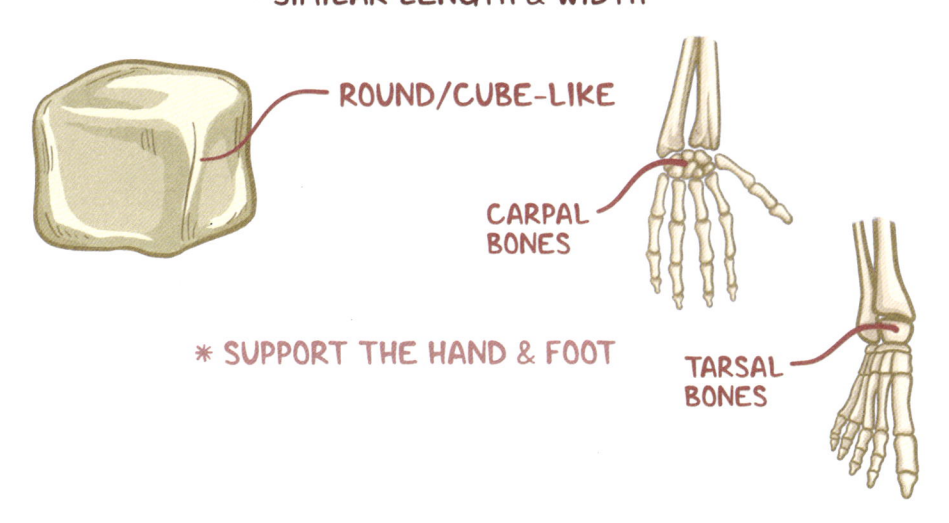

- ROUND/CUBE-LIKE
- CARPAL BONES
- TARSAL BONES

* SUPPORT THE HAND & FOOT

OSMOSIS.ORG 101

Flat bones are thin bones, and some of them are curved. They include bones of the skull, shoulder blades or scapulae, sternum, and ribs. Their main job is to serve as armor plating that protects vital organs like the brain, heart, and lungs **(Figure 10.5)**.

Sesamoid bones are embedded in the tendons. They're like giant sesame seeds in shape. Most of these bones are found in the metacarpal phalangeal joints in the hand and metatarsal phalangeal joints in the feet. The larger sesamoid bones include the pisiform bone in the wrist and the patella bone in the kneecap. These increase the angle between the bone and the muscle tendon, allowing more leverage for the muscles. The sesamoid bones also provide support and protect the tendon from wear and tear **(Figure 10.6)**.

Lastly, irregular bones are basically the misfits. They don't fit into any of the previous categories. These include the facial bones, mandible, vertebrae of the vertebral column, sacrum, and coccyx **(Figure 10.7)**.

Figure 10.5

* FLAT BONES
~ THIN/CURVED

* ARMOR PLATING
  - PROTECTS VITAL ORGANS

- SCAPULAE
- STERNUM
- SKULL
- RIBS

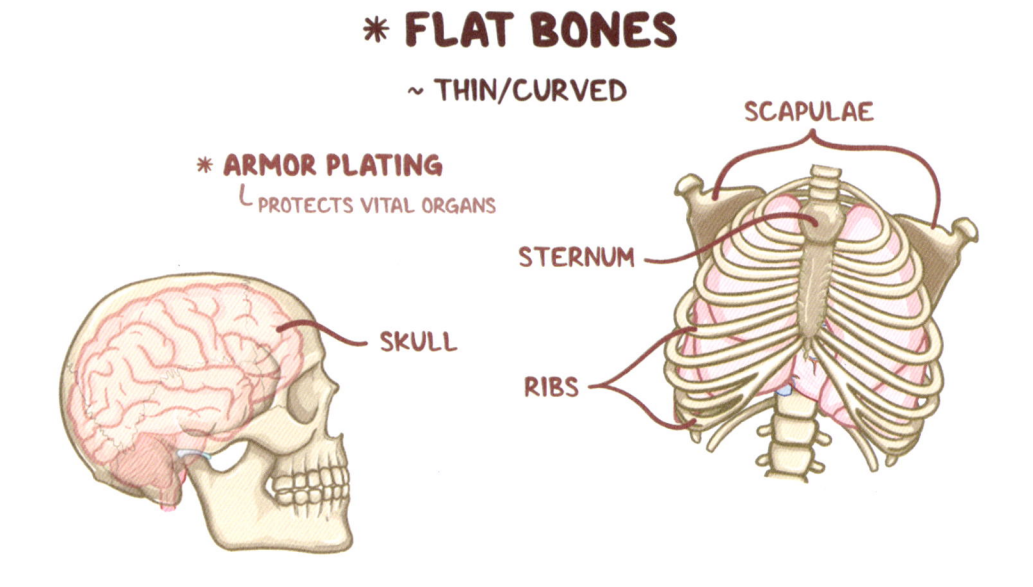

Figure 10.6

* SESAMOID BONES
~ IMBEDDED IN TENDONS
(SESAME SEEDS)

- PISIFORM
- PATELLA

* ↑ ANGLE BETWEEN BONE & TENDON
  - MORE LEVERAGE

* PROVIDE SUPPORT & PROTECT TENDON

Figure 10.7

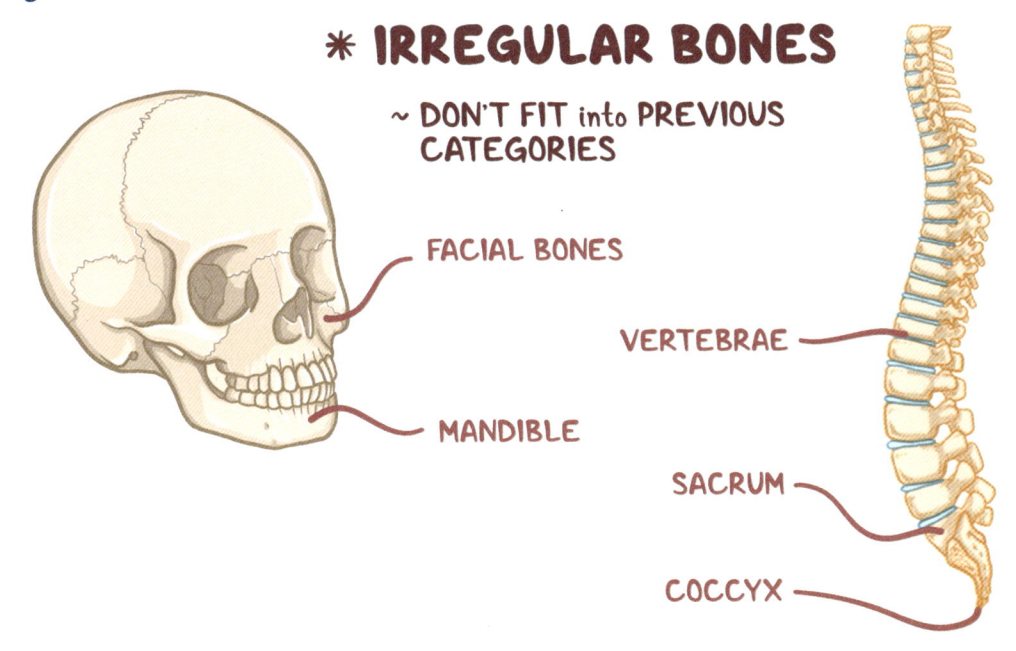

* IRREGULAR BONES

~ DON'T FIT into PREVIOUS CATEGORIES

- FACIAL BONES
- MANDIBLE
- VERTEBRAE
- SACRUM
- COCCYX

SURFACE STRUCTURES

Now, some bones have surface structures that help them function. For example, bones can have tubercles, which are small bumps that serve as an attachment site for muscles. A large tubercle is called a tuberosity. An example of this is the deltoid tuberosity on the humerus, which is where the deltoid muscle attaches to the bone **(Figure 10.8)**.

Figure 10.8

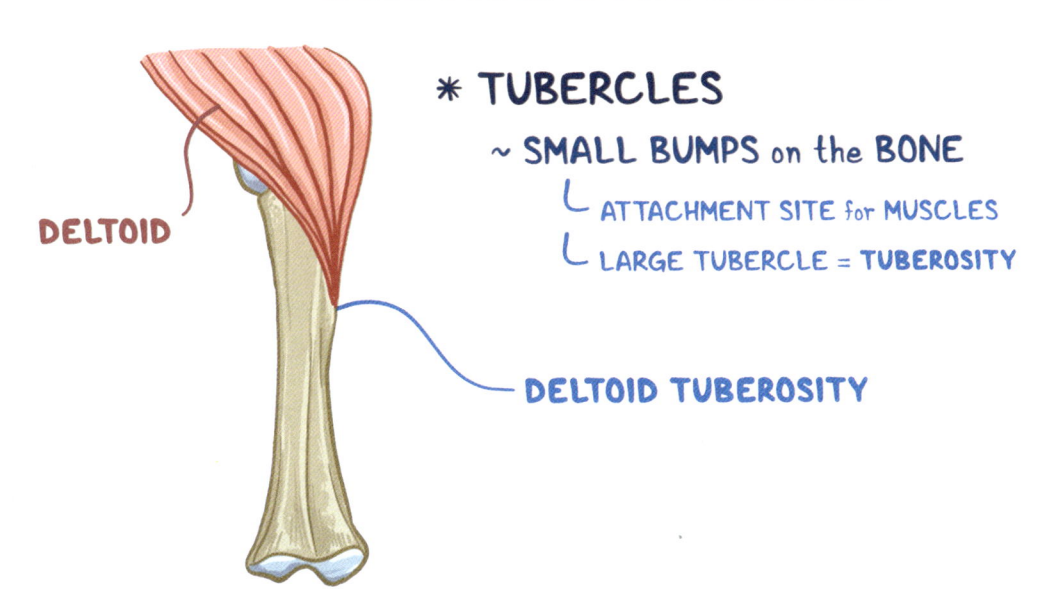

SURFACE STRUCTURES

- DELTOID

* TUBERCLES

~ SMALL BUMPS on the BONE
  - ATTACHMENT SITE for MUSCLES
  - LARGE TUBERCLE = TUBEROSITY

- DELTOID TUBEROSITY

Holes in the bone that allow blood vessels or nerves to pass through are called foramen. One example is the foramen magnum in the occipital bone of the skull, which allows the spinal cord to exit the skull **(Figure 10.9)**.

Bones can also have canals, which are tunnels within the bone that allow structures like blood vessels or nerves to travel through. An example of this is the optic canal in the sphenoid bone, which allows the optic nerve to travel from the brain to the eyes. Another name for a canal is a meatus, like the external auditory meatus of the ear, located in the temporal bone. The meatus allows sound to pass through to the eardrum **(Figure 10.10)**.

Figure 10.9

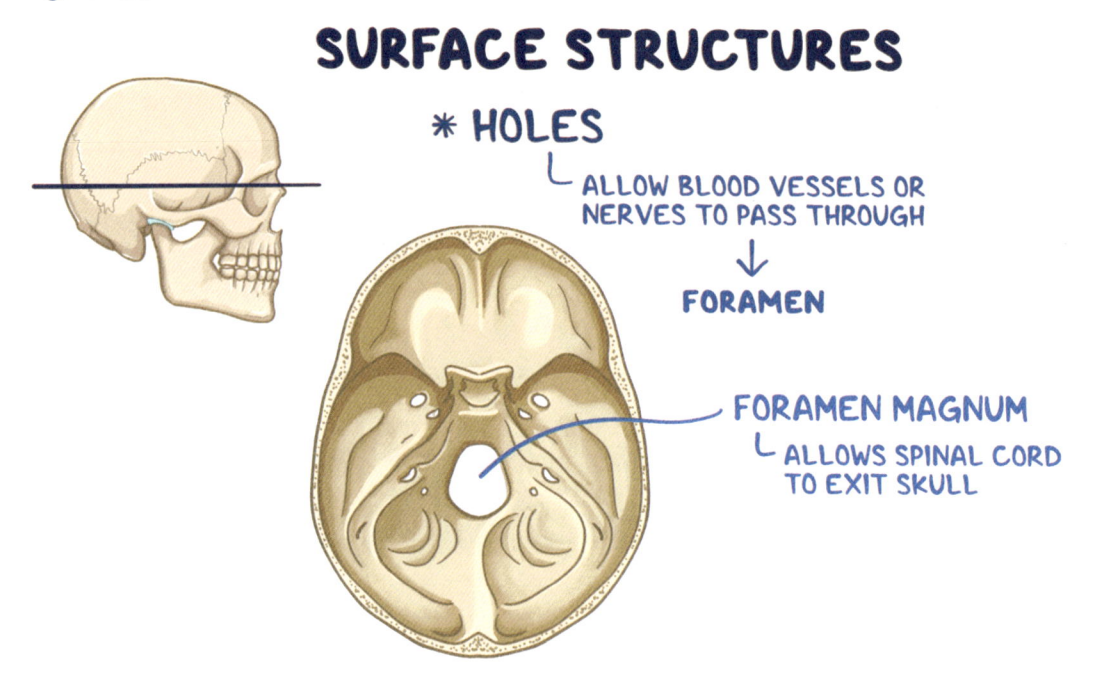

SURFACE STRUCTURES
* HOLES
  - ALLOW BLOOD VESSELS OR NERVES TO PASS THROUGH
  - FORAMEN
  - FORAMEN MAGNUM
    - ALLOWS SPINAL CORD TO EXIT SKULL

Figure 10.10

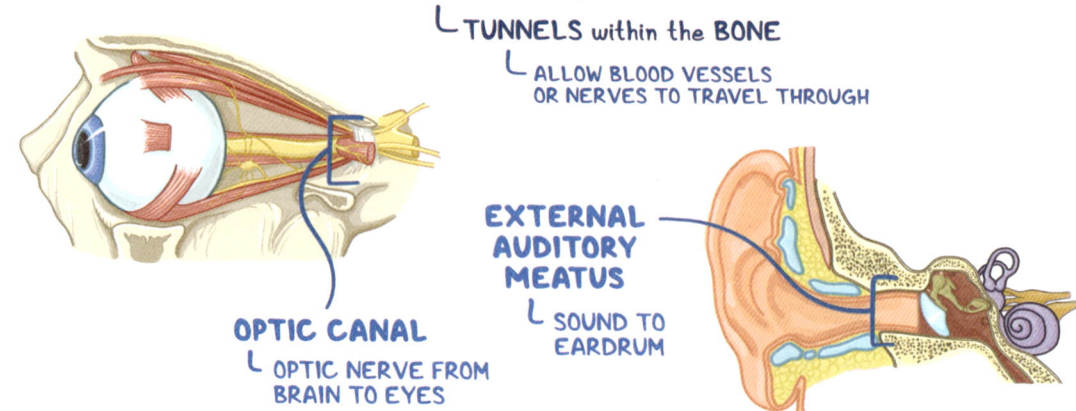

SURFACE STRUCTURES
* CANALS / MEATUS
  - TUNNELS within the BONE
  - ALLOW BLOOD VESSELS OR NERVES TO TRAVEL THROUGH
  - OPTIC CANAL
    - OPTIC NERVE FROM BRAIN TO EYES
  - EXTERNAL AUDITORY MEATUS
    - SOUND TO EARDRUM

Some bones have a fossa, which is a depression within the bone, where another structure rests. One example is the hypophyseal fossa, or sella turcica, on the sphenoid bone, which is like a tiny seat where the pituitary gland rests **(Figure 10.11)**.

Lastly, there are sinuses and cavities, which may be empty spaces within a bone or may be formed by multiple bones coming together. Examples include: the nasal cavity, which is formed by the maxilla, the nasal bone, and palatine bone, as well as the paranasal sinuses, like the maxillary sinus, within the maxillary bone **(Figure 10.12)**.

Figure 10.11

SURFACE STRUCTURES

* FOSSA
- DEPRESSION within the BONE
  - ANOTHER STRUCTURE RESTS

- HYPOPHYSEAL FOSSA (SELLA TURCICA)
- PITUITARY GLAND

Figure 10.12

SURFACE STRUCTURES

* SINUSES & CAVITIES
- EMPTY SPACES within a BONE
- FORMED by MULTIPLE BONES COMING TOGETHER

NASAL CAVITY
- MAXILLA
- NASAL BONE
- PALATINE BONE

MAXILLARY SINUS
- MAXILLARY BONE

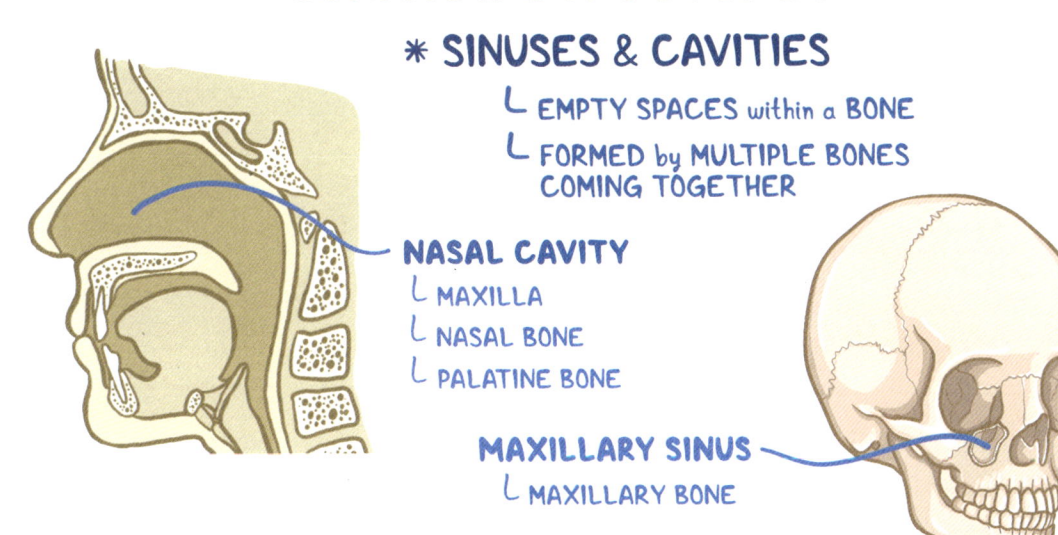

THE CORTICAL BONE

All bones share some similarities internally. For instance, if we look at a cross section of a bone, we can see two layers: first, a hard external layer known as the cortical bone; and, second, a softer internal layer of spongy bone, which looks like honeycombs and is known as the trabecular bone.

Let's examine the hard external layer first. The cortical bone is covered by a membrane of fibrous connective tissue called the periosteum, and that's where the muscles, tendons, and ligaments attach **(Figure 10.13)**. If we zoom in, we can see that the cortical bone has many pipe-like structures called osteons, which run through the length of the bone. Each pipe has an empty center called a haversian canal, which contains the nerves and blood vessels that supply the osteon **(Figure 10.14)**.

Adjacent osteons are connected to one another by horizontal channels called Volkmann's canals, which carry smaller blood vessels that branch from the main one. The thick walls of the osteon are made up of tightly packed, concentric layers of bone matrix. This bone matrix is made of type I collagen, which is further reinforced with hydroxyapatite—a mineral made of calcium and phosphate.

At the periphery of the osteon is a ring of cells called osteoblasts. These synthesize type I collagen and hydroxyapatite, creating new layers of matrix. Some of these osteoblasts become trapped in the new layers of matrix and mature into osteocytes within tiny cavities called lacunae. Osteocytes are less able to create bone matrix and, unlike osteoblasts, they can't multiply. Instead, osteocytes become mechanoreceptors that detect stress and damage. Mechanoreceptors help control the process of bone remodeling, which is when old bone is broken down and replaced with new bone **(Figure 10.15)**.

Dispersed among the osteoblasts are some larger cells called osteoclasts. Osteoclasts secrete enzymes to assist the breakdown of bone matrix, which releases the calcium and phosphate in the hydroxyapatite back into the blood. This is useful for bone remodeling, but it also comes in handy when there's low calcium level in the blood. In this way, the bones can be thought of as a storage sites for calcium **(Figure 10.16)**.

Figure 10.13

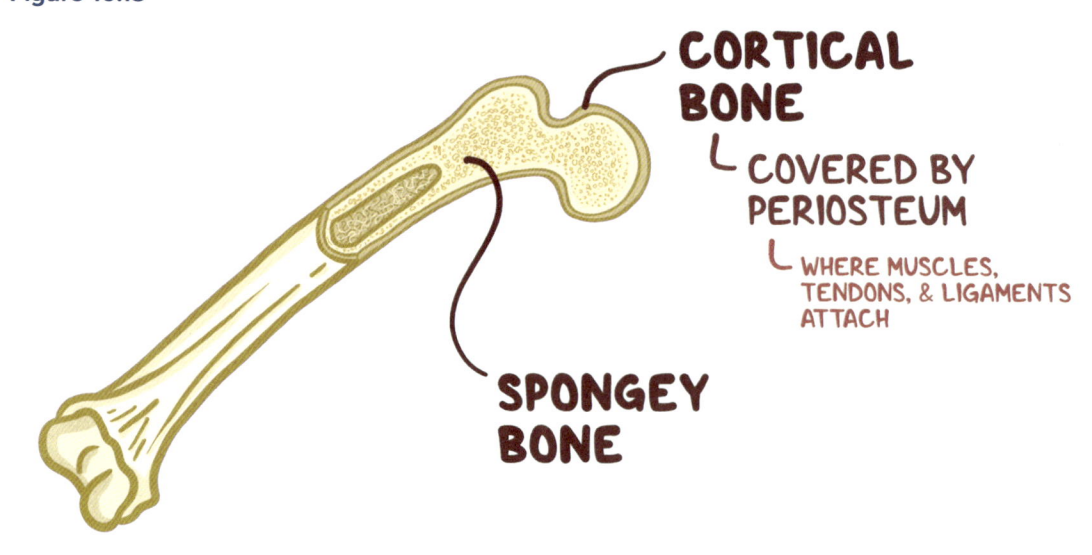

Chapter 10 The Skeletal System

Figure 10.14

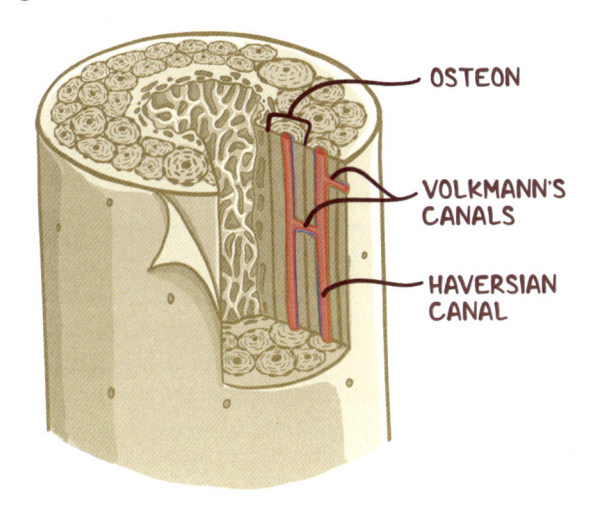

- OSTEON
- VOLKMANN'S CANALS
- HAVERSIAN CANAL

Figure 10.15

BONE MATRIX
└ TYPE I COLLAGEN
  ~ REINFORCED WITH **HYDROXYAPATITE**
    (Ca^{2+} & PO^-)

OSTEOBLASTS
└ SYNTHESIZE TYPE I COLLAGEN & HYDROXYAPATITE
  ↓
  NEW LAYERS OF MATRIX

OSTEOCYTES
└ LESS ABLE TO CREATE MATRIX
└ CAN'T MULTIPLY
→ MECHANORECEPTORS
  ~ DETECT STRESS & DAMAGE
  ~ CONTROL REMODELING

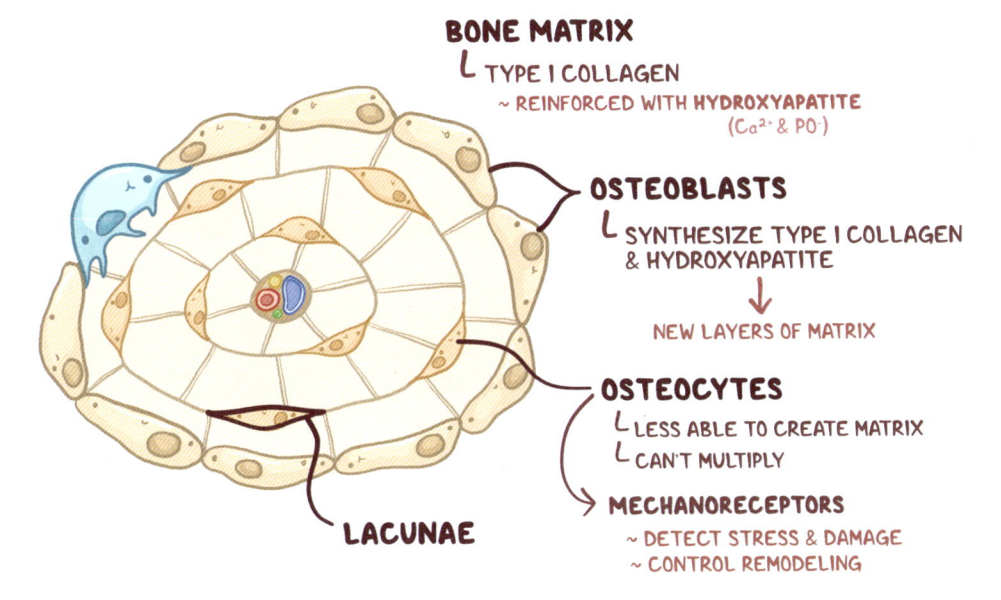

LACUNAE

Figure 10.16

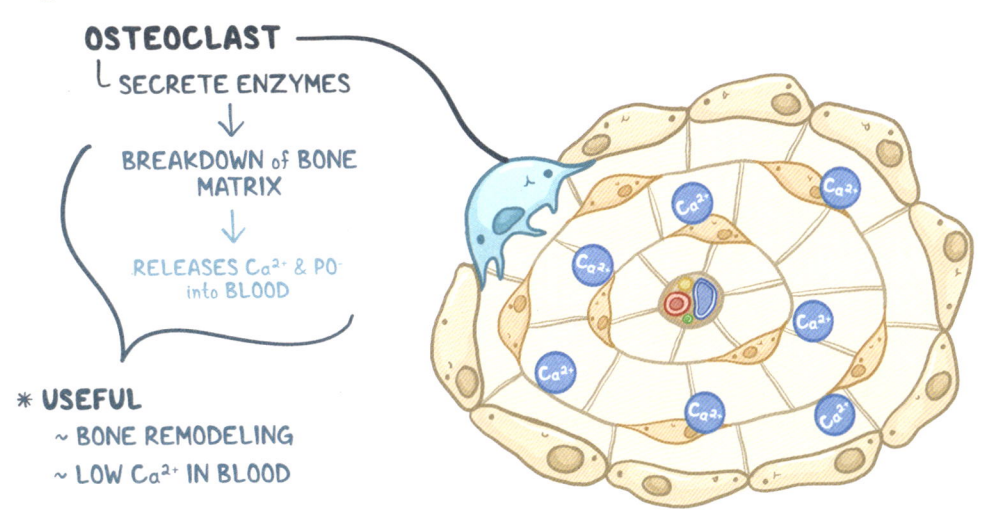

OSTEOCLAST
└ SECRETE ENZYMES
  ↓
  BREAKDOWN of BONE MATRIX
  ↓
  RELEASES Ca^{2+} & PO^- into BLOOD

✳ USEFUL
  ~ BONE REMODELING
  ~ LOW Ca^{2+} IN BLOOD

OSMOSIS.ORG 107

THE TRABECULAR BONE

Now, let's examine the softer internal layer of spongy bone. Under the tough cortical layer is the trabecular bone. The trabecular bone is composed of material similar to the cortical bone, but the organizational structure is far more loose. It has networks of branching rods called trabeculae. These make the spongy bone less dense and a great deal softer than the cortical bone. They also give the spongy bone its "hole-ridden" appearance—like a sponge **(Figure 10.17)**!

Within this layer is the bone marrow, which is composed of a mix of hematopoietic stem cells that eventually differentiate into red blood cells, white blood cells, and platelets. The marrow also contains adipocytes, or fat cells, which store fat—a great source of energy. Marrow can be divided into either red marrow, which contains mostly hematopoietic cells, or yellow marrow, which has a higher percentage of adipocytes **(Figure 10.18)**. In bones that form the appendicular skeleton, like long femur bones, the red marrow is mostly located at the tips. Meanwhile, the shaft of the bone contains a hollow medullary cavity filled with yellow marrow. In contrast, in bones that form the axial skeleton, there is no medullary cavity and, thus, they are mostly packed with red marrow **(Figure 10.19)**.

Figure 10.17

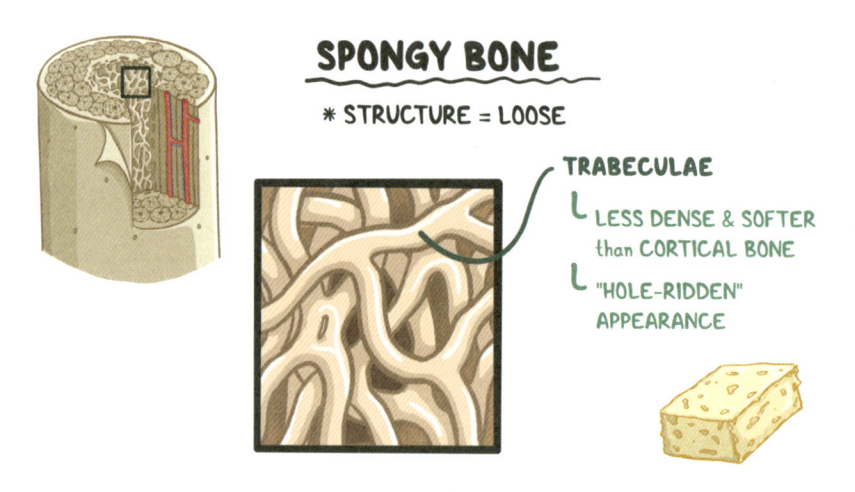

Figure 10.18

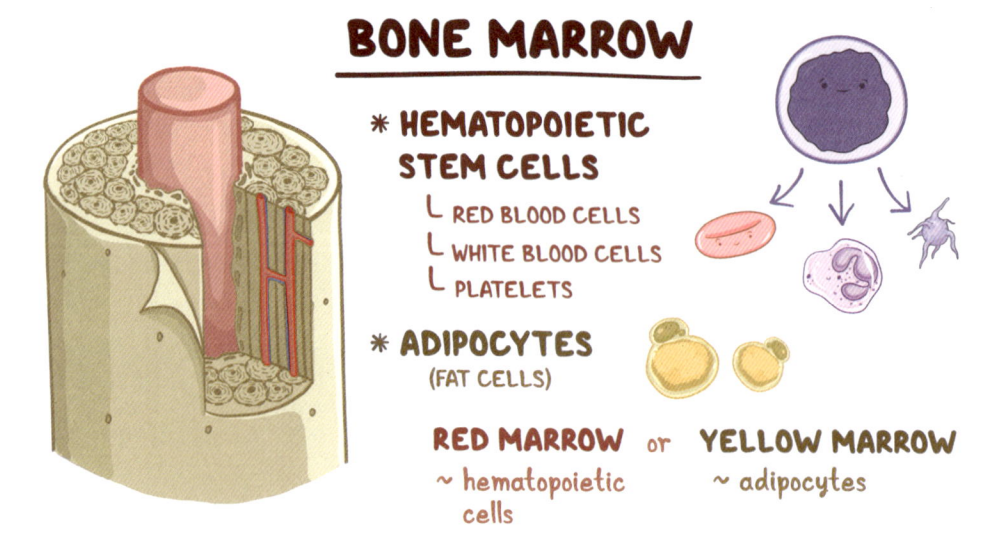

Chapter 10 The Skeletal System

Figure 10.19

BONE MARROW

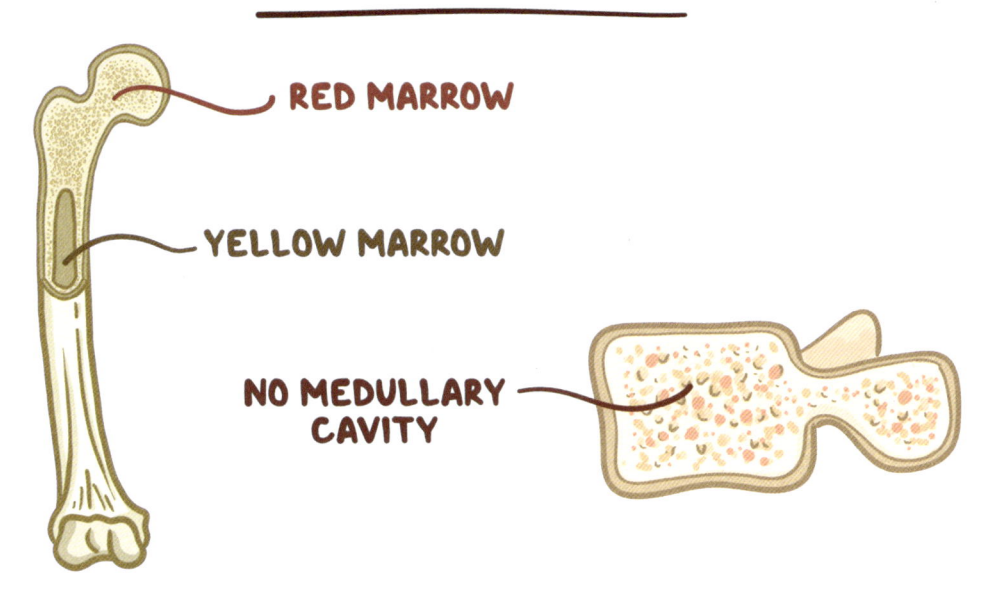

- RED MARROW
- YELLOW MARROW
- NO MEDULLARY CAVITY

SUMMARY

All right, as a quick recap, the human skeleton consists of approximately 206 bones, which can be divided into the axial and appendicular skeleton. There are long, short, flat, sesamoid, and irregular bones. Bones give shape to your body, provide support to your internal organs, and allow movement to occur. They also produce platelets, red blood cells, and white blood cells and they store calcium and phosphate. Each bone has an outer layer made of tough cortical bone and an inner layer made of soft spongy bone. Red bone marrow is found in the spongy bone and yellow marrow is found mainly in the medullary cavity of long bones **(Figure 10.20)**.

Figure 10.20

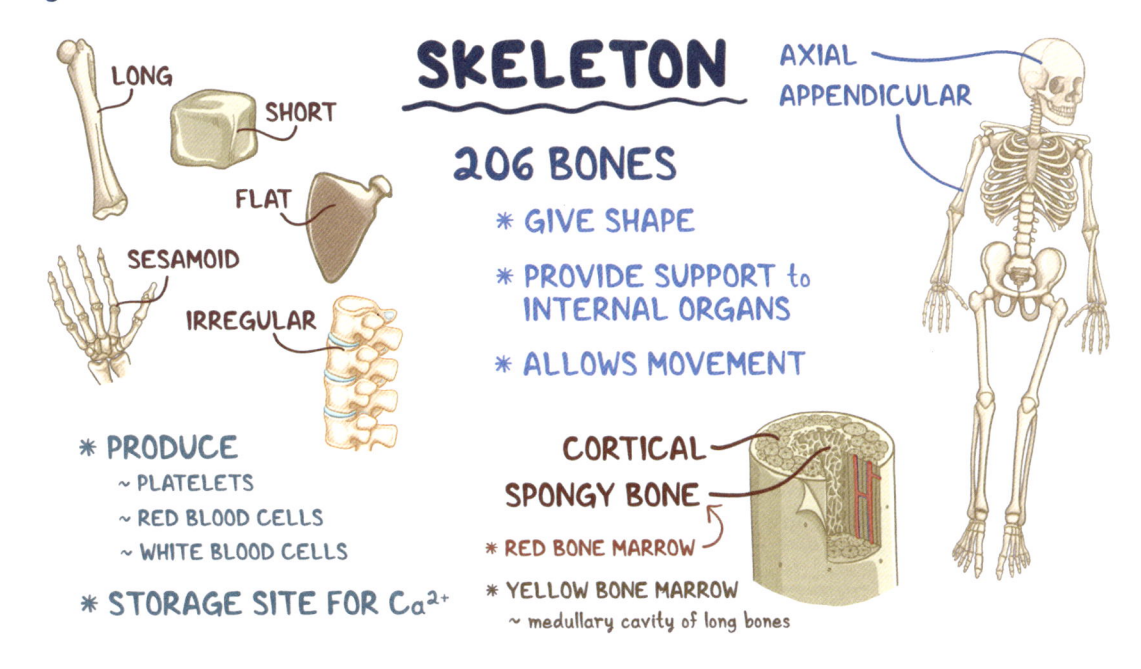

SKELETON

- LONG
- SHORT
- FLAT
- SESAMOID
- IRREGULAR

AXIAL
APPENDICULAR

206 BONES
* GIVE SHAPE
* PROVIDE SUPPORT to INTERNAL ORGANS
* ALLOWS MOVEMENT

* PRODUCE
  ~ PLATELETS
  ~ RED BLOOD CELLS
  ~ WHITE BLOOD CELLS
* STORAGE SITE FOR Ca^{2+}

CORTICAL
SPONGY BONE
* RED BONE MARROW
* YELLOW BONE MARROW
  ~ medullary cavity of long bones

OSMOSIS.ORG 109

THE INTEGUMENTARY SYSTEM

osms.it/integumentary_system

The skin makes up around 7% of our total body weight, making it the largest organ in the body. Admittedly, however, it's hard to imagine it as a single organ. The skin, along with its accessory structures like oil and sweat glands, makes up what is called the integumentary system. The integumentary system protects the body from infections, helps regulate body temperature, and contains nerve receptors that detect pain, sensation, and pressure **(Figure 11.1)**.

LAYERS OF THE SKIN: EPIDERMIS, DERMIS, & HYPODERMIS

The skin is divided into three layers: the epidermis, dermis, and hypodermis. The epidermis forms the thin outermost layer of skin. Underneath, is the thicker dermis layer that contains the nerves and blood vessels. And finally, there's the hypodermis, which is made of fat and connective tissue that anchors the skin to the underlying muscle **(Figure 11.2)**.

Figure 11.1

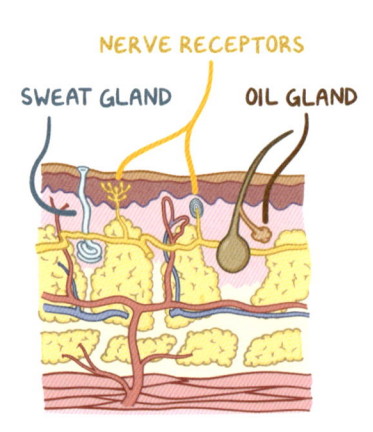

Figure 11.2

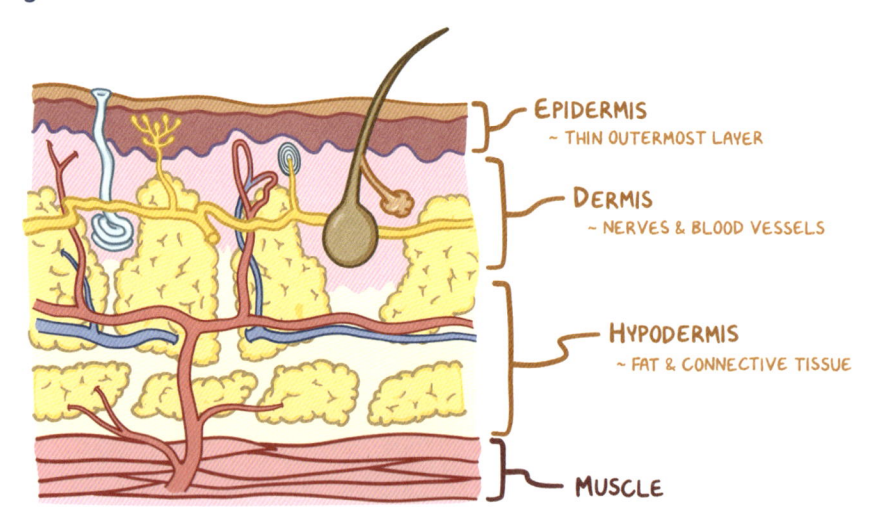

Chapter 11 The Integumentary System

EPIDERMIS

The epidermis itself is made of multiple layers of developing keratinocytes—flat pancake-shaped cells named for the keratin protein they're filled with **(Figure 11.3)**. Keratin is a fibrous protein that allows keratinocytes to protect themselves—from being destroyed, for instance, when you rub your hands through the sand at the beach. Keratinocytes also make and secrete glycolipids—where *glyco-* means sugar, and *lipid* means fat. Glycolipids help to prevent water from easily seeping into and out of the body **(Figure 11.4)**.

Keratinocytes start their life at the lowest layer of the epidermis called the stratum basale, or basal layer, which is made of a single layer of stem cells that continually divide and produce new keratinocytes. These new keratinocytes then migrate upwards to form the other layers of the epidermis. The stratum basale also contains another group of cells. These are the melanocytes, which secrete a protein pigment, or coloring substance, called melanin. Melanin is actually a broad term that constitutes several types of melanin found in people of differing skin color. These subtypes of melanin range in color from black to reddish yellow and their relative quantity defines a person's skin color.

When keratinocytes are exposed to the sun, they send a chemical signal to the melanocytes, which stimulates the melanocytes into making more melanin. The melanocytes move the melanin into small sacs called melanosomes, and these get taken up by newly formed keratinocytes. Melanin then acts as a natural sunscreen, because its protein structure disspitates, or scatters, UVB light. Without protection, UVB light can damage the DNA in the skin cells and lead to skin cancer. Darker types of melanin and greater quantities of this kind of melanin are produced by individuals living close to the equator because they typically get more sun exposure. Despite the potential for skin damage, UVB light is essential. It helps generate vitamin D, an important regulator of calcium absorption. Keratinocytes contain cholesterol precursor molecules that are activated by UVB into vitamin D **(Figure 11.5)**.

As keratinocytes in the stratum basale mature and lose the ability to divide, they migrate into the next layer, called the stratum spinosum, which is about eight to 10 cell layers thick. Keratinocytes in the stratum spinosum layer have tiny proteins on the membrane that look like tiny spines; these help the cells adhere to one another **(Figure 11.6)**. The stratum spinosum layer also has dendritic cells lurking around. These are star-shaped immune cells, and they are constantly on the patrol looking for invading microbes **(Figure 11.7)**.

Figure 11.3

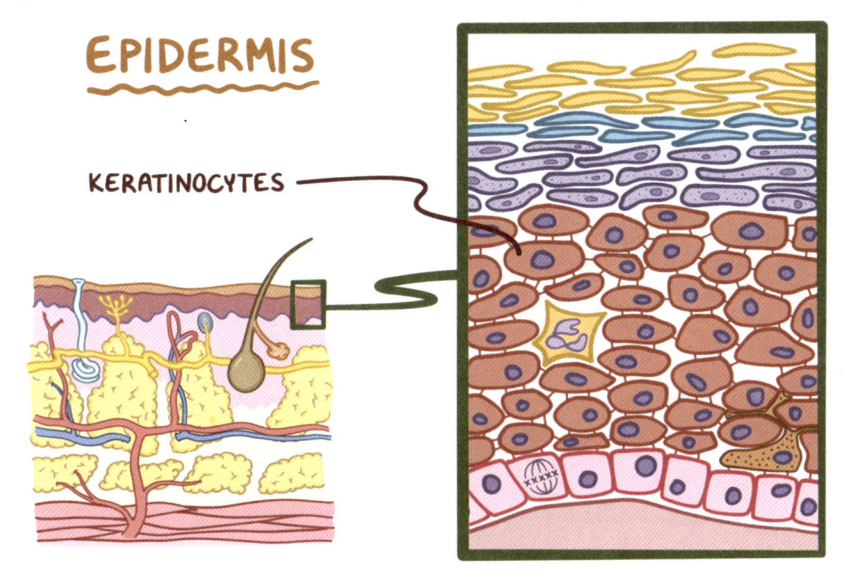

OSMOSIS.ORG 111

Figure 11.4

EPIDERMIS

KERATINOCYTES
* KERATIN PROTEIN
  └ FIBROUS PROTEIN
* MAKE & SECRETE GLYCOLIPIDS
  - SUGAR
  - FAT

STRATUM BASALE
* SINGLE LAYER of STEM CELLS
* CONTINUALLY DIVIDES
  └ PRODUCING NEW KERATINOCYTES

MELANOCYTE
* MELANIN
  ~ PIGMENT PROTEIN
  ~ BLACK to REDDISH YELLOW
  ~ NATURAL SUNSCREEN (SCATTERS UVB LIGHT)

Figure 11.5

~ DARKER MELANIN & GREATER QUANTITIES are PRODUCED by INDIVIDUALS LIVING CLOSER to the EQUATOR

~ UVB LIGHT HELPS US GENERATE VITAMIN D
  └ IMPORTANT REGULATOR of CALCIUM ABSORPTION

~ KERATINOCYTES CONTAIN CHOLESTEROL PRECURSORS
  → UVB LIGHT → VITAMIN D

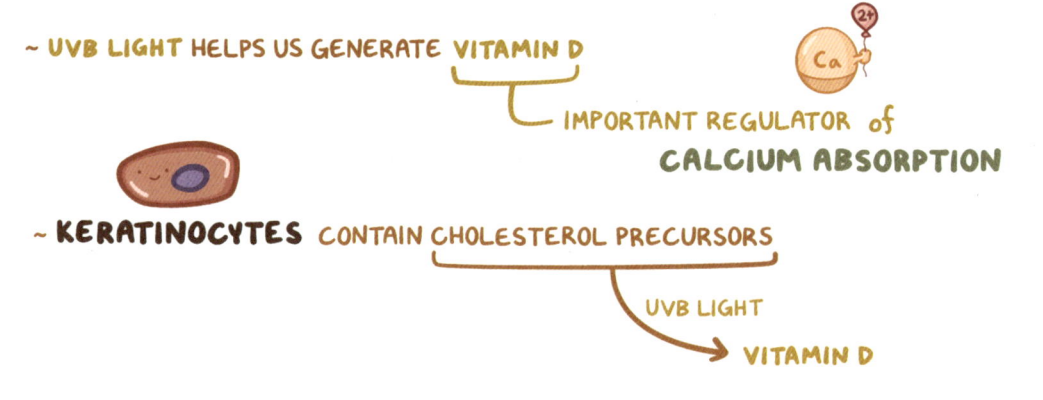

Figure 11.6

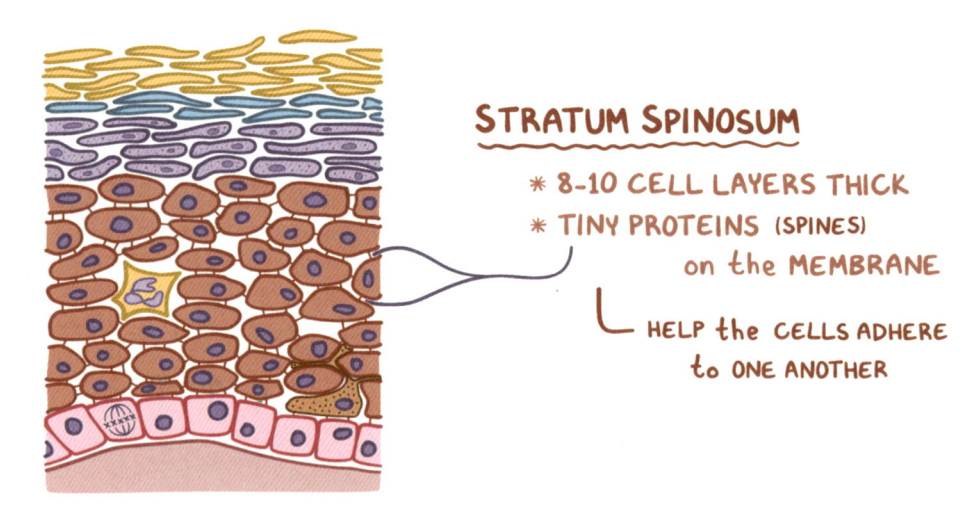

STRATUM SPINOSUM

* 8-10 CELL LAYERS THICK
* TINY PROTEINS (SPINES) on the MEMBRANE
  └ HELP the CELLS ADHERE to ONE ANOTHER

Chapter 11 The Integumentary System

The next layer is the stratum granulosum, which is three to five cell layers thick. Keratinocytes in this layer begin the process of keratinization. During this process, the keratinocytes flatten out and die. As a result, they create the epidermal skin barrier **(Figure 11.8)**. To achieve this, keratinocytes in the stratum granulosum layer produce large amounts of keratin precursor proteins and glycolipids, which remain within granules called keratohyalin granules and lamellar granules, respectively. Keratohyalin granules eventually begin to aggregate and cross-link, forming enormous bundles of keratin within the keratinocyte. Lamellar granules, on the other hand, get secreted and stick to the outer cell surface. This forms a sort of cement between the cells, making them more resistant to external forces and water loss. Over time, the intracellular organelles disintegrate and the cells flatten out and die **(Figure 11.9)**.

Keratinization leads to the development of the stratum lucidum layer, which is two to three cell layers thick. It is made up of translucent, dead keratinocytes that have secreted most of their lamellar granules. The stratum lucidum is only found in thick skin—on the palms of the hands and soles of the feet—because those areas need extra protection. The stratum lucidum is absent in thin skin, which covers the rest of the body **(Figure 11.10)**.

Finally, there's the stratum corneum, or the uppermost and thickest layer of the epidermis, which is like a wall of 20–30 cell layers. Picture this by imagining that the glycolipid is the cement and the dead keratinized cells are the bricks. The dead keratinocytes secrete natural antibiotics called defensins, which poke holes in bacteria. As new keratinocytes push up into the stratum corneum, older dead cells are sloughed off—forming skin flakes or dandruff **(Figure 11.11)**.

Figure 11.7

DENDRITIC CELLS

* STAR-SHAPED IMMUNE CELLS
* CONSTANTLY PATROLLING
  └ LOOKING for INVADING MICROBES

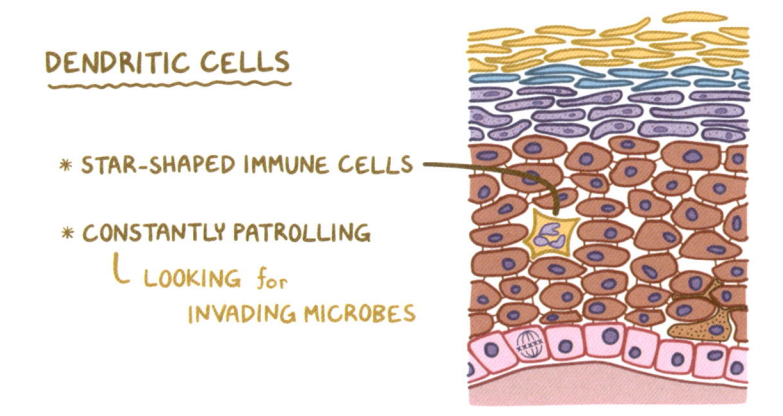

Figure 11.8

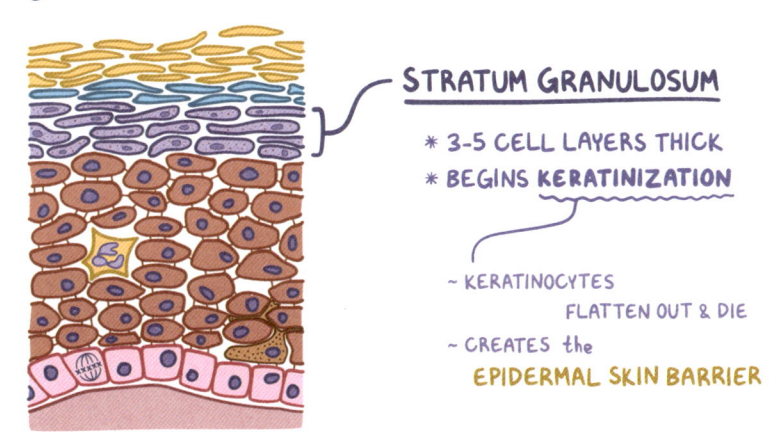

STRATUM GRANULOSUM

* 3-5 CELL LAYERS THICK
* BEGINS **KERATINIZATION**
  ~ KERATINOCYTES FLATTEN OUT & DIE
  ~ CREATES the EPIDERMAL SKIN BARRIER

Figure 11.9

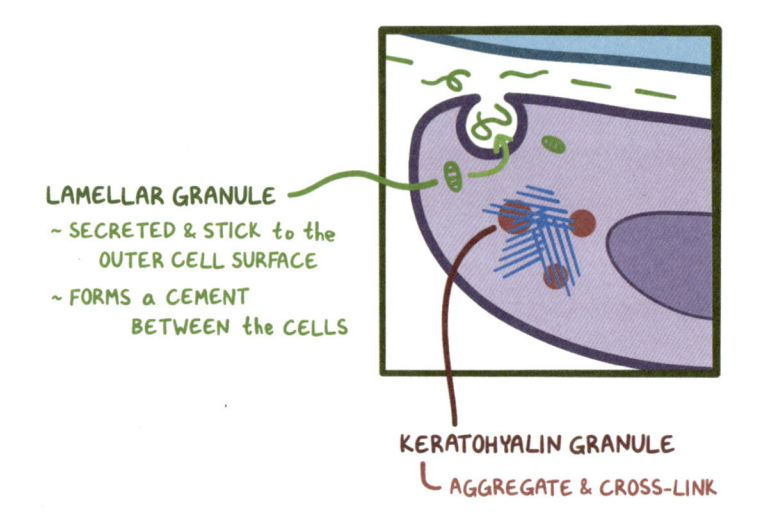

LAMELLAR GRANULE
- SECRETED & STICK to the OUTER CELL SURFACE
- FORMS a CEMENT BETWEEN the CELLS

KERATOHYALIN GRANULE
- AGGREGATE & CROSS-LINK

Figure 11.10

STRATUM LUCIDUM

* 2-3 CELL LAYERS THICK
* TRANSLUCENT, DEAD KERATINOCYTES

SECRETED MOST of their LAMELLAR GRANULES

* ONLY FOUND in THICK SKIN (e.g. PALMS & SOLES of the FEET)
* ABSENT in THIN SKIN

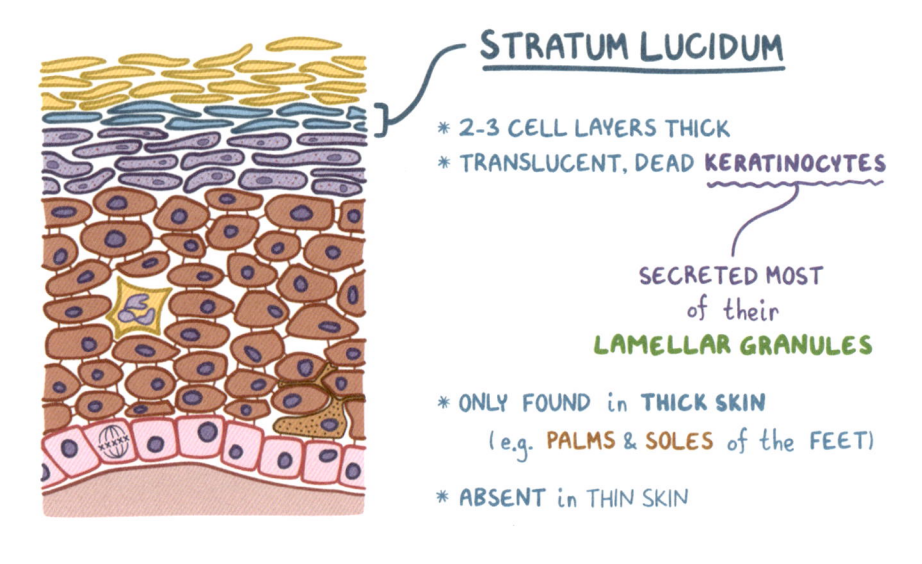

Figure 11.11

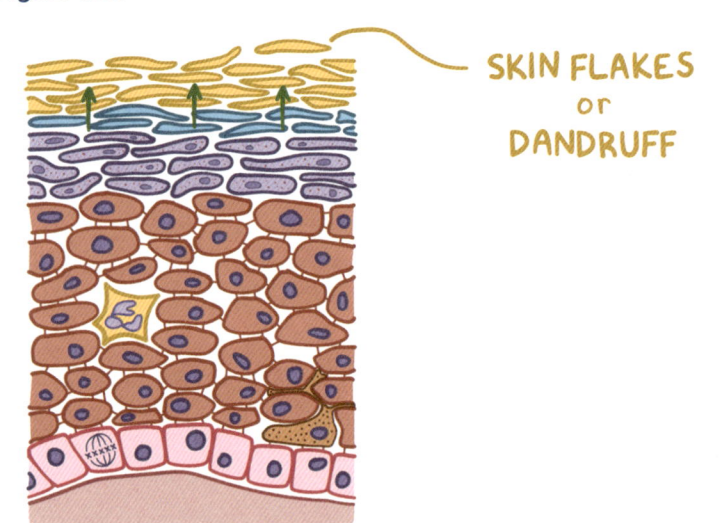

SKIN FLAKES or DANDRUFF

DERMIS

Now, the dermis lies below the stratum basale of the epidermis and it's much thicker than the epidermis **(Figure 11.12)**. The dermis is divided into two layers: a thin papillary layer below the stratum basale and a deeper reticular layer. The papillary layer contains fibroblasts, which produce a connective tissue protein called collagen. The fibroblasts are arranged in finger-like projections called papillae; each papillae contains blood vessels and nerve endings. One type of nerve ending found here is called a Meissner corpuscle. This is a disk-shaped structure that detects fine touch. It's what allows you to know exactly where a feather touches your arm. Another type of nerve found in the papillae are free nerve endings. These are dendrites that detect pain. The papillary layer also contains macrophages, which capture pathogens that make it past the epidermis. It's also the papillary layer that's responsible for our fingerprints. These are necessary for the gripping and sensing abilities of the fingers and feet. They also have the added benefit of making each of us as unique as snowflakes **(Figure 11.13)**!

Next is the reticular layer of the dermis. This layer is even thicker than the papillary layer. Like the papillary layer, the reticular layer contains fibroblasts with scattered macrophages. But the collagen in the reticular layer is packed very tightly together, making it excellent for tissue support. In addition, fibroblasts in the reticular layer secrete elastin—a stretchy protein that gives skin its flexibility. The reticular layer also contains the skin's accessory structures: oil and sweat glands, hair follicles, lymphatic vessels, and nerves, as well as all of the blood vessels that serve these tissues **(Figure 11.14)**. One type of nerve ending found in the reticular layer is the Pacinian corpuscle. This is an onion-shaped structure that detects pressure or vibration. It's what allows you to feel someone grabbing your arm **(Figure 11.15)**.

Since the reticular layer contains many blood vessels and sweat glands, it's also largely responsible for regulating temperature. When body temperature rises—as it might during a workout—the nervous system causes these blood vessels to dilate and the sweat glands to secrete sweat. Dilation of blood vessels brings a greater amount of blood closer to the skin surface, and this subsequently allows the skin surface to lose heat to outside environment. Heat is needed to evaporate the sweat that coats the skin's surface. In effect, heat is lost from the skin surface with every drop of sweat that evaporates. In contrast, when it's cold outside, blood vessels constrict and this diverts blood flow away from the skin. In this case, there's no sweat and body heat is conserved.

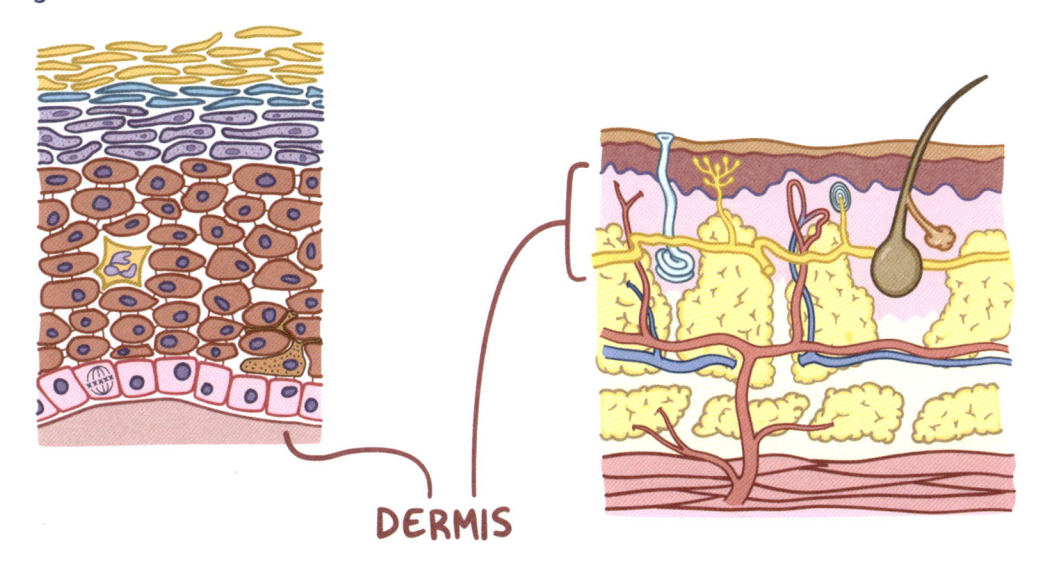

Figure 11.12

DERMIS

Figure 11.13

DERMIS

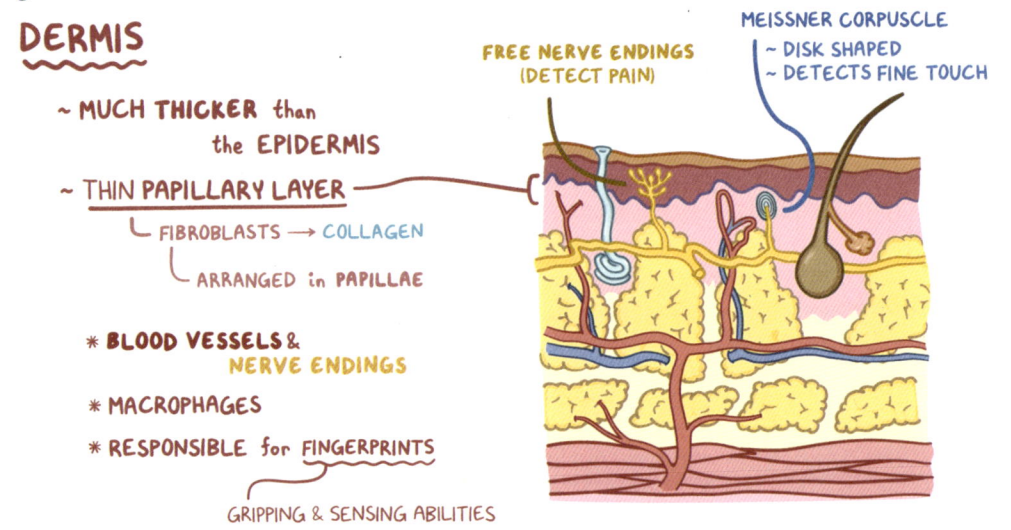

- ~ MUCH THICKER than the EPIDERMIS
- ~ THIN PAPILLARY LAYER
  - FIBROBLASTS → COLLAGEN
  - ARRANGED in PAPILLAE

* BLOOD VESSELS & NERVE ENDINGS
* MACROPHAGES
* RESPONSIBLE for FINGERPRINTS
  - GRIPPING & SENSING ABILITIES

FREE NERVE ENDINGS (DETECT PAIN)

MEISSNER CORPUSCLE
- DISK SHAPED
- DETECTS FINE TOUCH

Figure 11.14

SWEAT GLAND
OIL GLAND
HAIR FOLLICLE
NERVES

RETICULAR LAYER

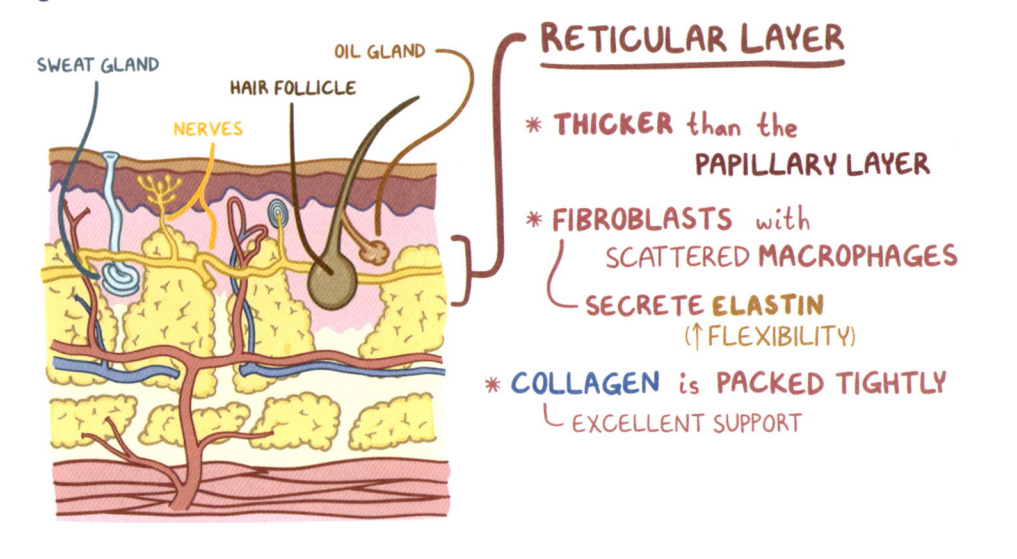

* THICKER than the PAPILLARY LAYER
* FIBROBLASTS with SCATTERED MACROPHAGES
  - SECRETE ELASTIN (↑FLEXIBILITY)
* COLLAGEN is PACKED TIGHTLY
  - EXCELLENT SUPPORT

Figure 11.15

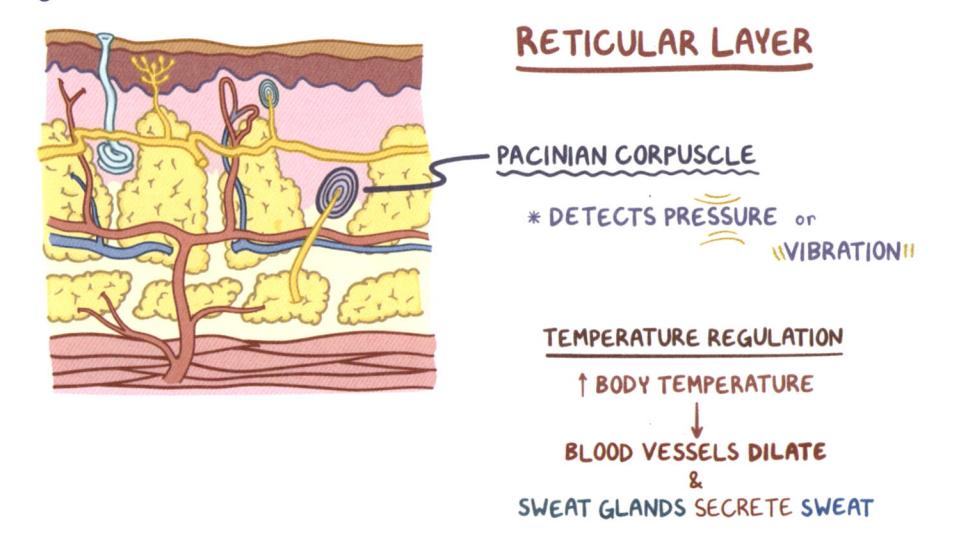

RETICULAR LAYER

PACINIAN CORPUSCLE

* DETECTS PRESSURE or VIBRATION

TEMPERATURE REGULATION

↑ BODY TEMPERATURE
↓
BLOOD VESSELS DILATE
&
SWEAT GLANDS SECRETE SWEAT

Chapter 11 The Integumentary System

Figure 11.16

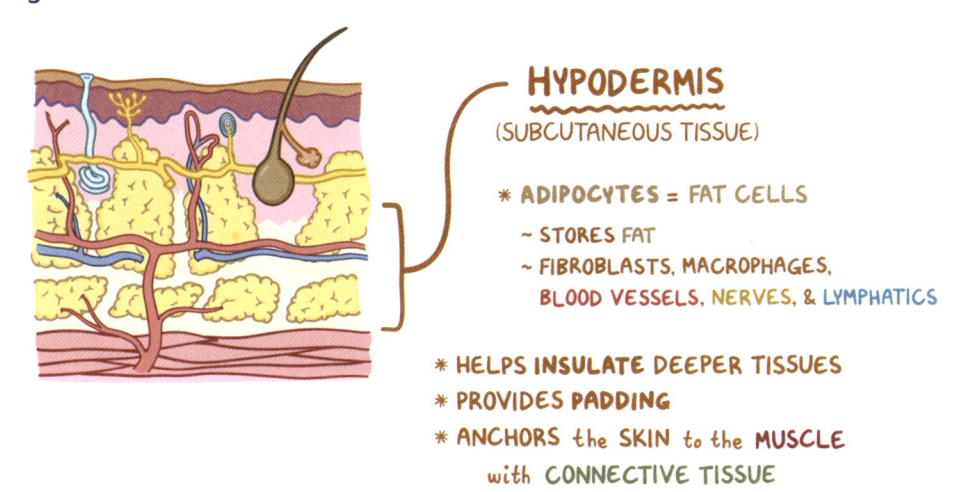

HYPODERMIS
(SUBCUTANEOUS TISSUE)

* **ADIPOCYTES** = FAT CELLS
  - STORES FAT
  - FIBROBLASTS, MACROPHAGES, BLOOD VESSELS, NERVES, & LYMPHATICS
* HELPS **INSULATE** DEEPER TISSUES
* PROVIDES **PADDING**
* **ANCHORS** the SKIN to the MUSCLE with CONNECTIVE TISSUE

HYPODERMIS

Finally, after the epidermis, and just below the dermis, there's the layer called the hypodermis, or subcutaneous tissue. This layer contains fat cells called adipocytes, which help store most of the fat in our body. It also contains fibroblasts, macrophages, blood vessels, nerves, and lymphatics. The hypodermis helps insulate deeper tissues, provides padding to the body, and anchors the skin to the muscle with connective tissue proteins like collagen **(Figure 11.16)**.

SUMMARY

All right, as a quick recap, the skin, or the integumentary system, is the largest organ of the body. The integumentary system is divided into three major components: the epidermis, dermis, and hypodermis. The epidermis is the most superficial layer and it's responsible for protection from pathogens and the environment, as well as for vitamin D production. The dermis lies below the epidermis and it controls temperature regulation, assists with sensation, and is responsible for the skin's color. Finally, the hypodermis lies below the dermis and provides a point of attachment for the skin to the deeper muscles **(Figure 11.17)**.

Figure 11.17

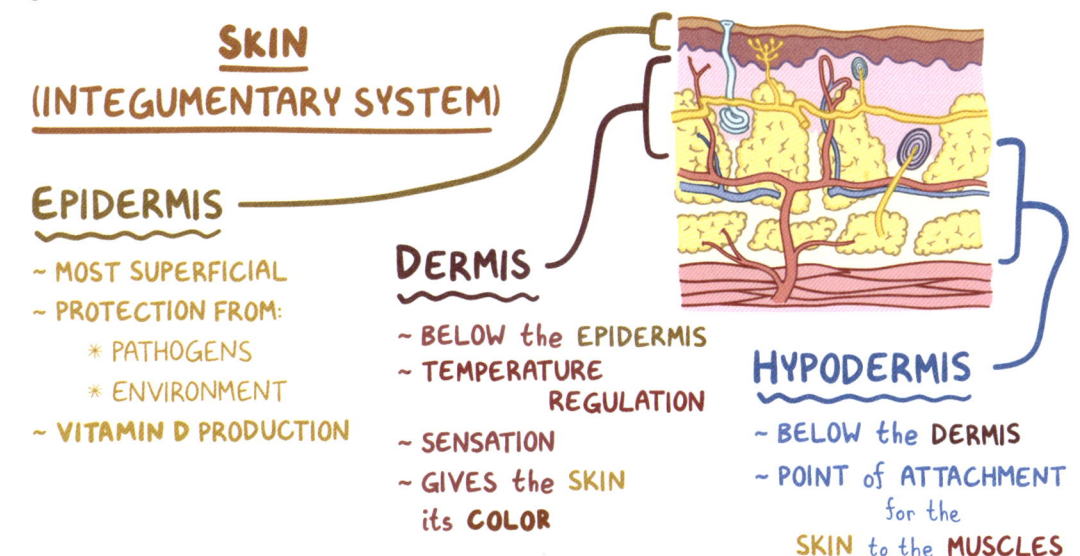

SKIN (INTEGUMENTARY SYSTEM)

EPIDERMIS
- MOST SUPERFICIAL
- PROTECTION FROM:
  * PATHOGENS
  * ENVIRONMENT
- VITAMIN D PRODUCTION

DERMIS
- BELOW the EPIDERMIS
- TEMPERATURE REGULATION
- SENSATION
- GIVES the SKIN its COLOR

HYPODERMIS
- BELOW the DERMIS
- POINT of ATTACHMENT for the SKIN to the MUSCLES

THE MALE REPRODUCTIVE SYSTEM

osms.it/male_reproductive_system

The male reproductive system includes internal and external organs and structures that help with reproduction. The external male sex organs are the penis, and below it, the scrotum. Inside the scrotum, there are the two testicles, or testes—the male gonads. Inside the body, there's a system of ducts through which sperm travel during ejaculation, as well as the male accessory sex glands, which secrete nourishing fluids for the travelling sperm **(Figure 12.1)**.

STRUCTURE OF THE TESTES

Now, the testes are two organs the size of small plums, that are located in a skin and muscle pouch called the scrotum. This pouch has a line called the scrotal raphe running down the middle, which separates it in two chambers, one for each testis. The scrotum hangs outside of the body but has several layers of muscles and fascia that keep the temperature of the testes about three degrees lower than body temperature, which is perfect for sperm production. When it's cold outside, the scrotal skin wrinkles and the scrotum elevates to bring the testes closer to the body to warm up. When it's warm outside, the scrotal skin loosens up, the scrotum lowers the testes away from the body, and heat is released through sweating **(Figure 12.2)**.

Figure 12.1

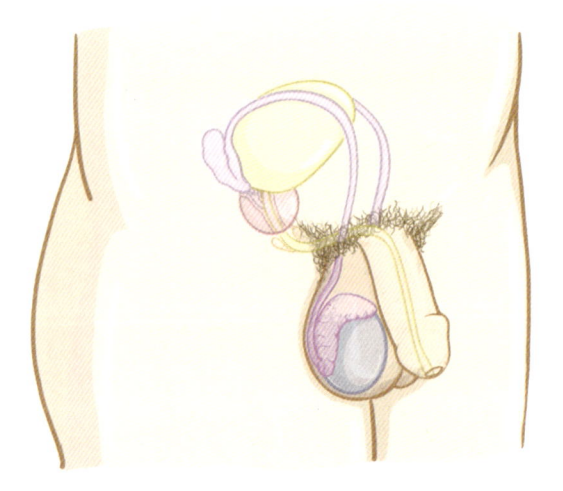

Chapter 12 The Male Reproductive System

The testes themselves are covered on the outside by the tunica albuginea—a white, fibrous layer. If we were to slice a testis open and look inside, we'd see that the tunica albuginea sends fibrous projections called septa towards the center of the testis. These septa partition each testis into about 250 lobules, and each lobule contains one to four seminiferous tubules, which are where sperm is synthesized. The seminiferous tubules come together and form a single straight tubule that exits the lobule and enters a small network of tubules called the rete testis. The rete testis is located in the center of the testis, in a region called the mediastinum testis, and consists of a small network of ducts that split up and come together again. Once the sperm make it through the rete testis, they go through the efferent ducts to the epididymis. The epididymis is a comma-shaped organ that also has a head, a body, and a tail, and curves along the posterior edge of each testis **(Figure 12.3)**.

Figure 12.2

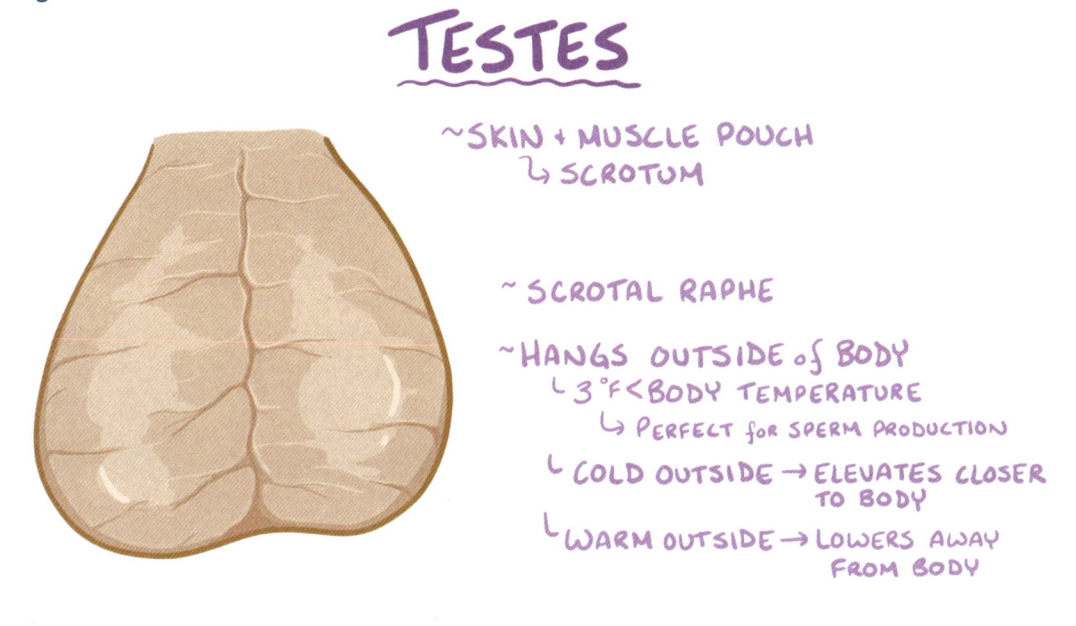

TESTES
- SKIN + MUSCLE POUCH
  - SCROTUM
- SCROTAL RAPHE
- HANGS OUTSIDE of BODY
  - 3°F < BODY TEMPERATURE
    - PERFECT for SPERM PRODUCTION
  - COLD OUTSIDE → ELEVATES CLOSER TO BODY
  - WARM OUTSIDE → LOWERS AWAY FROM BODY

Figure 12.3

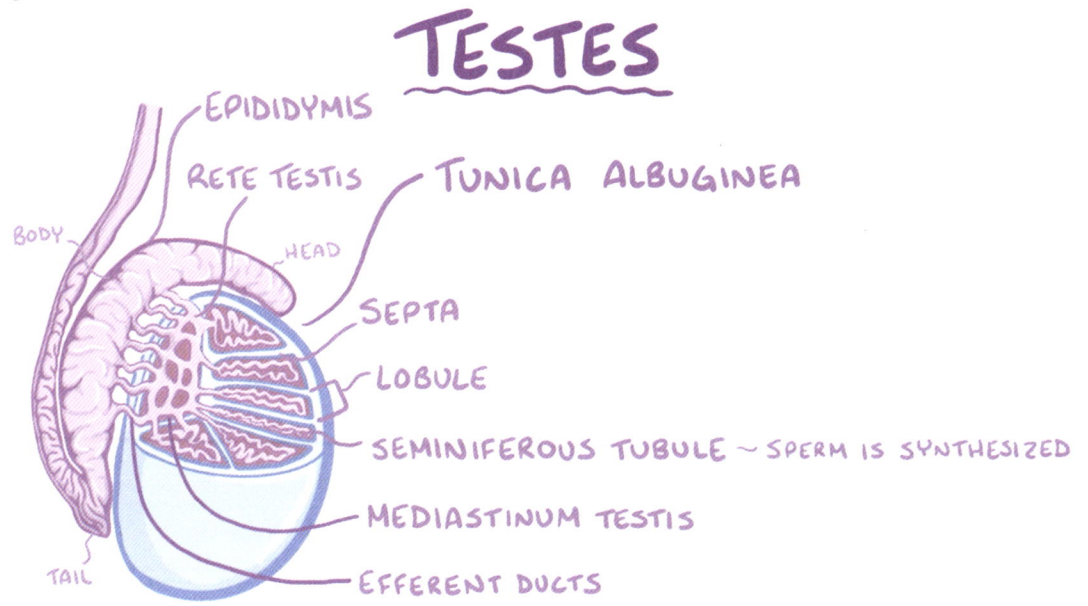

TESTES
- EPIDIDYMIS
- RETE TESTIS
- TUNICA ALBUGINEA
- BODY
- HEAD
- SEPTA
- LOBULE
- SEMINIFEROUS TUBULE ~ SPERM IS SYNTHESIZED
- MEDIASTINUM TESTIS
- TAIL
- EFFERENT DUCTS

SEMINIFEROUS TUBULES

Now let's zoom in on a single seminiferous tubule, which is the sperm factory. A seminiferous tubule has a thick wall of epithelial cells that surround a fluid-filled lumen—a bit like a garden hose. Outside the tubule, there's connective tissue with capillaries, as well as Leydig cells, which produce testosterone. The wall of the tubule is made up of three kinds of cells. At the periphery, there's the spermatogonia, which are the primordial sperm cells that begin dividing over and over in puberty, and which give rise to male gametes. Next, there are the spermatocytes, which migrate towards the lumen as they differentiate into sperm. Finally, there are Sertoli cells, which are large cells that extend from the margin all the way to the lumen of the tubule. Sertoli cells provide nutrients to developing sperm cells and contribute to the blood-testis barrier by only allowing certain molecules, like testosterone, into the seminiferous tubule **(Figure 12.4)**.

SPERMATOGENESIS

Sperm production, or spermatogenesis, begins in puberty under the command of the hypothalamus. The hypothalamus is a part of the brain that secretes gonadotropin-releasing hormone, or GnRH. That gonadotropin-releasing hormone travels to the nearby pituitary, which secretes two hormones of its own: luteinizing hormone, or LH, and follicle-stimulating hormone, or FSH, both of which travel to the gonads **(Figure 12.5)**.

Before puberty, gonadotropin-releasing hormone and, in turn, follicle stimulating hormone and luteinizing hormone, are secreted in low, constant amounts. At puberty, secretion of these hormones intensifies and becomes pulsatile— sometimes more of the hormone is released, and sometimes less of the hormone is released. Luteinizing hormone binds to Leydig cells and stimulates the production of testosterone, whereas follicle stimulating hormone binds to Sertoli cells, making them produce androgen-binding protein, or ABP, which allows more testosterone to cross the blood-testis barrier and enter the seminiferous tubule. So, it's the increased concentrations of follicle stimulating hormone, luteinizing hormone, and testosterone that really get spermatogenesis going.

Figure 12.4

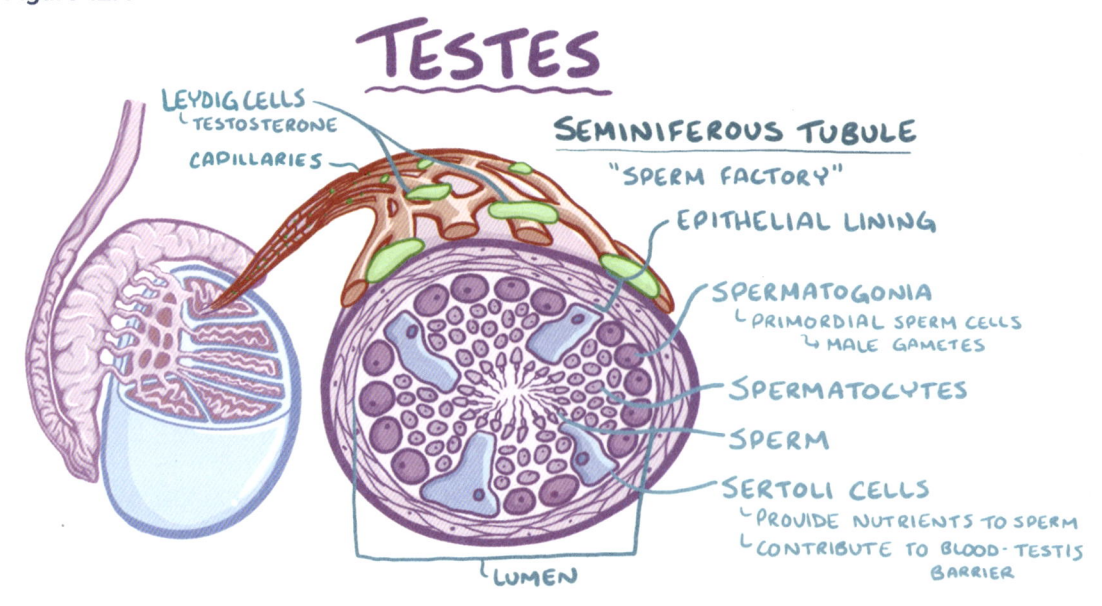

Chapter 12 The Male Reproductive System

Spermatogenesis starts with the spermatogonia, which are diploid cells, so they have 46 chromosomes, two of which are sex chromosomes—an X and a Y. For diploid spermatogonia to form haploid gametes, which only have 23 chromosomes, they first undergo mitosis followed by meiosis I and meiosis II. Through mitosis, a spermatogonium gives rise to two 46-chromosome daughter cells, one of which eventually becomes a primary spermatocyte, and the other of which becomes a spermatogonium. In this way the population of spermatogonia stays constant. The primary spermatocyte then undergoes meiosis while slowly moving towards the lumen of the seminiferous tubule, passing between two Sertoli cells that nourish it in the process. Meiosis I produces a pair of secondary spermatocytes, which are haploid cells that contain 23 chromosomes each, one of which is either an X or a Y chromosome. These secondary spermatocytes enter meiosis II and divide into two haploid spermatids, which also have 23 chromosomes, but only one chromatid—so the right number of chromosomes and the proper amount of DNA **(Figure 12.6)**.

Spermatids enter the lumen of the seminiferous tubule and undergo spermiogenesis, which is when they acquire a tail and turn into sperm. It takes roughly two months for spermatogonia to develop into sperm, and this process is regulated by various hormones. Sertoli cells secrete inhibin, which sends a negative feedback signal to the pituitary gland to reduce follicle-stimulating hormone production, and Leydig cells produce increasing levels of testosterone, which sends a negative feedback signal to the pituitary to reduce luteinizing hormone production. All in all, this keeps the production of sperm at around 100 million per day—easier to remember as a whole lot of swimmers **(Figure 12.7)**.

Sperm are made up of a few distinct parts. At the head is the acrosome, which contains enzymes that will help penetrate the oocyte, the female gamete. Then there's a middle piece, like a neck, which is loaded with mitochondria that provide the sperm with energy to move. Finally, there's the tail, which helps the sperm swim. But when they're inside the seminiferous tubules, the sperm haven't learnt how to wiggle their tails just yet. To learn this, they must exit the seminiferous tubules and go through the rest of the ducts inside the testis. The seminiferous tubules contract with a wave-like motion called peristalsis, and this motion moves the sperm through the straight tubules and into the rete testis, and eventually into the epididymis. Sperm enters the epididymis through its head region, and are stored for a few months in the body region where they mature. Here is where they begin to wag their tails and wait patiently for ejaculation **(Figure 12.8)**.

Figure 12.5

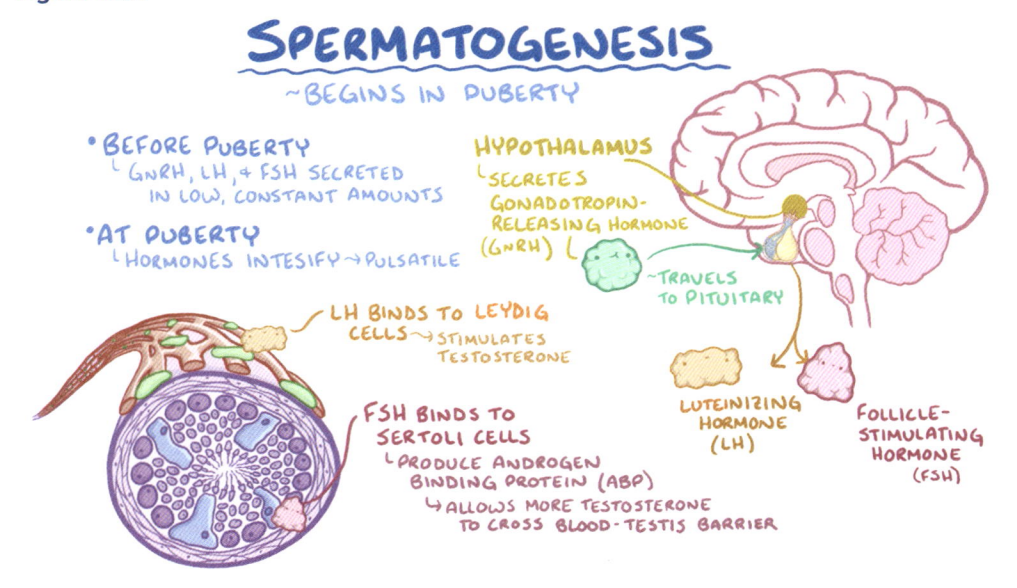

Figure 12.6

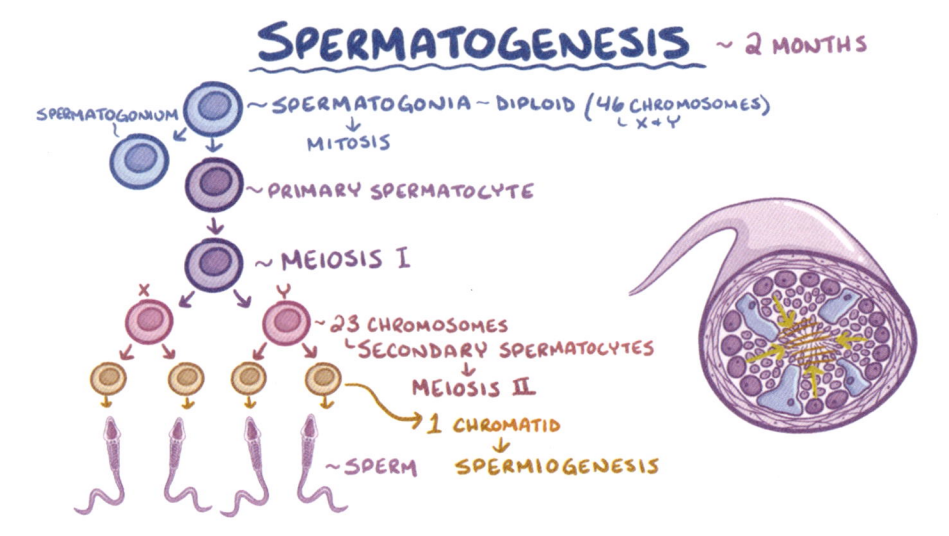

SPERMATOGENESIS ~ 2 MONTHS

- SPERMATOGONIUM
- SPERMATOGONIA ~ DIPLOID (46 CHROMOSOMES)
  - X + Y
- MITOSIS
- PRIMARY SPERMATOCYTE
- MEIOSIS I
- 23 CHROMOSOMES
  - SECONDARY SPERMATOCYTES
- MEIOSIS II
  - 1 CHROMATID
  - SPERMIOGENESIS
- SPERM

Figure 12.7

SPERMATOGENESIS

- SERTOLI CELLS
  - INHIBIN
  - NEGATIVE FEEDBACK
  - ↓↓ FSH PRODUCTION
- LEYDIG CELLS
  - ↑↑ TESTOSTERONE
  - NEGATIVE FEEDBACK
  - ↓↓ LH PRODUCTION

PRODUCTION of SPERM → 100 MILLION / DAY

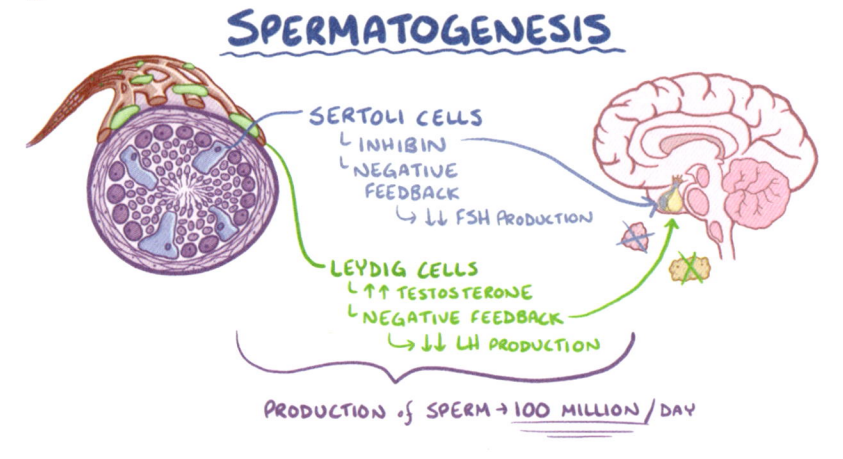

Figure 12.8

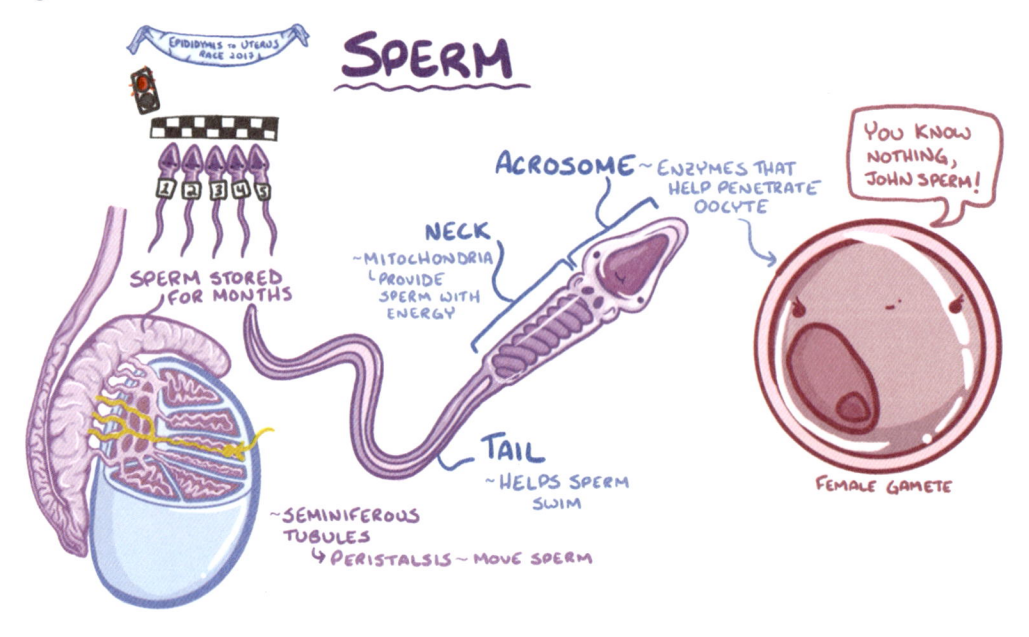

SPERM

EPIDIDYMIS to UTERUS RACE 2013

- SPERM STORED FOR MONTHS
- ACROSOME ~ ENZYMES THAT HELP PENETRATE OOCYTE
- NECK
  - MITOCHONDRIA
  - PROVIDE SPERM WITH ENERGY
- TAIL
  - HELPS SPERM SWIM
- SEMINIFEROUS TUBULES
  - PERISTALSIS ~ MOVE SPERM

"YOU KNOW NOTHING, JOHN SPERM!"

FEMALE GAMETE

Chapter 12 The Male Reproductive System

ERECTION AND EJACULATION

During ejaculation, the sperm that have matured exit through the tail of the epididymis and enter the vas deferens. The left and right vas deferens are two long tubes that are part of the spermatic cord on both sides, entering the pelvic cavity through the superficial inguinal ring. The left and right vas deferens go behind the bladder and descend along the posterior bladder wall. Here, they dilate in a region called the ampulla, before narrowing again to continue as the ejaculatory ducts, which empty out into the first portion of the urethra.

The seminal vesicles, which are a pair of male accessory sex glands, lie adjacent to the left and right ampulla of the vas deferens, and they make seminal fluid. This fluid is loaded with fructose, an energy source for the sperm. The seminal vesicles also empty out into the urethra at the ejaculatory ducts. Below the opening of the ejaculatory ducts, there's the second male accessory sex gland, the prostate, a walnut-sized gland that wraps around the urethra and makes prostatic fluid. Beneath the prostate, on either side of the urethra, there's a third pair of male accessory sex glands, called the bulbourethral glands. The bulbourethral glands make a thick, clear mucus that acts as a lubricant.

Together, the secretions of these glands nourish the sperm and protect them from the acidic vaginal environment, giving them a better chance at reaching and fertilizing an oocyte. All of these fluids and the sperm mix to form semen, which is ultimately ejaculated through the urethra **(Figure 12.9)**.

Now, the urethra is also the way urine exits the body, but during ejaculation, the bladder sphincter right above the prostate contracts, and that prevents urine from mixing with semen. Below the openings of the bulbourethral glands, the urethra is contained within the penis—so it's called the penile urethra. The penis ends with an enlarged tip, the glans penis, that has an opening called the external urethral orifice at its very tip, through which semen and urine are released outside the body **(Figure 12.10)**.

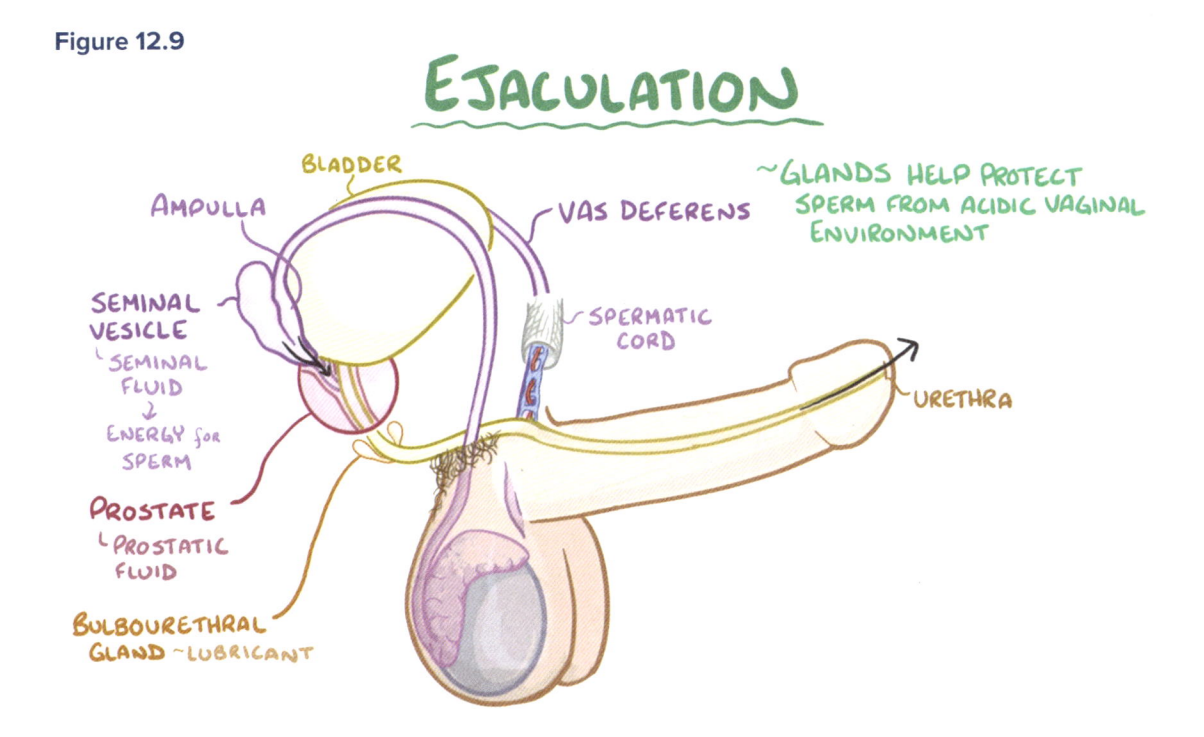

Figure 12.9

Around the glans penis, a cuff of loose skin makes up the foreskin, which is sometimes removed during a medical procedure called circumcision. On the inside, the penis is made up of three long cylindrical bodies of erectile tissue: the corpus spongiosum, which actually contains the urethra, and the two corpora cavernosa. The corpus spongiosum also has an internal part, called the bulb, through which the urethra enters the penis, and the corpora cavernosa attach all the way to the pelvic bones. Together, the internal parts of these erectile bodies make up the root of the penis, which is embedded in the perineum.

The erectile tissues are made up of a maze of vascular spaces that give a spongy appearance. These vascular spaces are lined with endothelial cells and surrounded by smooth muscle cells, and the entire erectile tissue is wrapped in a fibrous tissue layer called the tunica albuginea. During sexual arousal, the smooth muscle cells relax, and more blood flows inside the vascular spaces. The corpora cavernosa distend, and they press against the inextensible tunica albuginea, compressing the veins in the penis, so blood is unable to drain away. The corpus spongiosum has a more flexible tunica albuginea, and so becomes less turgid, avoiding compression of the penile urethra. With blood coming in but no blood leaving, there's local engorgement, which is called an erection. Erection can also happen during sleep, even without sexual arousal—a phenomenon called nocturnal penile tumescence **(Figure 12.11)**.

Figure 12.10

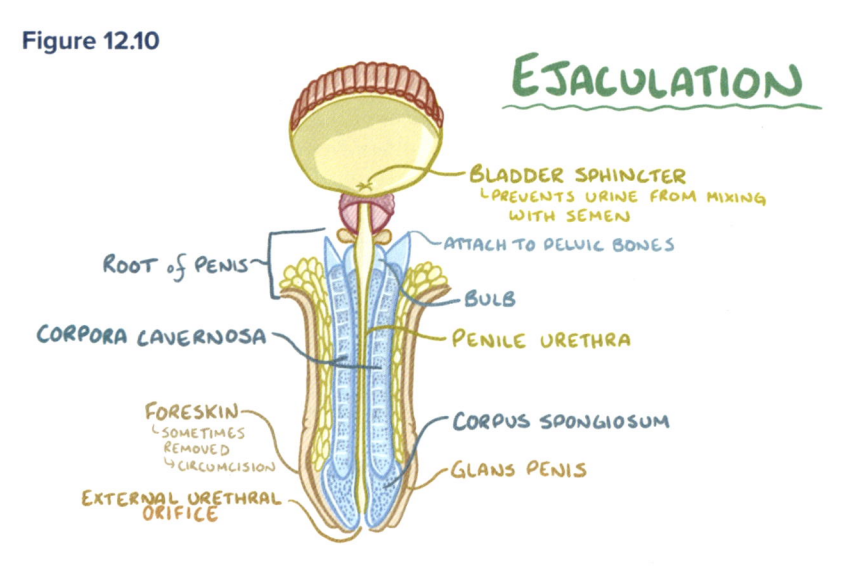

Figure 12.11

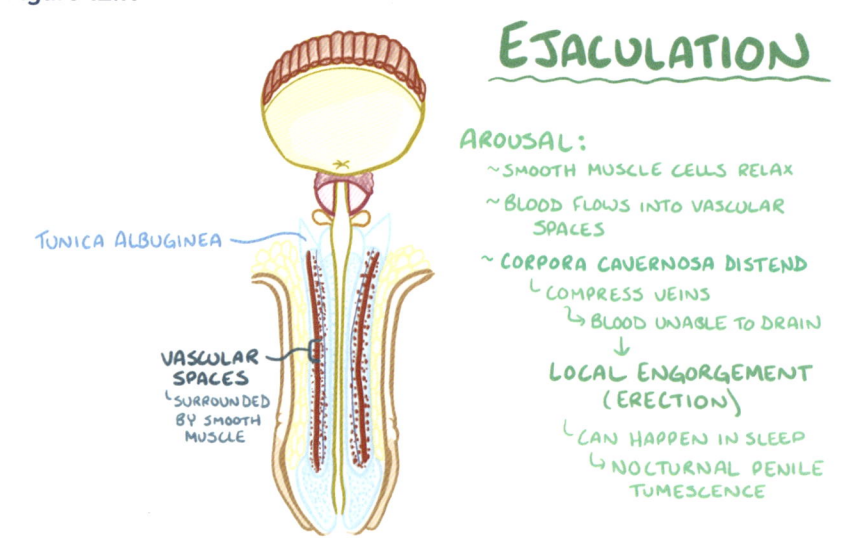

Chapter 12 The Male Reproductive System

SUMMARY

All right, as a quick recap... The male reproductive system consists of internal and external sex organs that help with the production, transport, and release of sperm—the male gametes. Sperm production begins at puberty and continues throughout the entire lifetime under the control of hypothalamic and pituitary hormones. Sperm goes to the epididymis for maturation and is released from the epididymis during ejaculation—traveling through a long and winding road of ducts along the way: the vas deferens, the ejaculatory ducts, and finally, the urethra, which opens at the tip of the penis **(Figure 12.12)**.

Figure 12.12

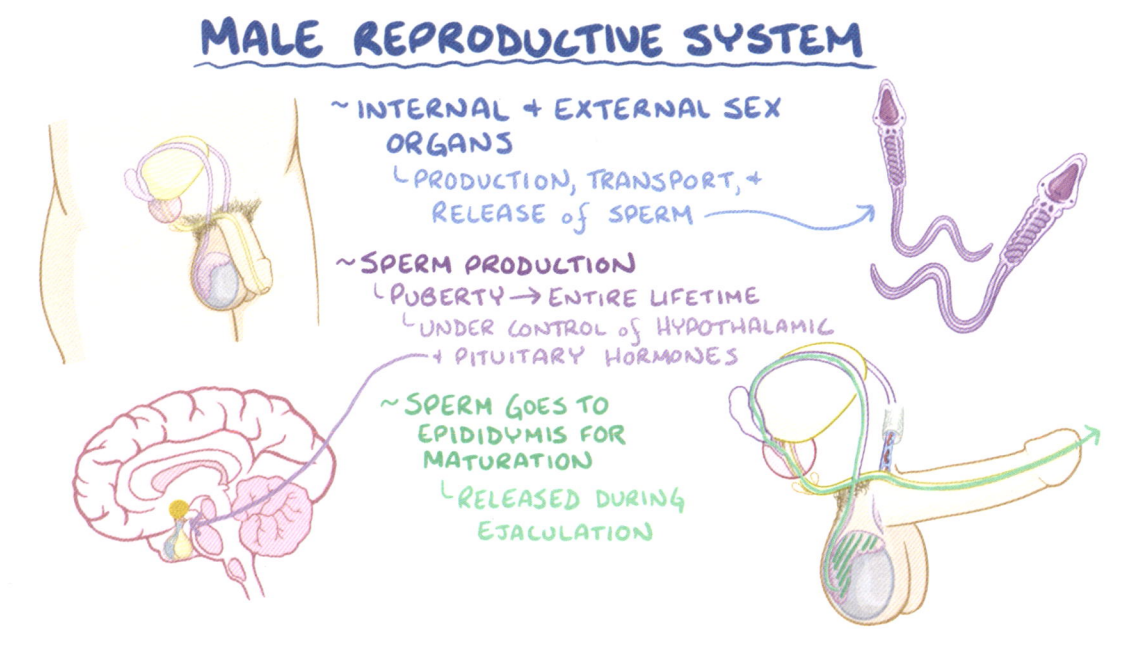

THE FEMALE REPRODUCTIVE SYSTEM

osms.it/female_reproductive_system

The female reproductive system includes all of the internal and external organs that help with reproduction. The internal sex organs are the ovaries, which are the female gonads, the fallopian tubes, which are two muscular tubes that connect the ovaries to the uterus, and the uterus, which is the strong muscular sack that a fetus can develop in. The neck of the uterus is called the cervix, and it protrudes into the vagina. At the opening of the vagina are the external sex organs, and these are usually just called the genitals and they're in the vulva region. They include the labia, the clitoris, and the mons pubis **(Figure 13.1)**.

THE OVARIES & OVARIAN FOLLICLES

The ovaries are a pair of white-ish organs about the size of walnuts. They're held in place, slightly above and on either side of the uterus and fallopian tubes by ligaments. Specifically, there's the broad ligament, the ovarian ligament, and the suspensory ligament. And the suspensory ligament is particularly important because the ovarian artery, ovarian vein, and ovarian nerve plexus pass through it to reach the ovary. If you slice the ovary open and look at it, there's an outer layer called the cortex, which has ovarian follicles scattered throughout it, and an inner layer called the medulla, which contains most of the blood vessels and nerves **(Figure 13.2)**.

At birth, the ovarian cortex has around two million follicles—that's roughly the population of Paris—and they're called primordial follicles. Each primordial follicle has a single immature sex cell called the primary oocyte at the core, and a layer of follicular cells surrounds this. The primary oocyte has 46 chromosomes, but eventually it has to turn into a gamete with only 23 chromosomes. To do this, the primary oocytes have to complete meiosis I, and in a person's lifetime only about 400 successfully do that **(Figure 13.3)**. This process of oocyte development follows that of follicular development, which can be broken into three stages.

Figure 13.1

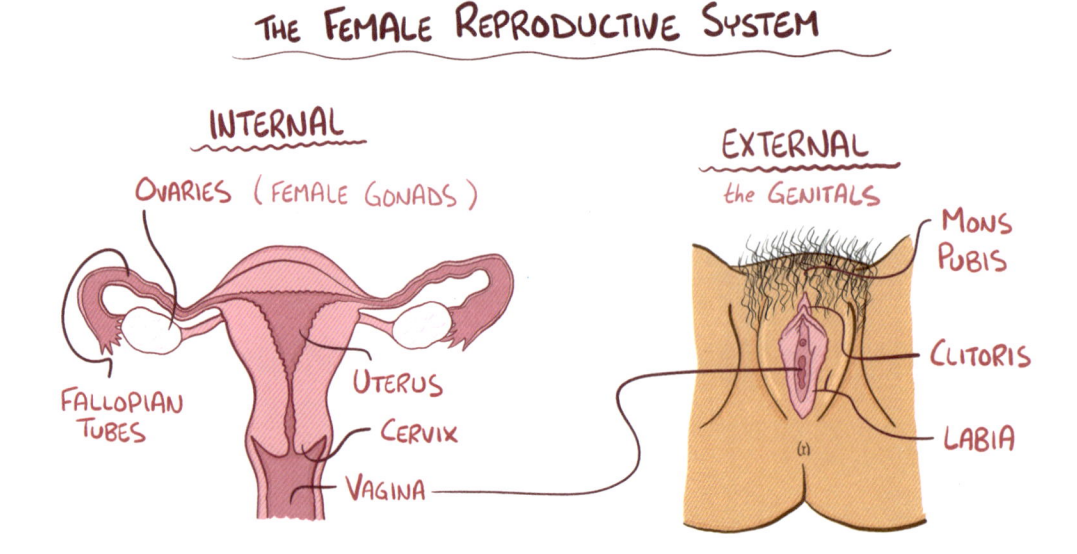

THE FEMALE REPRODUCTIVE SYSTEM

INTERNAL — OVARIES (FEMALE GONADS), FALLOPIAN TUBES, UTERUS, CERVIX, VAGINA

EXTERNAL — the GENITALS — MONS PUBIS, CLITORIS, LABIA

Chapter 13 The Female Reproductive System

The first stage lasts from infancy to puberty, and during this stage the primary oocyte remains stuck in the prophase step of meiosis I. So, in other words, the cell is living, but not dividing. Meanwhile, the primordial follicle turns into a primary follicle, meaning that the follicular cells surrounding the primary oocyte develop into granulosa cells **(Figure 13.4)**. The second stage of follicular development begins for a few lucky primary follicles with the first menstrual cycle in puberty, and a few more primary follicles go into the second stage with each subsequent menstrual cycle. In the second stage, the primary follicles develop into secondary and eventually tertiary, or graafian, follicles. In a secondary follicle, the primary oocyte is still in the prophase step of meiosis I, but now the follicle has additional layers of granulosa cells, as well as theca cells. Theca cells make androstenedione, a sex hormone precursor, and granulosa cells use the enzyme aromatase to convert it into estradiol, a member of the estrogen family **(Figure 13.5)**. In a graafian follicle, a central cavity called the antrum forms within the follicle, and the granulosa cells secrete a nourishing fluid for the primary oocyte directly into that antrum. The second stage takes roughly 70 to 85 days and results in a few fast-growing graafian follicles **(Figure 13.6)**. The third stage of follicular development starts when the graafian follicles are ready and occurs during the follicular phase of the menstrual cycle **(Figure 13.7)**.

Figure 13.2

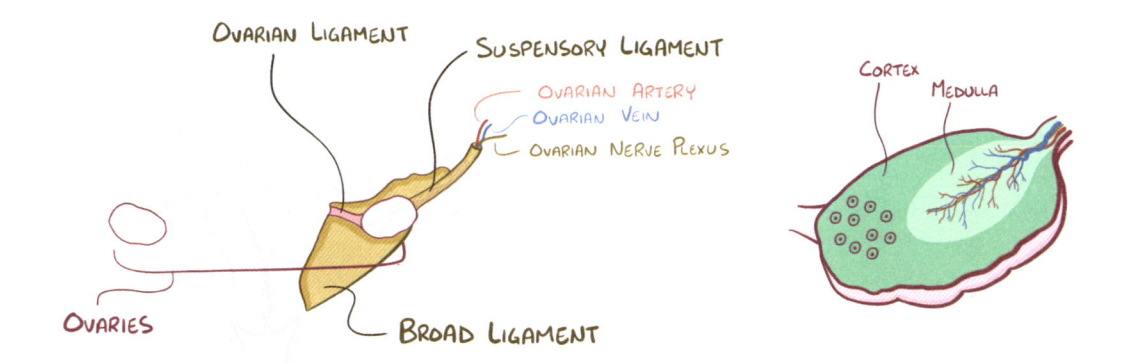

Figure 13.3

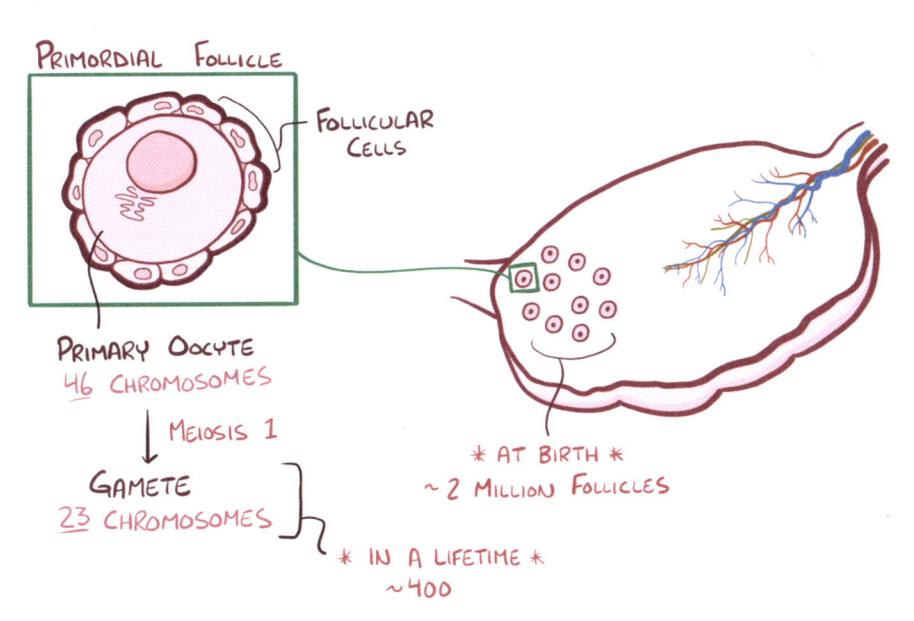

Figure 13.4

FIRST STAGE
INFANCY to PUBERTY

PRIMARY OOCYTE
STAYS in **PROPHASE** of MEIOSIS I

PRIMORDIAL FOLLICLE
(FOLLICULAR CELLS)
↓
PRIMARY FOLLICLE
(GRANULOSA CELLS)

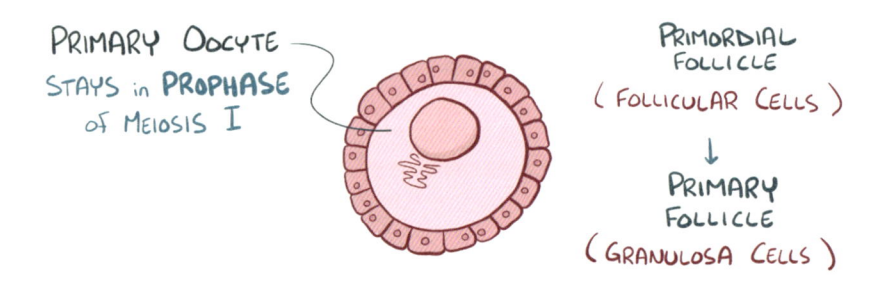

Figure 13.5

SECOND STAGE
a **FEW** PRIMARY FOLLICLES ENTER EACH MENSTRUAL CYCLE

PRIMARY FOLLICLES
↓
SECONDARY FOLLICLES
↓
TERTIARY FOLLICLES
(GRAAFIAN FOLLICLES)

SECONDARY FOLLICLE
- PRIMARY OOCYTE IS STILL IN PROPHASE
- MORE GRANULOSA CELLS
- THECA CELLS
  └ ANDROSTENEDIONE
       ↓ IN GRANULOSA CELLS
         AROMATASE
    ESTRADIOL

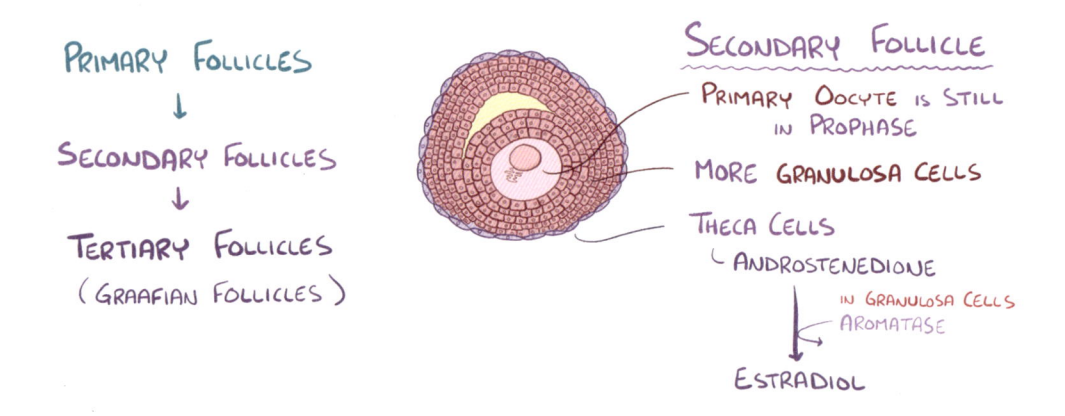

Figure 13.6

SECOND STAGE ~70-85 DAYS
a **FEW** PRIMARY FOLLICLES ENTER EACH MENSTRUAL CYCLE

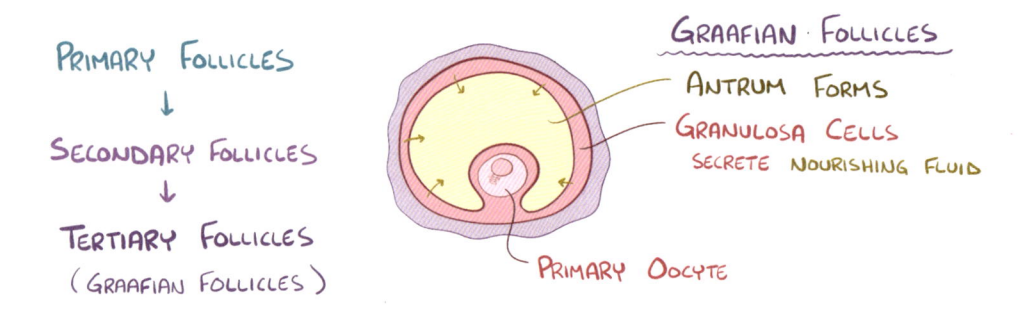

PRIMARY FOLLICLES
↓
SECONDARY FOLLICLES
↓
TERTIARY FOLLICLES
(GRAAFIAN FOLLICLES)

GRAAFIAN FOLLICLES
- ANTRUM FORMS
- GRANULOSA CELLS SECRETE NOURISHING FLUID
- PRIMARY OOCYTE

Figure 13.7

THIRD STAGE
BEGINS WHEN GRAAFIAN FOLLICLES ARE READY
OCCURS DURING FOLLICULAR PHASE

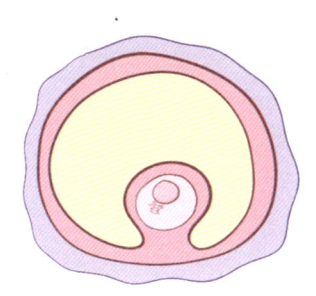

THE MENSTRUAL CYCLE & OVULATION

So let's briefly switch gears and go over the highlights of the menstrual cycle to put that follicular phase into context. The menstrual cycle starts on the first day of menstrual bleeding and lasts 28 days on average. Assuming a 28-day cycle, the follicular phase makes up the first two weeks of the menstrual cycle, and the luteal phase, the last two weeks. These two phases are separated by ovulation, which is when the follicle ruptures and releases an oocyte that is ready to be fertilized. This usually occurs on day 14 of a 28 day cycle **(Figure 13.8)**.

The menstrual cycle is ultimately controlled by the hypothalamus, which is at the base of the brain. Before puberty, the hypothalamus constantly secretes small amounts of a hormone called gonadotropin-releasing hormone, or GnRH. That gonadotropin-releasing hormone travels to the nearby pituitary, which secretes two hormones of its own: follicle-stimulating hormone, or FSH, and luteinizing hormone, or LH.

Once puberty hits, the hypothalamus starts to secrete gonadotropin-releasing hormone in pulses, sometimes more and sometimes less, and pituitary follicle-stimulating hormone and luteinizing hormone make the ovarian follicles develop. The amount of gonadotropin-releasing hormone can be mapped out like a wave over time, and the frequency and amplitude of the waves of gonadotropin-releasing hormone determine how much follicle-stimulating hormone and luteinizing hormone get produced by the pituitary.

Luteinizing hormone binds to luteinizing hormone receptors on theca cells and they make progesterone and androstenedione. Follicle-stimulating hormone binds to follicle-stimulating hormone receptors on granulosa cells and they make aromatase and, as a consequence, estrogen. Serum levels of estrogen and progesterone act as feedback for the command center in the brain, which adjusts its hormone production according to the phases of the menstrual cycle **(Figure 13.9)**.

During the follicular phase of each menstrual cycle, the few fast-growing graafian follicles enter the third stage of development. Pituitary follicle-stimulating hormone makes the follicles grow and the granulosa cells produce more estrogen. In addition to estrogen, the granulosa cells also secrete a hormone called activin, which stimulates follicle-stimulating hormone production, as well as binding to follicle-stimulating hormone receptors, and the activity of granulosa cell aromatase as well **(Figure 13.10)**.

Figure 13.8

THE MENSTRUAL CYCLE

* STARTS: FIRST DAY OF BLEEDING
* LASTS: AVERAGE OF 28 DAYS

FOLLICULAR PHASE
* FIRST TWO WEEKS *

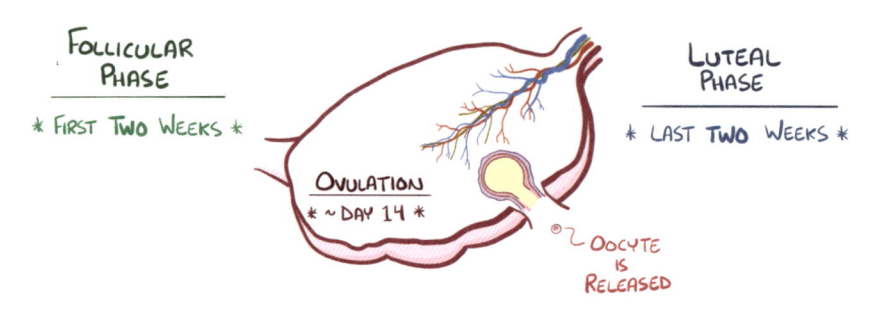

OVULATION
* ~ DAY 14 *

Oocyte is Released

LUTEAL PHASE
* LAST TWO WEEKS *

Figure 13.9

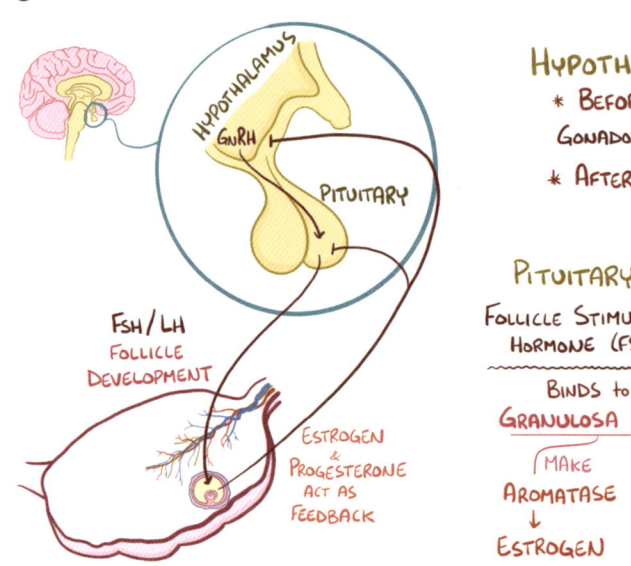

HYPOTHALAMUS
* BEFORE PUBERTY: CONSTANTLY SECRETES GONADOTROPIN RELEASING HORMONE (GnRH)
* AFTER PUBERTY: GnRH IS RELEASED IN PULSES

FSH/LH → FOLLICLE DEVELOPMENT

ESTROGEN & PROGESTERONE ACT AS FEEDBACK

PITUITARY

FOLLICLE STIMULATING HORMONE (FSH)
BINDS to GRANULOSA CELLS
MAKE AROMATASE ↓ ESTROGEN

LUTEINIZING HORMONE (LH)
BINDS to THECA CELLS
MAKE PROGESTERONE & ANDROSTENEDIONE

Figure 13.10

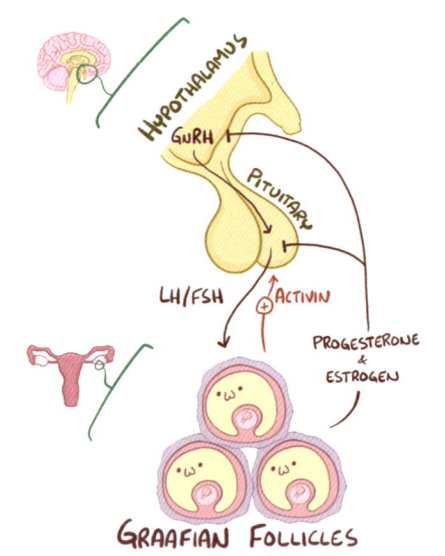

FOLLICULAR PHASE

* A FEW GRAAFIAN FOLLICLES ENTER the THIRD STAGE of DEVELOPMENT

* FSH MAKES:
  1. FOLLICLES GROW
  2. GRANULOSA CELLS
     - PRODUCE MORE ESTROGEN
     - SECRETE ACTIVIN
       ○ STIMULATES FSH PRODUCTION
       ○ BINDS FSH RECEPTORS IN GRANULOSA CELLS

MORE AROMATASE → MORE ESTROGEN

LH/FSH, ACTIVIN, PROGESTERONE & ESTROGEN

GRAAFIAN FOLLICLES

Chapter 13 The Female Reproductive System

Early in the follicular phase, a small rise in follicle-stimulating hormone, leads to a large increase in estrogen. However, estrogen acts a negative feedback signal—that is, it tells the pituitary to secrete less follicle-stimulating hormone and luteinizing hormone. Less follicle-stimulating hormone means that there is only enough left to stimulate one follicle. The follicle that has the most follicle-stimulating hormone receptors hoards most of this hormone, and becomes the dominant follicle **(Figure 13.11)**. It usually takes about a week for a dominant follicle to get selected, and after that happens, the rest of the follicles regress and die off. The dominant follicle keeps secreting estrogen for the rest of the follicular phase. The steady increase in estrogen makes the pituitary more responsive to the pulsatile action of hypothalamic gonadotropin-releasing hormone. When blood estrogen levels reach 200 picograms/milliliter, dominant follicle estrogen becomes a positive feedback signal—that is, it makes the pituitary secrete a whole lot of follicle-stimulating hormone and luteinizing hormone in response to gonadotropin-releasing hormone. This triggers the primary oocyte within the dominant follicle to finally complete meiosis I and turn into a secondary oocyte, which has 23 chromosomes **(Figure 13.12)**. The dominant follicle completes its third stage of development in a blaze of glory called ovulation. That's when the nearly two centimeter sized follicle ruptures and releases the tiny secondary oocyte into the fallopian tube. The secondary oocyte stops in metaphase of meiosis II, and waits for fertilization as the menstrual cycle transitions into the luteal phase **(Figure 13.13)**.

The luteal phase makes up the second half of the menstrual cycle, week 3 and week 4 of the 4-week cycle. Right after ovulation, while the luteinizing hormone levels are still high, the remains of the follicle turn into the corpus luteum, which is made up of luteinized granulosa and theca cells. Luteinized granulosa cells secrete inhibin, which inhibits the pituitary gland from making follicle-stimulating hormone. Without follicle-stimulating hormone, estrogen levels fall, and the amount of luteinizing hormone goes back to the level before ovulation. Luteinized theca cells respond to the low luteinizing hormone concentrations after ovulation by producing more progesterone. So, overall, this means that progesterone surpasses estrogen as the dominant hormone during the luteal phase of the menstrual cycle **(Figure 13.14)**. If fertilization occurs—meaning if a sperm meets the secondary oocyte—then the corpus luteum continues making progesterone until the placenta forms. If fertilization doesn't happen, then the corpus luteum stops making hormones after approximately 10 days, becomes fibrotic, and is called the corpus albicans **(Figure 13.15)**.

Figure 13.11

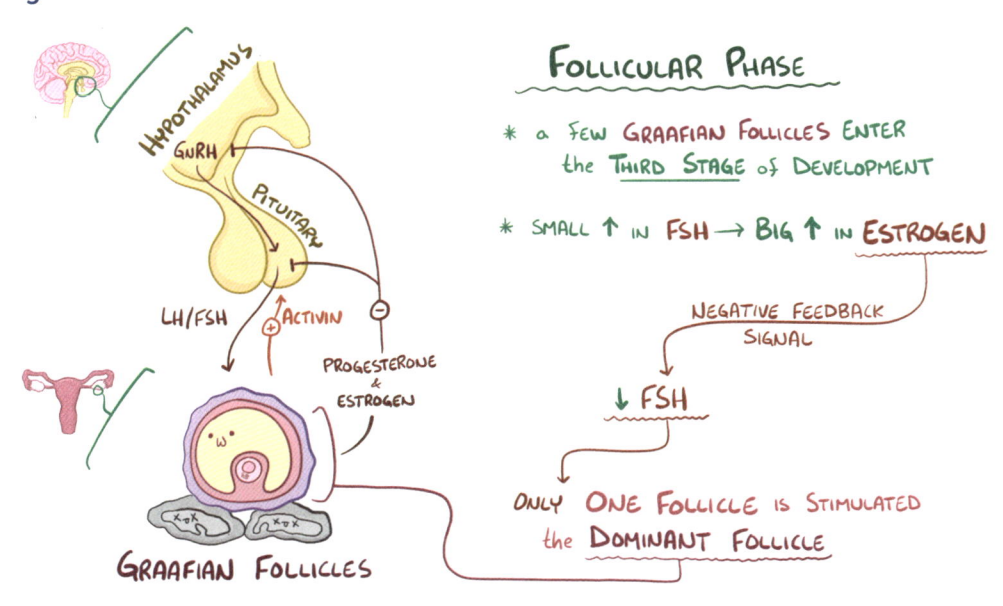

Figure 13.12

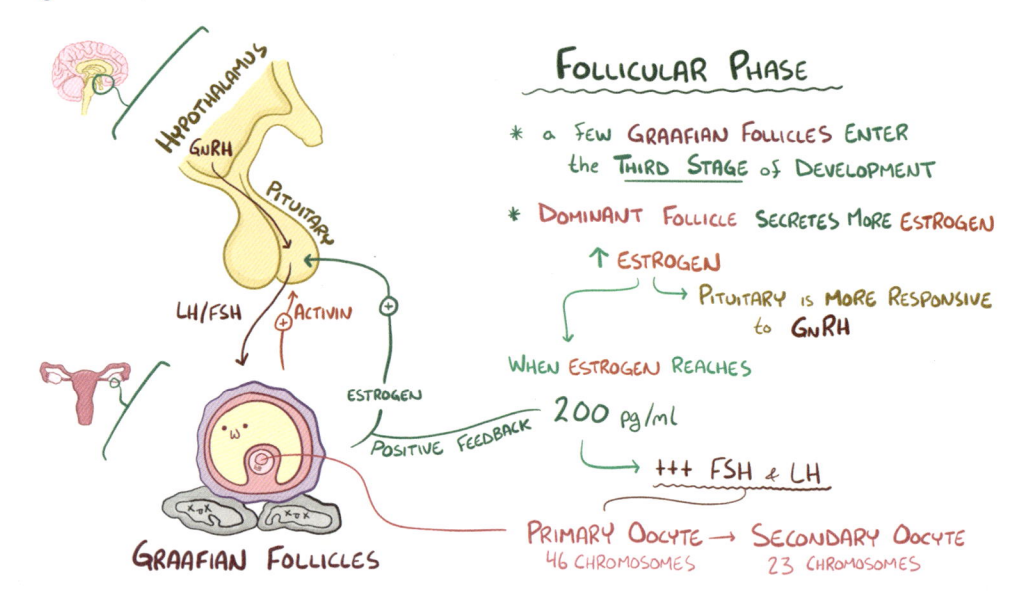

Follicular Phase

* a few GRAAFIAN FOLLICLES ENTER the THIRD STAGE of DEVELOPMENT
* DOMINANT FOLLICLE SECRETES MORE ESTROGEN

↑ ESTROGEN
→ PITUITARY is MORE RESPONSIVE to GnRH

WHEN ESTROGEN REACHES 200 pg/ml
→ +++ FSH & LH

PRIMARY OOCYTE → SECONDARY OOCYTE
46 CHROMOSOMES   23 CHROMOSOMES

Figure 13.13

Follicular Phase

* a few GRAAFIAN FOLLICLES ENTER the THIRD STAGE of DEVELOPMENT
* DOMINANT FOLLICLE SECRETES MORE ESTROGEN

↑ ESTROGEN
→ PITUITARY is MORE RESPONSIVE to GnRH

WHEN ESTROGEN REACHES 200 pg/ml
→ +++ FSH & LH

PRIMARY OOCYTE → SECONDARY OOCYTE
46 CHROMOSOMES   23 CHROMOSOMES

OVULATION 2cm

SECONDARY OOCYTE
* to FALLOPIAN TUBE
* STOPS in METAPHASE of MEIOSIS 2

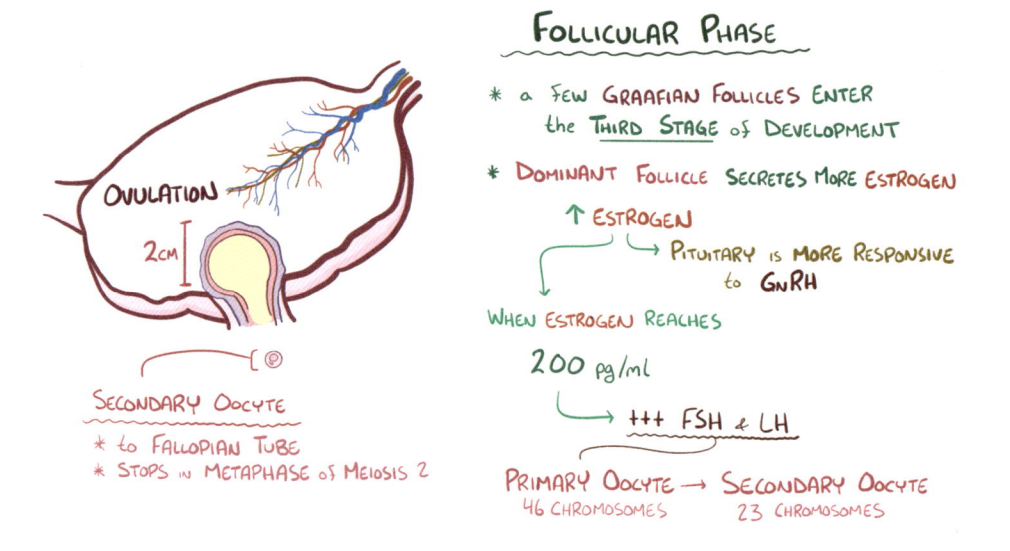

Figure 13.14

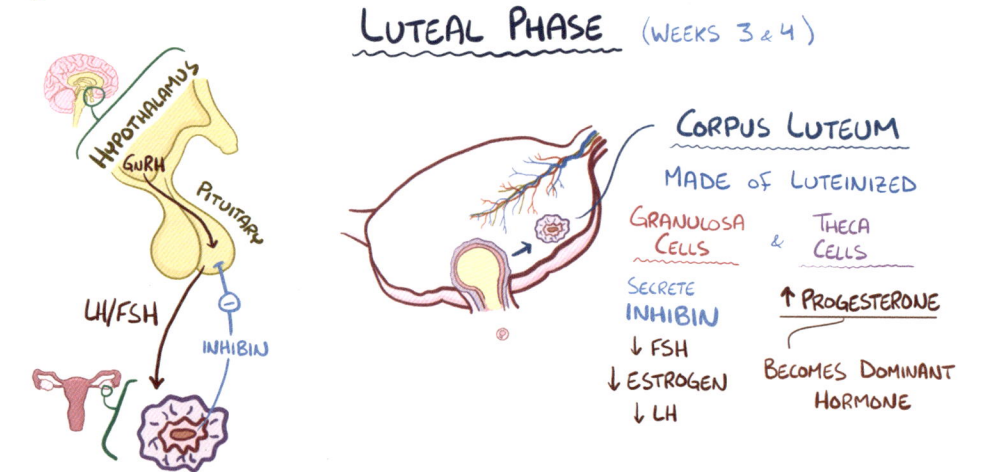

Luteal Phase (WEEKS 3 & 4)

CORPUS LUTEUM
MADE of LUTEINIZED
GRANULOSA CELLS & THECA CELLS

SECRETE INHIBIN
↓ FSH
↓ ESTROGEN
↓ LH

↑ PROGESTERONE
BECOMES DOMINANT HORMONE

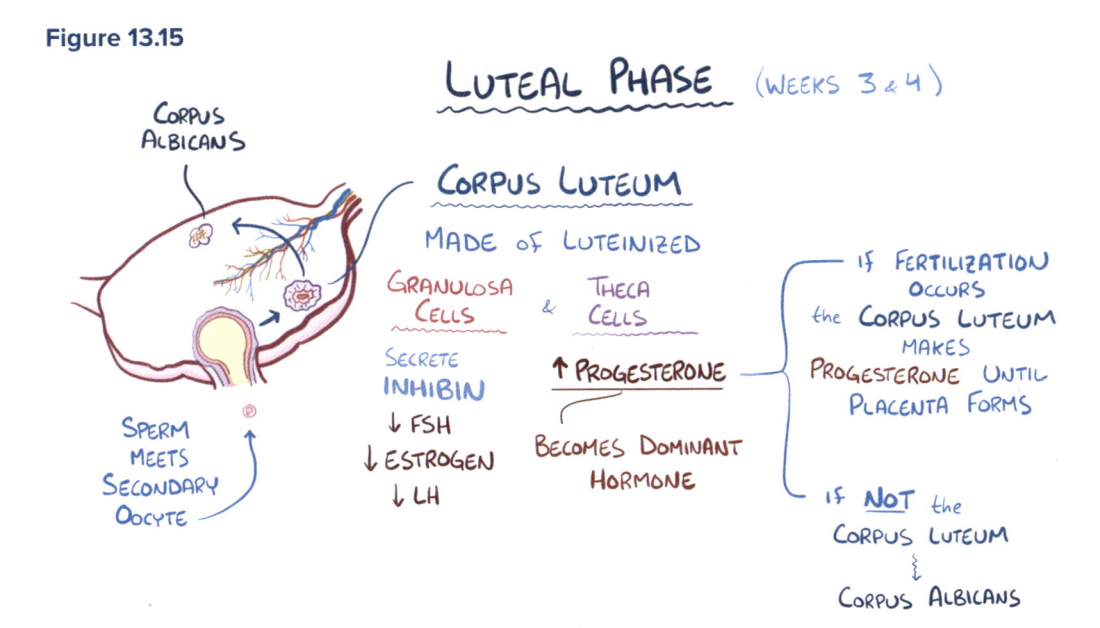

Chapter 13 The Female Reproductive System

Figure 13.15

LUTEAL PHASE (WEEKS 3 & 4)

CORPUS ALBICANS

CORPUS LUTEUM
MADE OF LUTEINIZED
GRANULOSA CELLS & THECA CELLS

SECRETE INHIBIN
↓ FSH
↓ ESTROGEN
↓ LH

↑ PROGESTERONE
BECOMES DOMINANT HORMONE

SPERM MEETS SECONDARY OOCYTE

IF FERTILIZATION OCCURS the CORPUS LUTEUM MAKES PROGESTERONE UNTIL PLACENTA FORMS

IF **NOT** the CORPUS LUTEUM → CORPUS ALBICANS

THE FALLOPIAN TUBES

After ovulation, the secondary oocyte makes a very quick journey through the peritoneal space and lands in the fallopian tube. The first part of the fallopian tube that the oocyte encounters is the fimbriae, which are the finger-like projections that surround the ovary and guide the secondary oocyte into the fallopian tube. Next is the infundibulum, where fertilization happens between the secondary oocyte and the sperm—this is the magical spot where they meet. Then there's the ampullar region, which curves around the ovary, and finally the isthmus region, which opens into the uterine cavity. On the outside, the fallopian tubes are covered by peritoneum, and supported by the mesosalpinx, which is part of the broad ligament. On the inside, the fallopian tubes have smooth muscle with an inner lining that has ciliated cells that slowly sweep the secondary oocyte or zygote towards the uterus **(Figure 13.16)**.

THE UTERUS

The uterus is a hollow organ that sits behind the urinary bladder and in front of the rectum. The top of the uterus above the openings of the fallopian tubes is called the fundus, and the region below the openings is called the uterine body. The uterus tapers down into the uterine isthmus and finally the cervix, which protrudes into the vagina. The cervix has a superior opening up top, and an inferior opening down below, both of which have mucus plugs to keep the uterus closed off except during menstruation and right before ovulation to allow sperm to reach the secondary oocyte. The uterus is anchored to the sacrum by utero-sacral ligaments, to the anterior body wall by round ligaments, and it's supported laterally by cardinal ligaments as well as the mesometrium, which is part of the broad ligament **(Figure 13.17)**.

The wall of the uterus has three layers: the perimetrium, which is a layer continuous with the lining of the peritoneal cavity, the myometrium, which is made of smooth muscle that contracts during childbirth to help push the baby out, and the endometrium, a mucosal layer, that undergoes monthly cyclic changes. During the follicular phase of the menstrual cycle, the endometrium thickens in case fertilization occurs, and during the luteal phase, spiral arteries emerge to bring more nutrients to support the thick endometrium. If fertilization doesn't occur, the spiral arteries collapse, and the superficial layers of the endometrium die. During menstruation or menstrual bleeding, that dead tissue is removed or sloughed off of the uterus through the vagina **(Figure 13.18)**.

Figure 13.16

FALLOPIAN TUBES

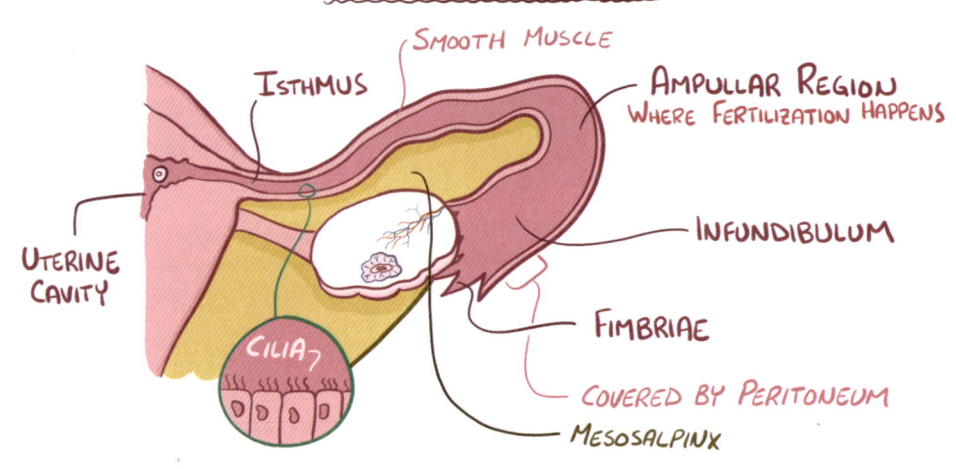

- SMOOTH MUSCLE
- ISTHMUS
- AMPULLAR REGION — WHERE FERTILIZATION HAPPENS
- INFUNDIBULUM
- FIMBRIAE
- COVERED BY PERITONEUM
- MESOSALPINX
- UTERINE CAVITY
- CILIA

Figure 13.17

UTERUS

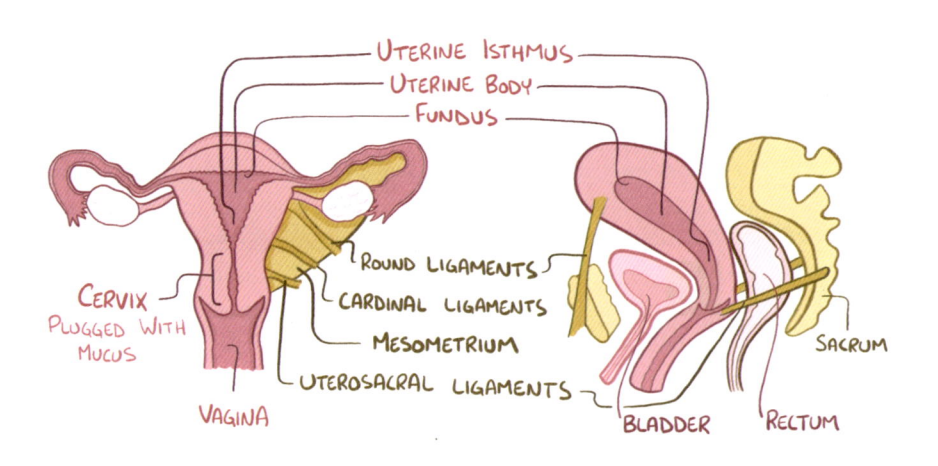

- UTERINE ISTHMUS
- UTERINE BODY
- FUNDUS
- ROUND LIGAMENTS
- CARDINAL LIGAMENTS
- MESOMETRIUM
- UTEROSACRAL LIGAMENTS
- CERVIX — PLUGGED WITH MUCUS
- VAGINA
- BLADDER
- RECTUM
- SACRUM

Figure 13.18

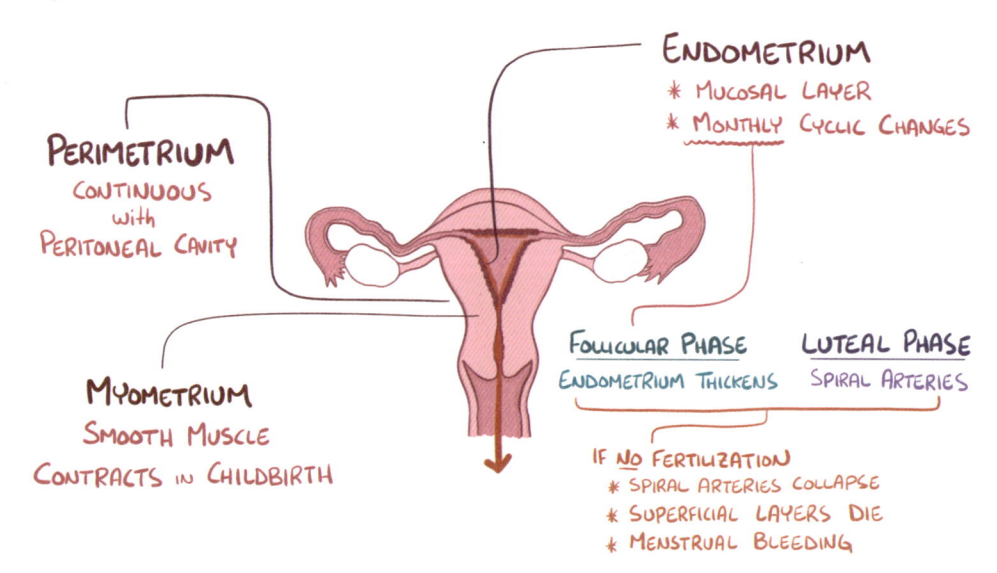

- **ENDOMETRIUM**
  * MUCOSAL LAYER
  * MONTHLY CYCLIC CHANGES
- **PERIMETRIUM** — CONTINUOUS WITH PERITONEAL CAVITY
- **MYOMETRIUM** — SMOOTH MUSCLE CONTRACTS IN CHILDBIRTH
- **FOLLICULAR PHASE** — ENDOMETRIUM THICKENS
- **LUTEAL PHASE** — SPIRAL ARTERIES
- IF NO FERTILIZATION
  * SPIRAL ARTERIES COLLAPSE
  * SUPERFICIAL LAYERS DIE
  * MENSTRUAL BLEEDING

Chapter 13 The Female Reproductive System

Figure 13.19

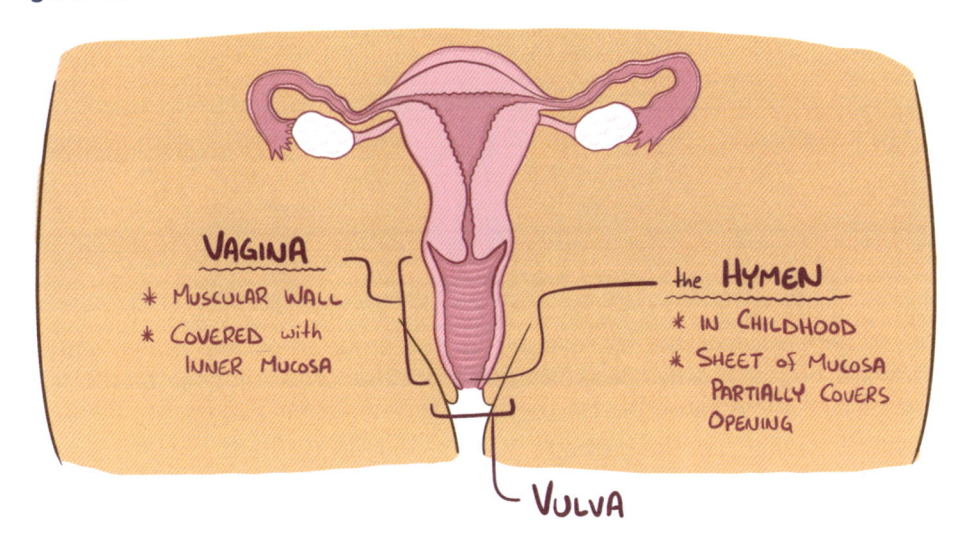

VAGINA
* Muscular wall
* Covered with inner mucosa

the HYMEN
* In childhood
* Sheet of mucosa partially covers opening

VULVA

Figure 13.20

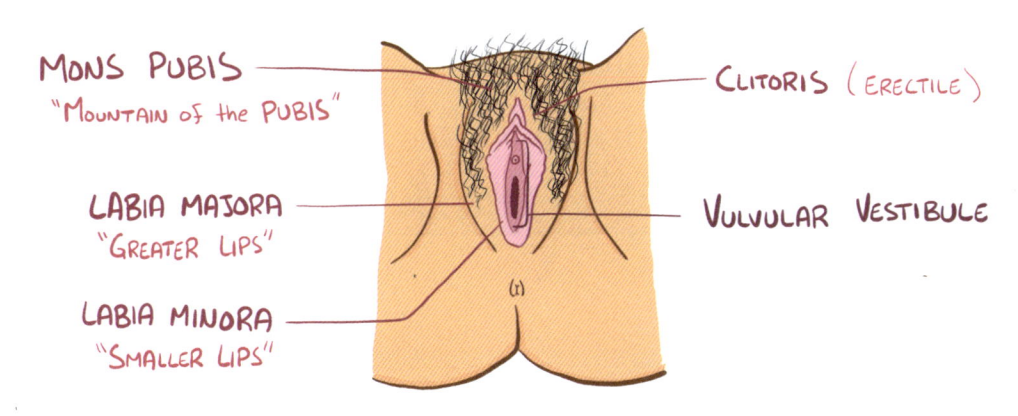

THE EXTERNAL SEX ORGANS (THE VULVA)

MONS PUBIS
"Mountain of the Pubis"

CLITORIS (ERECTILE)

LABIA MAJORA
"Greater Lips"

VULVULAR VESTIBULE

LABIA MINORA
"Smaller Lips"

Figure 13.21

THE FEMALE REPRODUCTIVE SYSTEM

INTERNAL

FALLOPIAN TUBES

UTERUS
* Where pregnancy develops

OVARIES
* ♀ Gonads
* Produce:
  └ Ova
  └ Sex Hormones

VAGINA
* the Birth Canal

EXTERNAL

MONS PUBIS
CLITORIS
LABIA

OSMOSIS.ORG 135

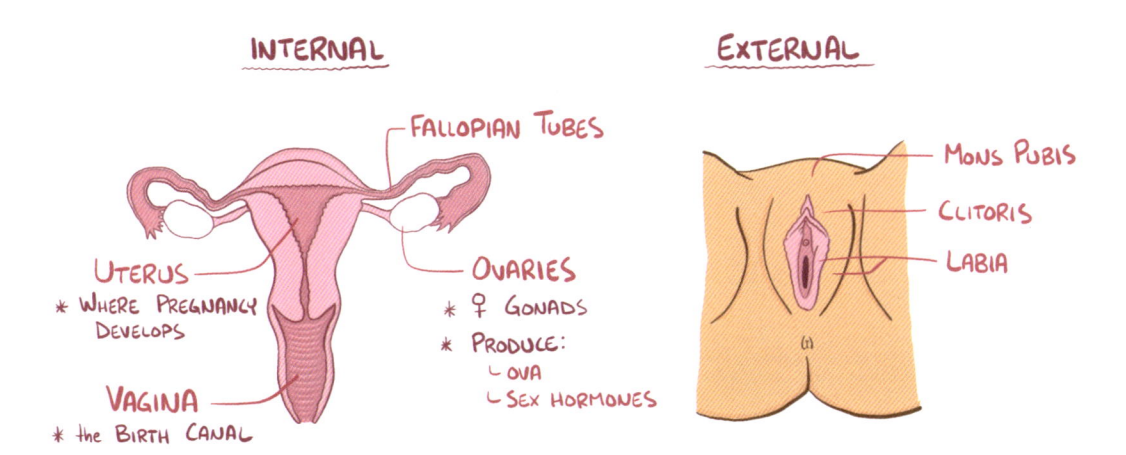

THE VAGINA

The vagina has a muscular wall and is covered by an inner mucosa with ridges that run along it. The vagina is the passageway for the baby during childbirth, and it opens up into the vulva. In childhood, a thin sheet of vaginal mucosa called the hymen partially covers the vaginal opening, and it can break because of exercise, the use of tampons, or sexual intercourse **(Figure 13.19)**.

THE VULVA

The external sex organs, together referred to as the vulva, are the labia majora (or greater lips), labia minora (or smaller lips), the mons pubis, or the mountain of the pubis, and the clitoris, a small erectile organ that develops from the same embryonic tissue as the male penis. It is hooded by a skin fold called the clitoral hood. Both the labia majora and the mons pubis become covered in pubic hair during puberty. The labia majora cover the labia minora, and between the two labia minora there is a space called the vulvar vestibule that includes the opening of the vagina and the the urethral opening **(Figure 13.20)**.

SUMMARY

All right, so as a quick recap… The female reproductive system consists of internal sex organs, including the ovaries, the fallopian tubes, the uterus and the vagina, as well as external sex organs such as the labia, the mons pubis and the clitoris. The ovaries are the female gonads, and they produce the ova, as well as the female sex hormones. Both the ovaries and the uterus are subject to the pulsatile hormonal activity of the hypothalamus and pituitary glands. The uterus is where pregnancy develops, and the baby comes into the world through the birth canal, or the vagina, that connects the internal and external sex organs **(Figure 13.21)**.

THE NERVOUS SYSTEM

osms.it/nervous_system

The nervous system is involved in nearly everything we do: how we see, how we walk, and how we talk. The nervous system is divided into two main parts: the central nervous system, which consists of the brain and the spinal cord; and the peripheral nervous system, which is further divided into the somatic and autonomic nervous systems.

AFFERENT & EFFERENT DIVISIONS

Broadly speaking, the nervous system can be split into two divisions: an afferent division and an efferent division. The afferent division brings sensory information from the outside into the central nervous system. This division includes visual receptors, auditory receptors, chemoreceptors, and somatosensory—or touch—receptors.

In contrast, the efferent division brings motor information from the central nervous system to the peripheral nervous system. Ultimately, this results in the contraction of skeletal muscles to trigger movement through the somatic nervous system, as well as the contraction of smooth muscles to trigger activity of the internal organs through the autonomic nervous system **(Figure 14.1)**.

NERVOUS SYSTEM CELLS

The nervous system is made up of two main types of cells: neurons and glial cells. Neurons are the main cells of the nervous system. They're composed of a cell body, which contains all the cell's organelles. When there's a group of neuron cell bodies in the central nervous system, the whole thing is called a nucleus, whereas a group of neuron cell bodies located outside of the central nervous system is called a ganglion.

Figure 14.1

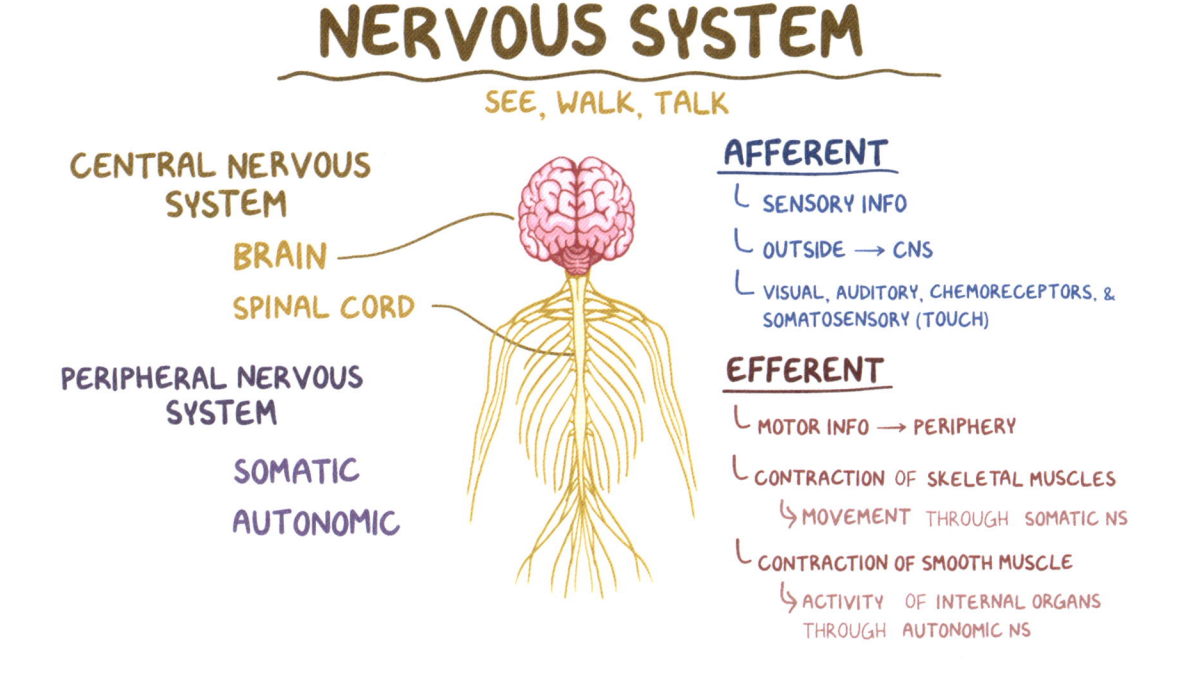

Neurons contain nerve fibers that extend out from the neuron cell body. These may be dendrites, which receive signals from other neurons, or axons, which send signals to other neurons. The point at which two neurons come together is called a synapse, and this is the point at which one end of an axon releases neurotransmitters, relaying the signal to the dendrites or directly to the cell body of the next neuron in the series. To trigger the release of neurotransmitters, neurons use an electrical signal that races down the axon. This is known as the action potential.

To help speed up that electrical signal, the axons are intermittently wrapped by a fatty protective sheath called myelin. This myelin comes from glial cells: the oligodendrocytes in the central nervous system, or the Schwann cells in the peripheral nervous system. Another type of glial cells are the astrocytes, which are only present in the central nervous system. Astrocytes lend structural and metabolic support to neurons. They also act as resident immune cells, and help seal and nourish the blood-brain barrier **(Figure 14.2)**.

The blood-brain barrier consists of tight junctions that connect endothelial cells, which line the capillaries in the brain. These tight junctions seal off the spaces between the endothelial cells. They're surrounded by basement membrane and astrocytes, which further strengthen the barrier. Think of the blood-brain barrier as the brain's bouncer, a highly selective membrane that turns bacteria—and other large, shady-looking molecules that are floating around in the blood— away at the door, while letting in nutrients like water, oxygen, glucose, and smaller, fat-soluble molecules **(Figure 14.3)**.

CENTRAL NERVOUS SYSTEM: THE BRAIN

The brain has several regions: the cerebrum, diencephalon, cerebellum, and brainstem. Let's begin with the cerebrum, which is divided into two cerebral hemispheres. The right cerebral hemisphere receives afferent fibers and sends efferent fibers to the left side of your body, while the left cerebral hemisphere receives afferent fibers and sends efferent fibers to the right side of your body. If we look at a cross section of the cerebrum, we would see two areas: the outermost area is the grey matter, or cerebral cortex, and is made up of billions of neuron cell bodies; and the innermost area is the white matter and is made up of the axons that come off of all of those neurons **(Figure 14.4)**.

Figure 14.2

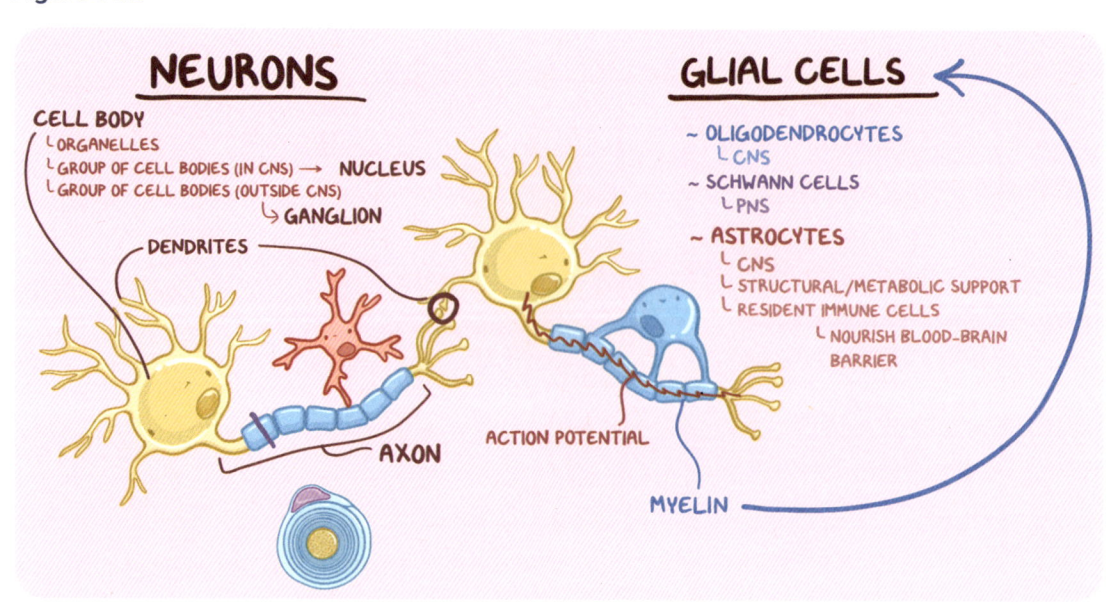

Chapter 14 The Nervous System

Figure 14.3

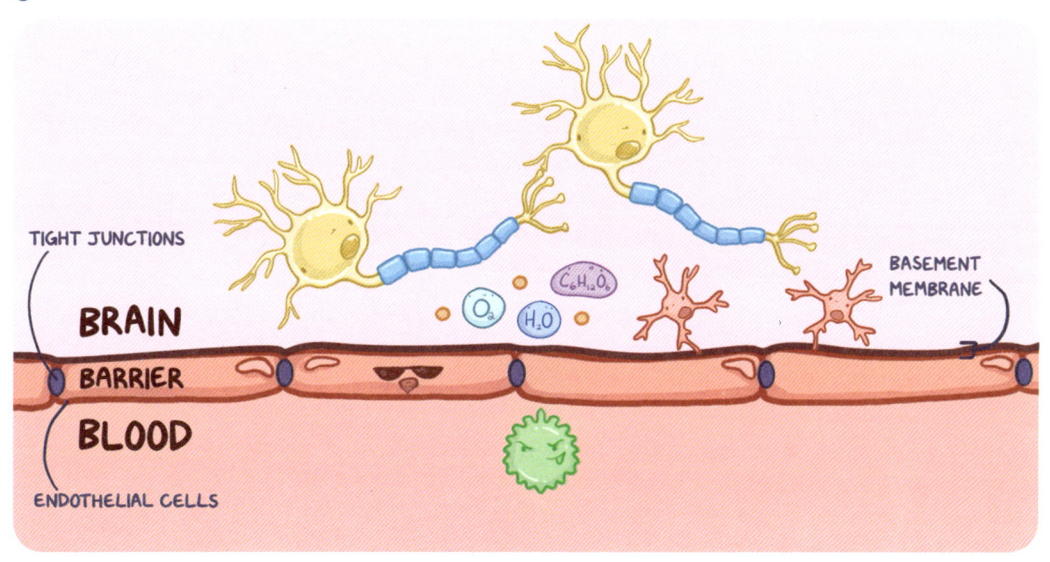

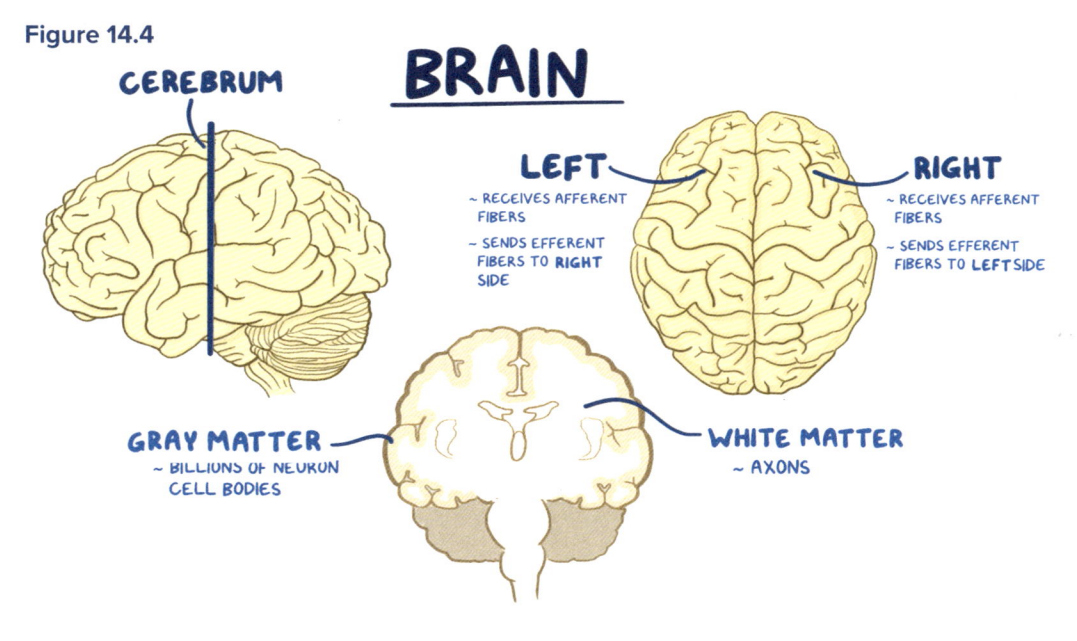

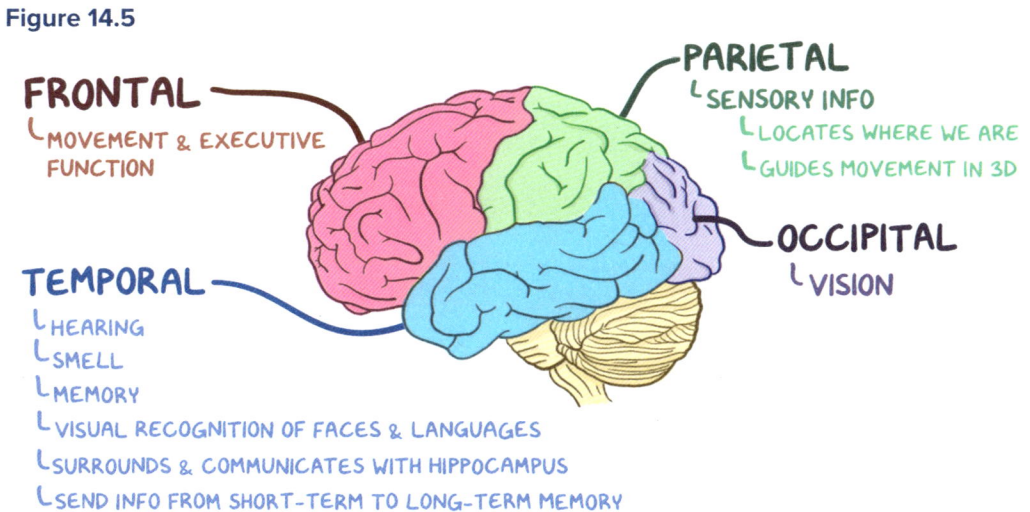

- TIGHT JUNCTIONS
- BRAIN
- BARRIER
- BLOOD
- ENDOTHELIAL CELLS
- BASEMENT MEMBRANE

Figure 14.4

BRAIN

CEREBRUM

LEFT
- ~ RECEIVES AFFERENT FIBERS
- ~ SENDS EFFERENT FIBERS TO RIGHT SIDE

RIGHT
- ~ RECEIVES AFFERENT FIBERS
- ~ SENDS EFFERENT FIBERS TO LEFT SIDE

GRAY MATTER
- ~ BILLIONS OF NEURON CELL BODIES

WHITE MATTER
- ~ AXONS

Figure 14.5

FRONTAL
- MOVEMENT & EXECUTIVE FUNCTION

PARIETAL
- SENSORY INFO
  - LOCATES WHERE WE ARE
  - GUIDES MOVEMENT IN 3D

OCCIPITAL
- VISION

TEMPORAL
- HEARING
- SMELL
- MEMORY
- VISUAL RECOGNITION OF FACES & LANGUAGES
- SURROUNDS & COMMUNICATES WITH HIPPOCAMPUS
- SEND INFO FROM SHORT-TERM TO LONG-TERM MEMORY

OSMOSIS.ORG 139

The cerebral cortex is divided into the frontal lobe, parietal lobe, temporal lobe, and the occipital lobe. The frontal lobe controls movement and executive function—your ability to make decisions. The parietal lobe processes sensory information, which allows you to locate exactly where you are physically and guides your movements in a three-dimensional space. The temporal lobe plays a role in hearing, smell, and memory, as well as in the visual recognition of faces and languages. The temporal lobe surrounds and communicates with the hippocampus and helps send information from short-term to long-term memory. Finally, there's the occipital lobe, which is primarily responsible for vision **(Figure 14.5)**.

Within the white matter are deeper subcortical—meaning they're below the cortex—structures. These include the internal capsule and the basal ganglia. You can think of the internal capsule as a highway that allows information to flow through the neurons entering and leaving the cerebral cortex **(Figure 14.6)**. The basal ganglia is actually two deep structures: the pallidum and the striatum, with the striatum further divided into the caudate nucleus and the putamen. The striatum receives input from the cerebral cortex about a desired movement. it then sends output to the other basal ganglia structures to control smooth movement. This is accomplished by inhibiting undesired movements. For example, when you walk, you have to move one leg at a time. When one leg steps forward, the other leg is inhibited by the basal ganglia so that it's stationary. It's the basal ganglia that prevents you from falling each time you take a step **(Figure 14.7)**!

Figure 14.6

Figure 14.7

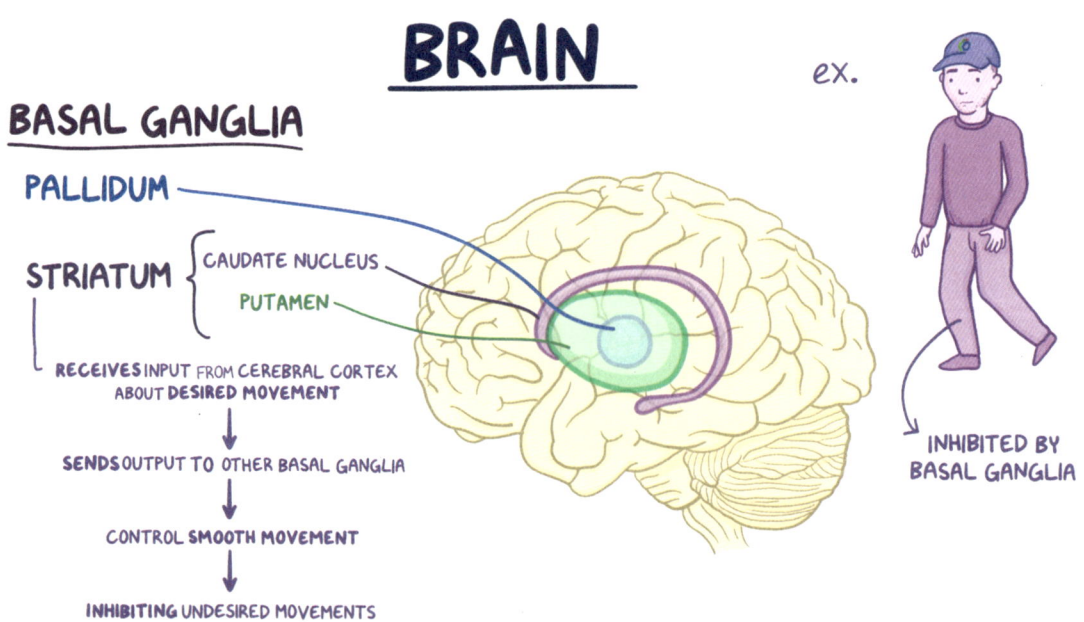

Chapter 14 The Nervous System

Let's examine the next region of the brain: the diencephalon, which is composed of an upper part, the thalamus, and a lower part, the hypothalamus. The thalamus is a collection of nuclei—millions of nerve cell bodies—that process the sensory information coming in from the body to the cerebral cortex. These nuclei also process the motor information travelling from the cerebral cortex to the body. The hypothalamus is a small region that does a variety of things. It regulates body temperature and the sleep-wake cycle, as well as eating and drinking.

To achieve all of this, the hypothalamus regulates the release of the major endocrine hormones. It sends signals to the pituitary, a pea-sized gland that hangs by a stalk from the base of the brain. The pituitary can be divided into two parts: the anterior and posterior pituitary. The pituitary gland produces and secretes hormones when it receives signals from the hypothalamus. Together, they form the hypothalamic-pituitary axis **(Figure 14.8)**.

Now, let's examine the cerebellum, which sits at the base of the skull. The cerebellum helps with coordinating movement, precision, and balance. The cerebellum receives sensory input about body position from the spinal cord and receives motor input from the brain. It integrates these two sets of information to help fine-tune motor activity and store it as muscle memory—which is why you never forget how to ride a bike **(Figure 14.9)**.

Figure 14.8

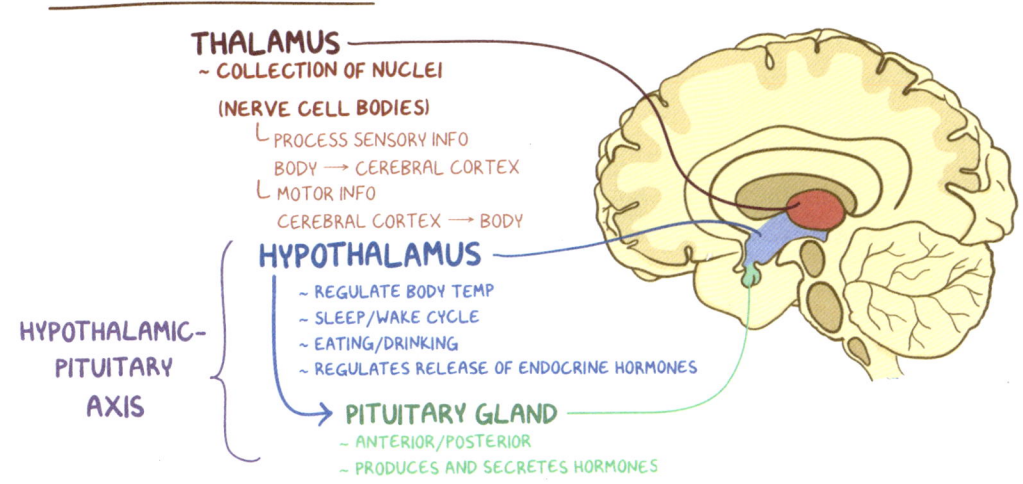

Figure 14.9

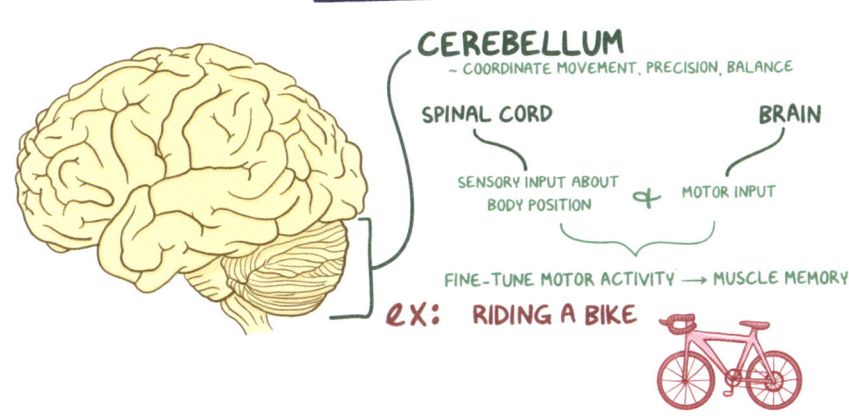

OSMOSIS.ORG 141

Finally, we have the brainstem, which is located in front of the cerebellum and connects to the spinal cord. The brainstem is made up of three parts: the midbrain, pons, and medulla. The midbrain is the uppermost part and participates in vision, hearing, motor control, the sleep-wake cycle, and consciousness. The pons is the middle part and contains nuclei that control facial expressions and sensation, as well as body equilibrium and posture. The medulla is the lower part and contains nuclei that help regulate blood pressure, breathing, swallowing, coughing, vomiting, and digestion **(Figure 14.10)**.

CENTRAL NERVOUS SYSTEM: THE SPINAL CORD

The spinal cord is a long rod of nervous tissue that extends down from the brainstem to the lumbar region of the vertebral column. Information travels up the spinal cord through afferent or sensory fibers and down the spinal cord through efferent or motor fibers. If we take a cross-section of the spinal cord, we'll find white matter on the outside, which contains the afferent and efferent fibers, and grey matter on the inside, which contains the nerve cell bodies. These nerve cell bodies are arranged in three grey columns, or horns, that look a bit like a butterfly. The three pairs of grey horns are divided into anterior or ventral horns, posterior or dorsal horns, and lateral horns **(Figure 14.11)**.

The anterior or ventral horns receive information from the motor cortex of the brain and send this information to the skeletal muscles in order to trigger voluntary movement. The posterior or dorsal horns take sensory information from the outside world and send it to the sensory cortex of the brain. Sensory information includes pressure, vibration, fine touch, and proprioception—the awareness of one's bodily position in space. Finally, there are the lateral horns, which are mainly involved with the sympathetic division of the autonomic motor system. These help regulate processes like urination, digestion, and heart rate **(Figure 14.12)**.

The spinal cord is responsible for coordinating reflexes, which are fast involuntary responses to a stimulus. Think, for example, of your last check-up and the moment your doctor tested your reflexes by giving your knee a sharp tap. Involuntary responses are the result of sensory neurons that synapse in the spinal cord, rather than in the brain. Shorter distance means faster signal!

Now, zooming in even closer, we see that both the brain and spinal cord are covered by meninges, which are three protective layers. The inner layer of the meninges is the pia mater, the middle layer is the arachnoid mater, and the outer layer is the dura mater. These first two layers, the pia and arachnoid mater, form the subarachnoid space, which houses the cerebrospinal fluid, or CSF. CSF is a clear, watery liquid which is pumped around the spinal cord and brain, cushioning them from impact and bathing them in nutrients **(Figure 14.13)**.

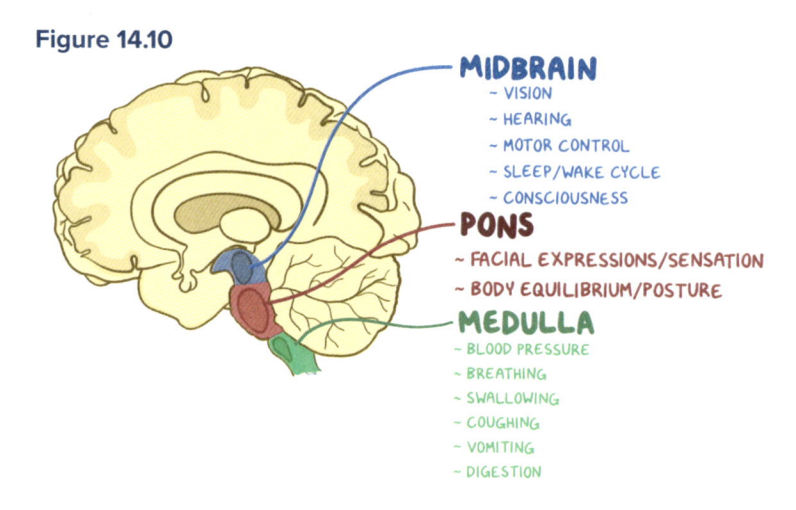

Figure 14.10

MIDBRAIN
- VISION
- HEARING
- MOTOR CONTROL
- SLEEP/WAKE CYCLE
- CONSCIOUSNESS

PONS
- FACIAL EXPRESSIONS/SENSATION
- BODY EQUILIBRIUM/POSTURE

MEDULLA
- BLOOD PRESSURE
- BREATHING
- SWALLOWING
- COUGHING
- VOMITING
- DIGESTION

Chapter 14 The Nervous System

Figure 14.11

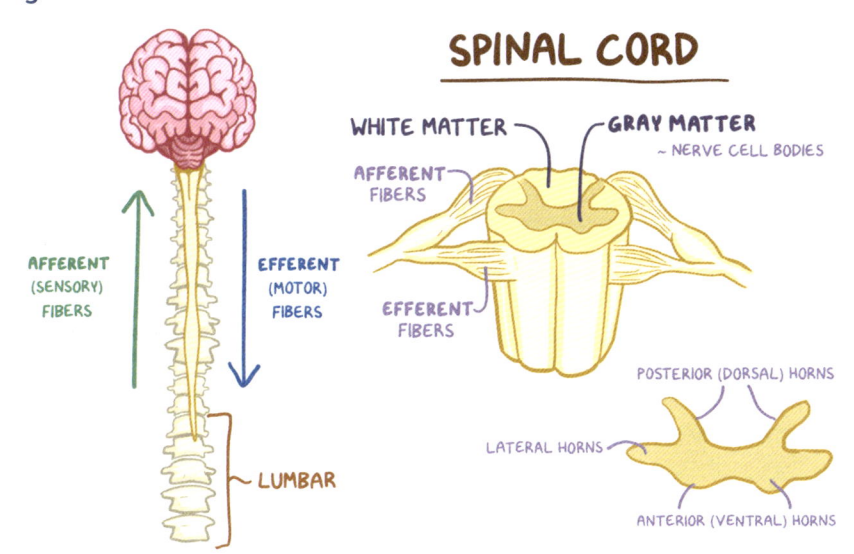

SPINAL CORD

- WHITE MATTER
  - AFFERENT FIBERS
  - EFFERENT FIBERS
- GRAY MATTER
  - ~ NERVE CELL BODIES

AFFERENT (SENSORY) FIBERS
EFFERENT (MOTOR) FIBERS
LUMBAR

- POSTERIOR (DORSAL) HORNS
- LATERAL HORNS
- ANTERIOR (VENTRAL) HORNS

Figure 14.12

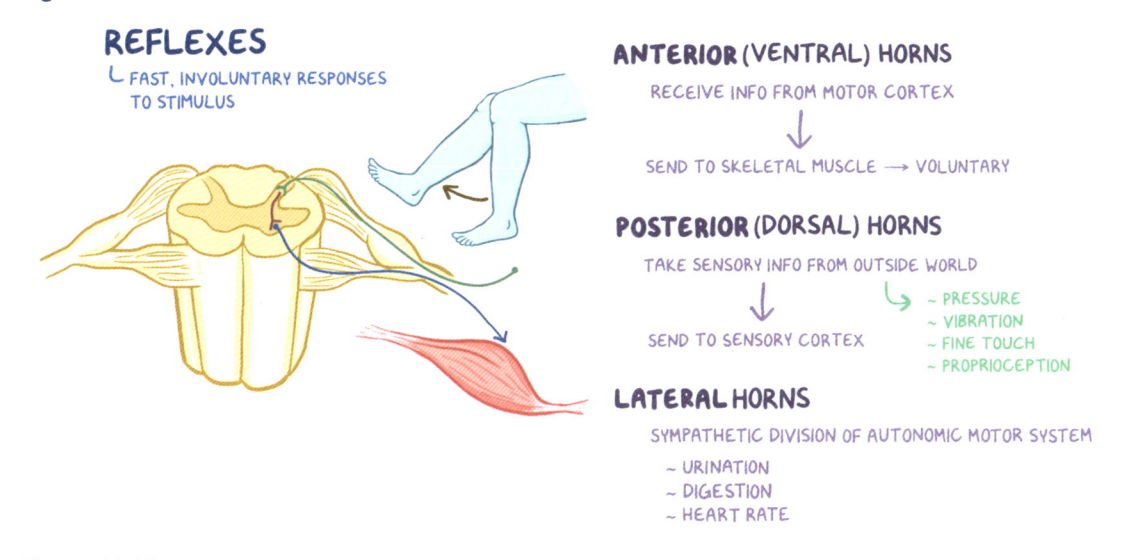

REFLEXES
└ FAST, INVOLUNTARY RESPONSES TO STIMULUS

ANTERIOR (VENTRAL) HORNS
RECEIVE INFO FROM MOTOR CORTEX
↓
SEND TO SKELETAL MUSCLE → VOLUNTARY

POSTERIOR (DORSAL) HORNS
TAKE SENSORY INFO FROM OUTSIDE WORLD
↓
SEND TO SENSORY CORTEX
  ↳ ~ PRESSURE
    ~ VIBRATION
    ~ FINE TOUCH
    ~ PROPRIOCEPTION

LATERAL HORNS
SYMPATHETIC DIVISION OF AUTONOMIC MOTOR SYSTEM
  ~ URINATION
  ~ DIGESTION
  ~ HEART RATE

Figure 14.13

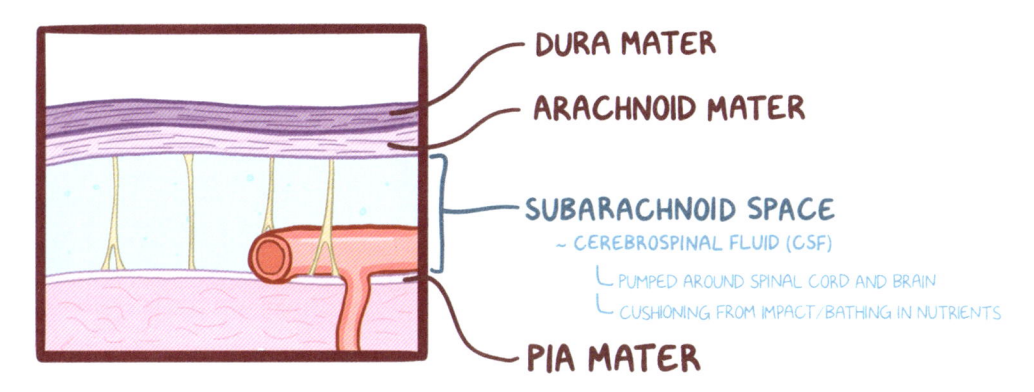

MENINGES
~ PROTECTIVE LAYERS OF THE BRAIN

- DURA MATER
- ARACHNOID MATER
- SUBARACHNOID SPACE
  ~ CEREBROSPINAL FLUID (CSF)
    └ PUMPED AROUND SPINAL CORD AND BRAIN
    └ CUSHIONING FROM IMPACT/BATHING IN NUTRIENTS
- PIA MATER

OSMOSIS.ORG 143

PERIPHERAL NERVOUS SYSTEM

The peripheral nervous system consists of nerves, which are enclosed bundles of axons, that connect the central nervous system to every other part of the body **(Figure 14.14)**.

There are twelve cranial nerve pairs that exit the skull and innervate the head and neck. The first two emerge from the cerebrum: the cranial nerve I, called the olfactory nerve, and cranial nerve II, called the optic nerve. The remaining cranial nerves emerge from different parts of the brainstem. Cranial nerve III, called the oculomotor nerve, and cranial nerve IV, called the trochlear nerve, emerge from the midbrain. Cranial nerve V, called the trigeminal nerve, cranial nerve VI, called the abducens nerve, cranial nerve VII, called the facial nerve, and cranial nerve VIII, called the vestibulocochlear nerve, emerge from the pons. And finally, cranial nerve IX, called the glossopharyngeal nerve, cranial nerve X, called the vagus nerve, cranial nerve XI, called the accessory nerve, and cranial nerve XII, called the hypoglossal nerve, all emerge from the medulla. The cranial nerves are numbered based on their front-to-back position when viewing the brain—with the exception of cranial nerves XI and XII, which are inverted **(Figure 14.15)**.

There are also 31 pairs of spinal nerves, which exit various regions of the spinal cord and innervate the rest of the body. There are eight pairs of cervical nerves, 12 pairs of thoracic nerves, five pairs of lumbar nerves, five pairs of sacral nerves, and one pair of coccygeal nerves **(Figure 14.16)**.

SOMATIC NERVOUS SYSTEM

The peripheral nervous system is divided into the somatic and autonomic nervous systems. The somatic nervous system is made up of afferent or sensory nerves, which have axons that carry sensory information from the peripheral tissues, like the skin, back to the cell bodies in the posterior horns of the spinal cord. The somatic nervous system also contains efferent or motor nerves, which have axons that carry motor information from the cell bodies in the anterior horns of the spinal cord to the neuromuscular junction, where these axons come into contact with the skeletal muscle cells **(Figure 14.17)**.

Figure 14.14

PERIPHERAL NERVOUS SYSTEM

- BUNDLES OF AXONS
- ~ CONNECT CENTRAL NERVOUS SYSTEM TO EVERY PART OF THE BODY

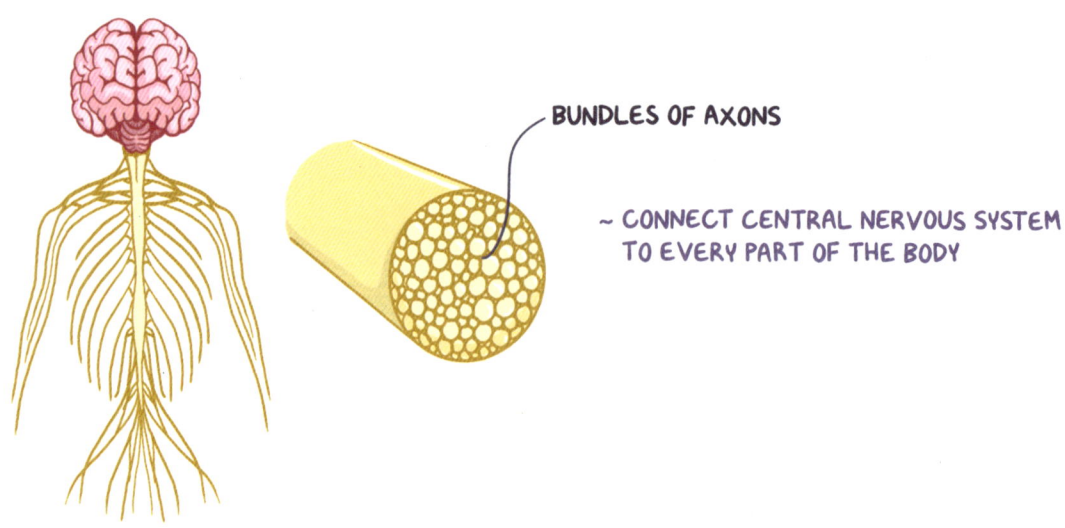

Figure 14.15

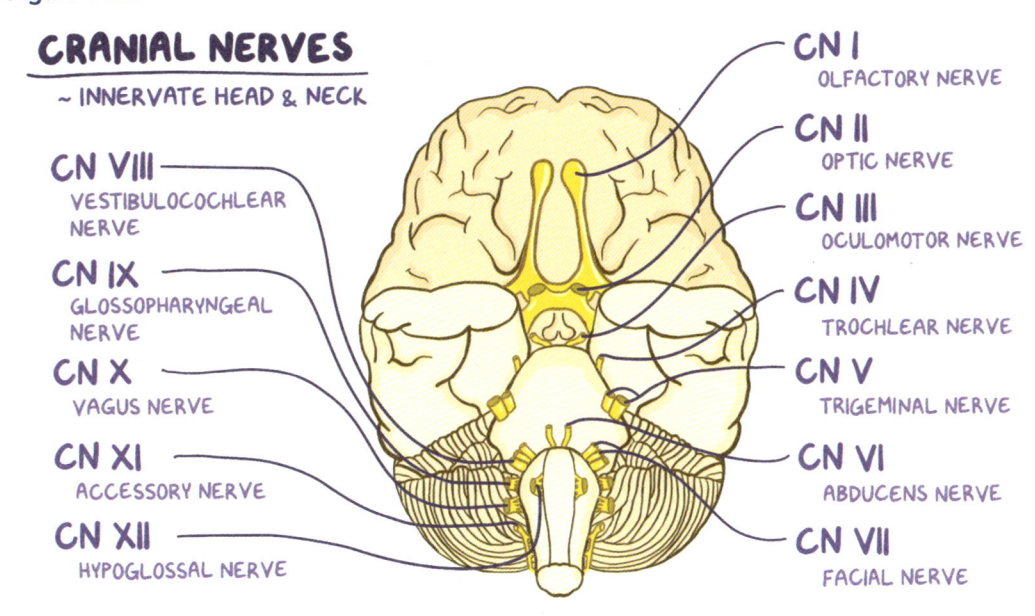

CRANIAL NERVES
~ INNERVATE HEAD & NECK

- CN VIII — VESTIBULOCOCHLEAR NERVE
- CN IX — GLOSSOPHARYNGEAL NERVE
- CN X — VAGUS NERVE
- CN XI — ACCESSORY NERVE
- CN XII — HYPOGLOSSAL NERVE
- CN I — OLFACTORY NERVE
- CN II — OPTIC NERVE
- CN III — OCULOMOTOR NERVE
- CN IV — TROCHLEAR NERVE
- CN V — TRIGEMINAL NERVE
- CN VI — ABDUCENS NERVE
- CN VII — FACIAL NERVE

Figure 14.16

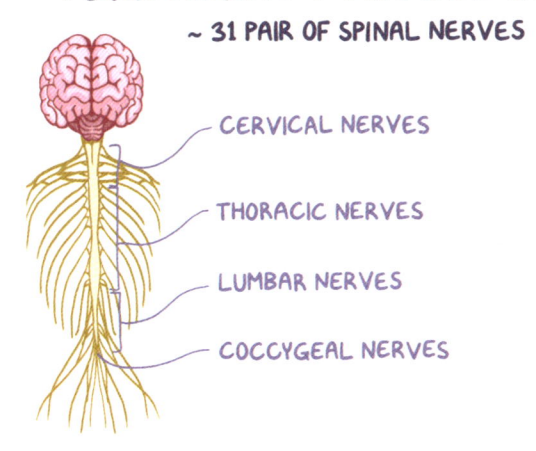

PERIPHERAL NERVOUS SYSTEM
~ 31 PAIR OF SPINAL NERVES

- CERVICAL NERVES
- THORACIC NERVES
- LUMBAR NERVES
- COCCYGEAL NERVES

Figure 14.17

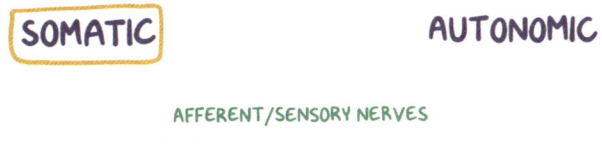

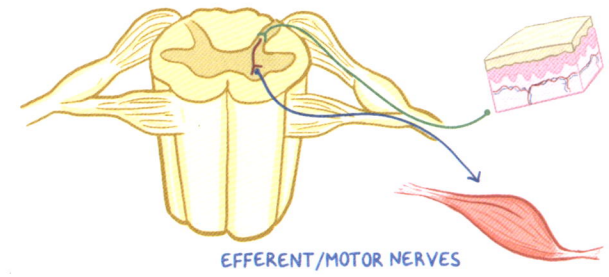

PERIPHERAL NERVOUS SYSTEM

SOMATIC   AUTONOMIC

AFFERENT/SENSORY NERVES

EFFERENT/MOTOR NERVES

Figure 14.18

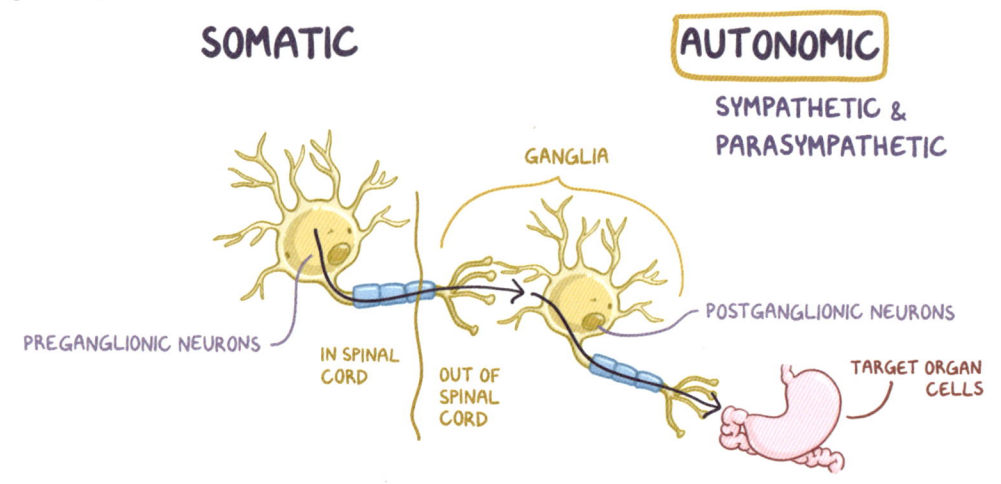

SOMATIC

AUTONOMIC

SYMPATHETIC & PARASYMPATHETIC

GANGLIA

PREGANGLIONIC NEURONS

IN SPINAL CORD

OUT OF SPINAL CORD

POSTGANGLIONIC NEURONS

TARGET ORGAN CELLS

Figure 14.19

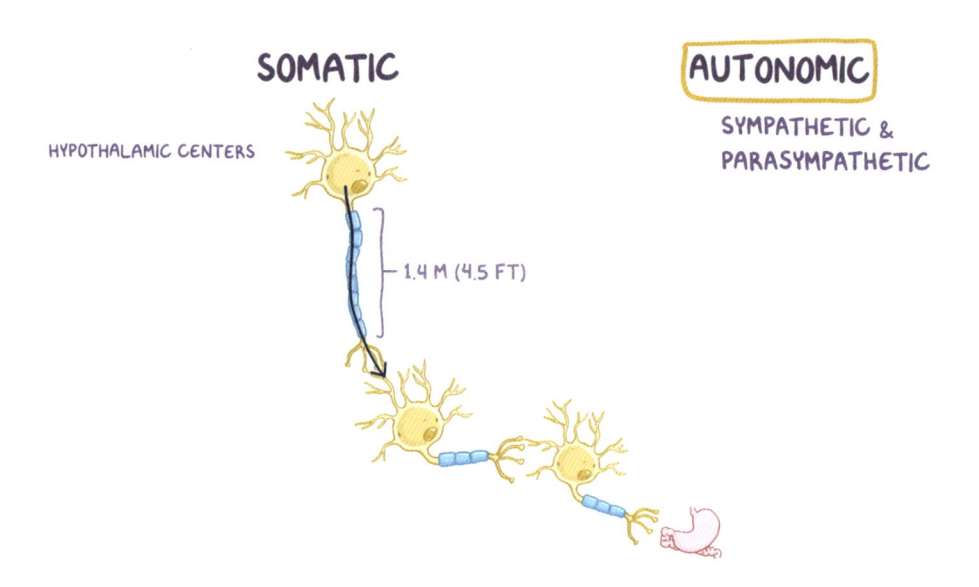

SOMATIC

AUTONOMIC

SYMPATHETIC & PARASYMPATHETIC

HYPOTHALAMIC CENTERS

1.4 M (4.5 FT)

Figure 14.20

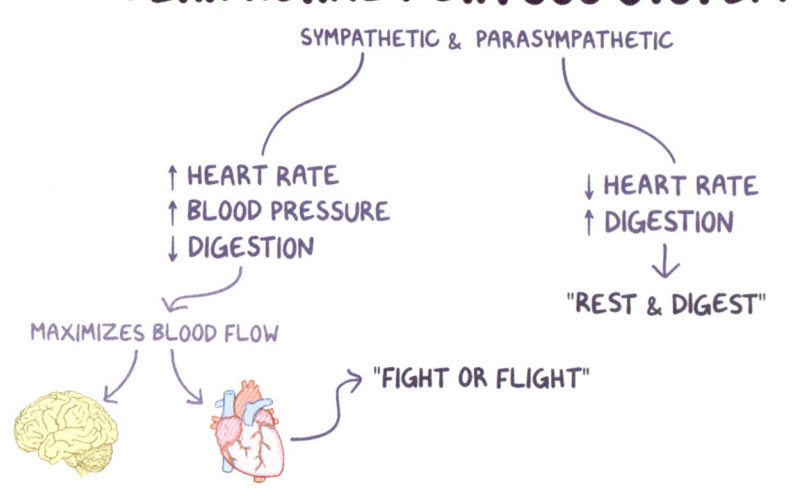

PERIPHERAL NERVOUS SYSTEM

SYMPATHETIC & PARASYMPATHETIC

↑ HEART RATE
↑ BLOOD PRESSURE
↓ DIGESTION

↓ HEART RATE
↑ DIGESTION

"REST & DIGEST"

MAXIMIZES BLOOD FLOW

"FIGHT OR FLIGHT"

146 OSMOSIS.ORG

Chapter 14 The Nervous System

AUTONOMIC NERVOUS SYSTEM

The autonomic nervous system, which is made up of both the sympathetic and parasympathetic nervous system, includes a relay of two neurons: preganglionic neurons, which have their cell bodies in nuclei throughout the spinal cord in the lateral horns; and postganglionic neurons, which have their cells bodies in ganglia out of the spinal cord. Axons of preganglionic neurons exit the spinal cord to reach the ganglia and synapse with postganglionic neurons. Then, the axons of postganglionic neurons exit the ganglia to reach the organs and synapse with the target organ cells **(Figure 14.18)**. Signals for the autonomic nervous system start in some hypothalamic centers. Hypothalamic neurons have really long axons—up to 1.4 meters, or 4.5 feet—and they carry signals all the way down to the spinal cord nuclei where they synapse with preganglionic neuron cell bodies **(Figure 14.19)**.

The sympathetic and parasympathetic nervous systems have opposite effects on the body. The sympathetic nervous system controls functions like increasing the heart rate and blood pressure, as well as slowing digestion. All of this maximizes blood flow to the muscles and brain, which enables your decision to either face a threat or run away from it—the fight-or-flight response! In contrast, the parasympathetic nervous system slows the heart rate and stimulates digestion. These effects can be summarized as: rest and digest **(Figure 14.20)**!

SUMMARY

All right, as a quick recap, the nervous system includes the following: the central nervous system, which is made up of the brain and spinal cord; and the peripheral nervous system, which is made up of all the nerves that connect the central nervous system to the muscles and organs. The spinal cord is the pathway through which afferent and efferent fibers travel to connect the brain and peripheral nervous system. Finally, the peripheral nervous system can be divided into: the somatic nervous system, which controls our skeletal muscles; and the autonomic nervous system, which is further divided into the sympathetic and the parasympathetic systems, which control smooth muscles and glands **(Figure 14.21)**.

Figure 14.21

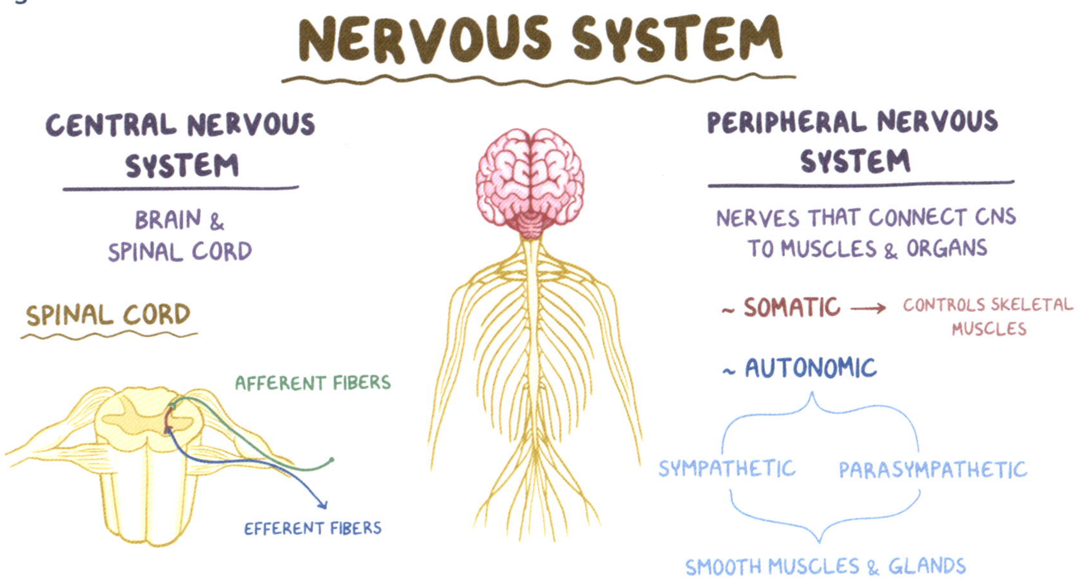

OSMOSIS.ORG 147

THE EAR

osms.it/ear_anatomy

Our ears have two main functions: they help us hear and keep our balance in physical space. They're made up of three parts: the outer ear, the middle ear, and the inner ear. The first part, the outer ear, consists of the part you see—and maybe even hang earrings on—the pinna, as well as the ear canal. The second part, the middle ear, is a tiny chamber that houses even tinier ear bones: the malleus, incus, and stapes. The third part, the inner ear, contains the cochlea, a special structure that converts sound waves into electrical impulses for the brain, and the semicircular canals which assist us with balance **(Figure 15.1)**.

Figure 15.1

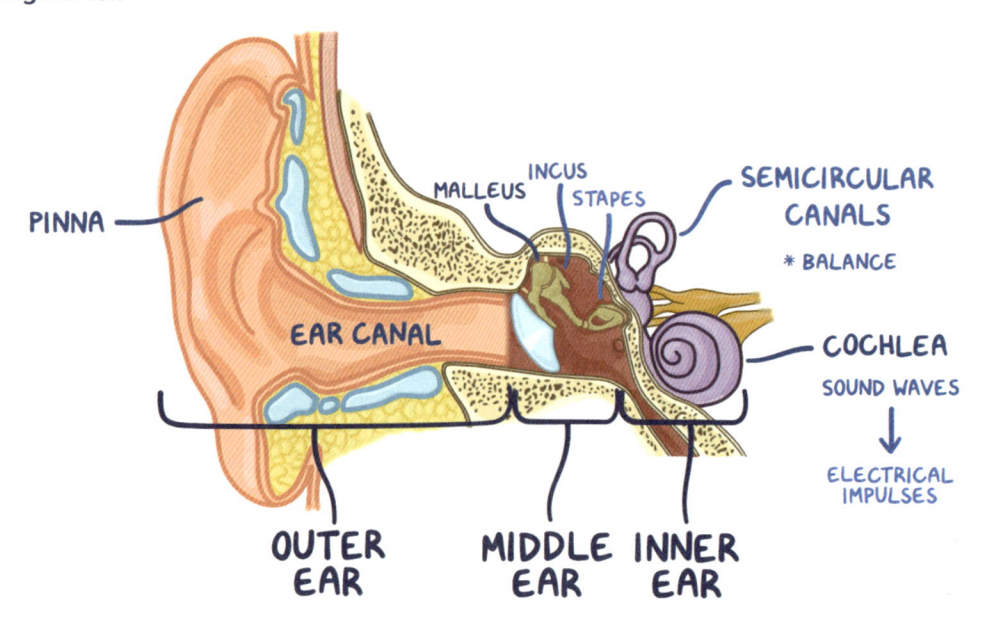

Figure 15.2

EXTERNAL EAR

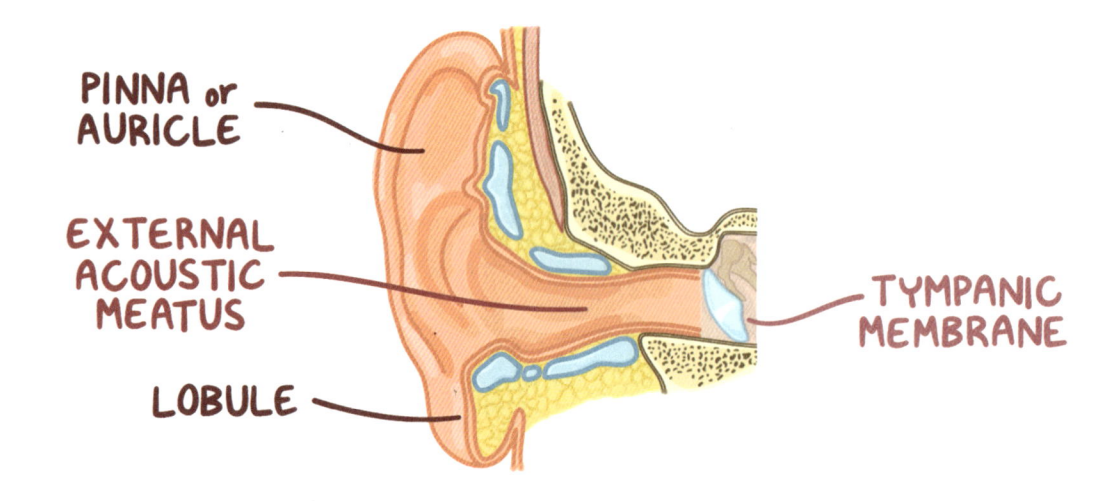

OUTER EAR

Let's start with the external ear. The pinna, also called the auricle, is made up of cartilage that gives our ears their various shapes and sizes. It also has a fleshy bit at the bottom, called the ear lobe or lobule. The pinna directs sound waves towards the opening of the ear canal.

The ear canal, or the external acoustic meatus, is a short curved tube that burrows through the temporal bone for about 1 inch—or 2.5 centimeters—and ends at the tympanic membrane **(Figure 15.2)**. On the inside, the ear canal is covered by skin, along with hair follicles and ceruminous glands. These glands secrete cerumen—that sticky, yellow-ish, earwax. Cerumen helps prevents foreign objects or even tiny insects—a creepy thought!—from entering and damaging the tympanic membrane. Be thankful for that earwax **(Figure 15.3)**!

The tympanic membrane, also called the eardrum, is a thin, translucent membrane that separates the external ear from the middle ear. It's shaped a bit like a cone, protruding slightly into the middle ear. When sound waves reach the eardrum, it vibrates and transmits those vibrations to the tiny bones in the middle ear **(Figure 15.4)**.

MIDDLE EAR

Now, the middle ear is an air-filled cavity inside the temporal bone, shaped like a tiny chamber with four walls, a floor, and roof. The eardrum makes up the lateral wall of this cavity. Opposite the eardrum is the medial, or internal wall, that separates the middle ear from the inner ear. The internal wall has two windows: an oval window above and a round window below. The two other walls of the middle ear are the posterior wall, in the back, and the anterior wall, in the front. The posterior wall has an opening called the mastoid antrum. It connects the middle ear with the mastoid cavity within the temporal bone. The anterior wall has an opening for the eustachian tube, which connects the middle ear to the nasopharynx. The eustachian tube has three main functions: equalizing pressure across the tympanic membrane, protecting the middle ear from the reflux of fluids travelling up from the nasopharynx, and clearing out middle ear secretions. The roof of the middle ear, called the epitympanic recess, is dome-shaped. And finally, to complete our picture of the middle chamber, the floor of the middle ear is a thin layer of bone that sits right above the jugular vein **(Figure 15.5)**.

Inside the middle ear chamber, there are three tiny bones arranged from the eardrum to the oval window: the malleus, incus, and stapes—named after their resemblance to a hammer, an anvil, and stirrups, respectively. The "handle" of the malleus rests on the eardrum, and the base of the stapes rests on the oval window. When the eardrum vibrates, the vibrations are transmitted from the malleus, to the incus, then to the stapes, and finally to the oval window, which transfers the vibrations to the inner ear **(Figure 15.6; Figure 15.7)**.

Figure 15.3

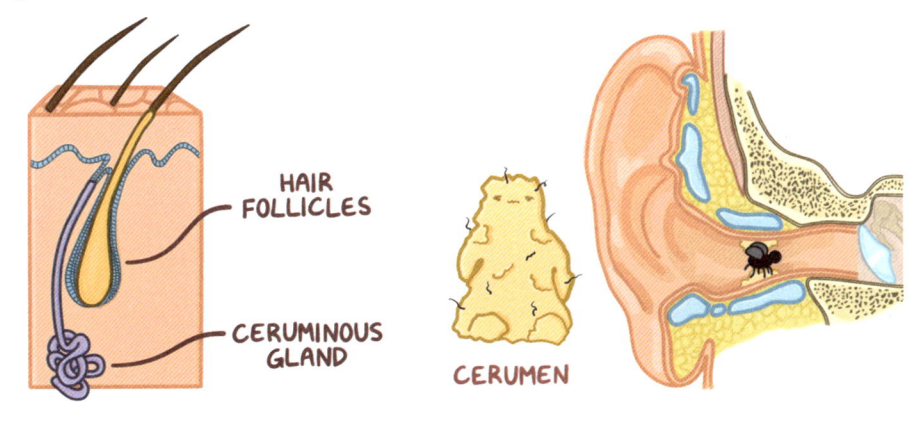

Figure 15.4

SOUND WAVES

TYMPANIC MEMBRANE

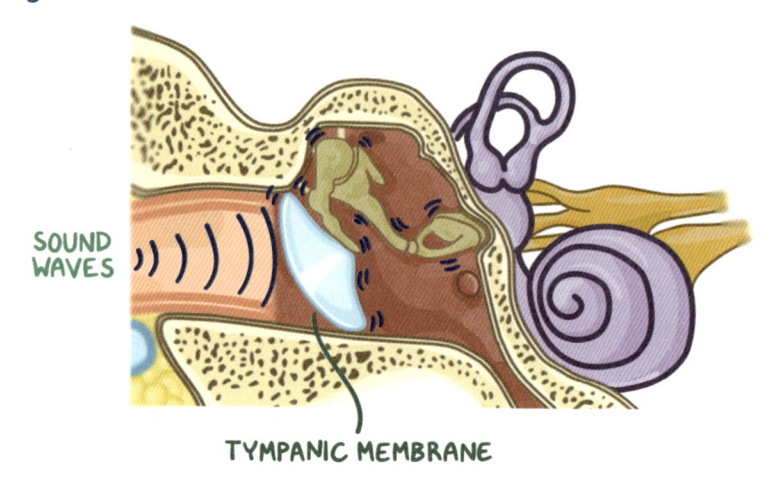

Figure 15.5

MIDDLE EAR

* AIR-FILLED CAVITY
* INSIDE TEMPORAL BONE

- ROOF EPITYMPANIC RECESS
- MASTOID ANTRUM
- POSTERIOR WALL
- EARDRUM LATERAL WALL
- OVAL WINDOW
- INTERNAL WALL
  - SEPARATES MIDDLE & INNER EAR
- ANTERIOR WALL
- FLOOR
- ROUND WINDOW

1. EQUALIZES PRESSURE across TYMPANIC MEMBRANE
2. PROTECTS from REFLUX of FLUIDS from NASOPHARYNX
3. CLEARS OUT MIDDLE EAR SECRETIONS

EUSTACHIAN TUBE
  - CONNECTS to NASOPHARYNX

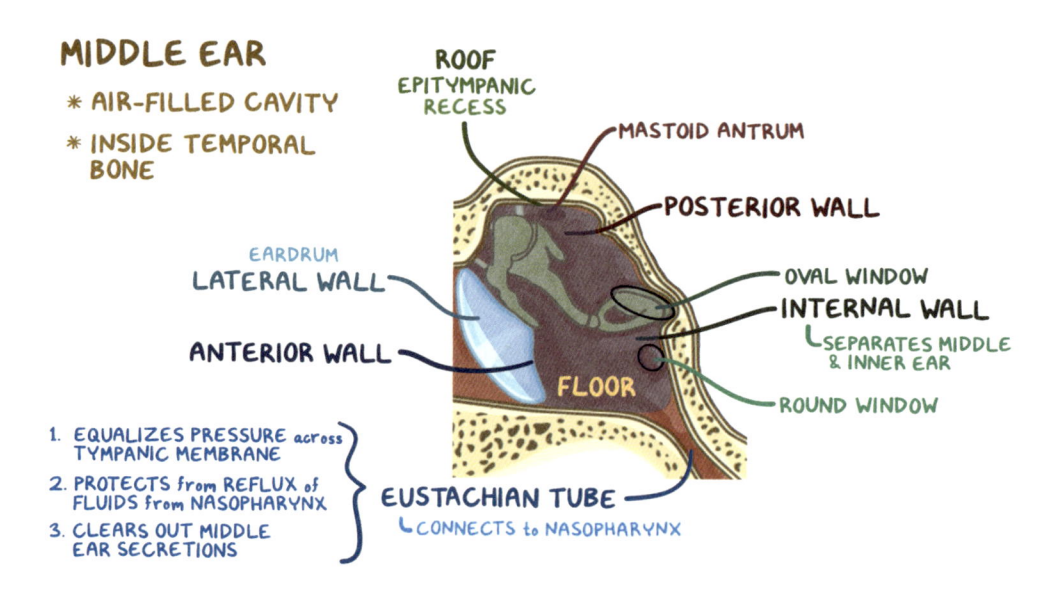

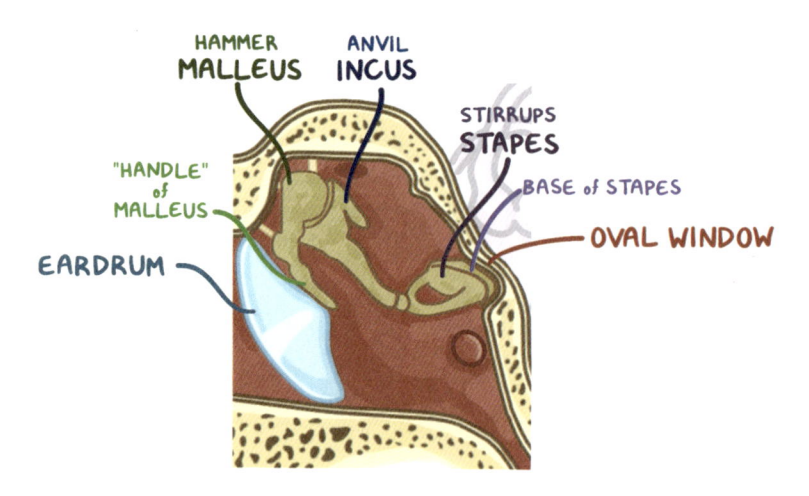

Figure 15.6

MIDDLE EAR CHAMBER

- HAMMER MALLEUS
- ANVIL INCUS
- STIRRUPS STAPES
- "HANDLE" of MALLEUS
- BASE of STAPES
- EARDRUM
- OVAL WINDOW

Figure 15.7

MIDDLE EAR CHAMBER

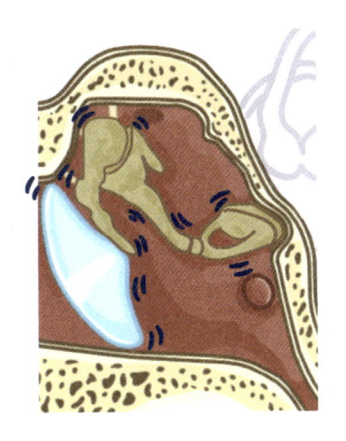

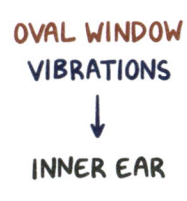

OVAL WINDOW VIBRATIONS
↓
INNER EAR

INNER EAR

The inner ear, sometimes called the labyrinth, is a marvelous bit of anatomical engineering. On the outside, the inner ear has a tough bony shell—the bony labyrinth. Inside the bony labyrinth is the membranous labyrinth. Now, both of these are filled with fluid: the bony labyrinth contains a fluid called perilymph, while the membranous labyrinth contains endolymph. The bony and membranous labyrinth make up the structure of all three parts of the inner ear: the vestibule, cochlea, and semicircular canals. Think of the first part, the vestibule, as a hallway that leads us to the remaining two rooms: one room containing the cochlea, towards the front of our head, that deals with hearing; and a second room containing the three semicircular canals, towards the back, that plays a role in balance. The movement of perilymph and endolymph within this labyrinth forms the basis for both hearing and balance **(Figure 15.8)**.

The cochlea is shaped like a snail's shell. If we take a cross-section of the inside, we'll find three parts: from top to bottom, the scala vestibuli, cochlear duct, and scala tympani. The scala vestibuli is connected to the middle ear through the oval window and contains perilymph. The cochlear duct is filled with endolymph and houses the organ of Corti—the mastermind of our hearing sense, which contains our hearing receptors, or hair cells. Finally, the scala tympani is connected to the middle ear through the round window and it contains perilymph **(Figure 15.9)**.

But how does this help me hear, you ask? Let's say your kitten starts to meow for food at 6:00 AM—even though her bowl is still half full, of course. When she meows, the sound vibrations travel through the external ear and the ossicles in the middle ear. When the foot of the stapes beats against the oval window, it transfers the vibrations over to the perilymph inside the scala vestibuli, forcing the fluid into motion. This motion transmits to the organ of Corti inside the cochlear duct. The hearing receptors convert the vibrations into an electrical impulse and the electrical impulse is sent to the brain via the auditory branch of the cranial nerve VIII. Meanwhile, the perilymph inside the scala tympani is also set in motion. This makes the round window bulge back out towards the middle ear, relieving pressure **(Figure 15.10)**.

Now your brain knows the cat is meowing, and you want to get out of bed and feed it. But even the tiniest movement, like removing your head from the pillow, engages the second part of your inner ear, the vestibular apparatus. The vestibular apparatus has two parts: the first part is the three semicircular canals; and the second part includes both the utricle and saccule, which each deal with different aspects of balance **(Figure 15.11)**.

Figure 15.8

INNER EAR - LABYRINTH

- SEMICIRCULAR CANALS ~ BALANCE
- MEMBRANOUS LABYRINTH ~ FILLED with ENDOLYMPH
- VESTIBULE
- BONY LABYRINTH ~ FILLED with PERILYMPH
- COCHLEA ~ HEARING

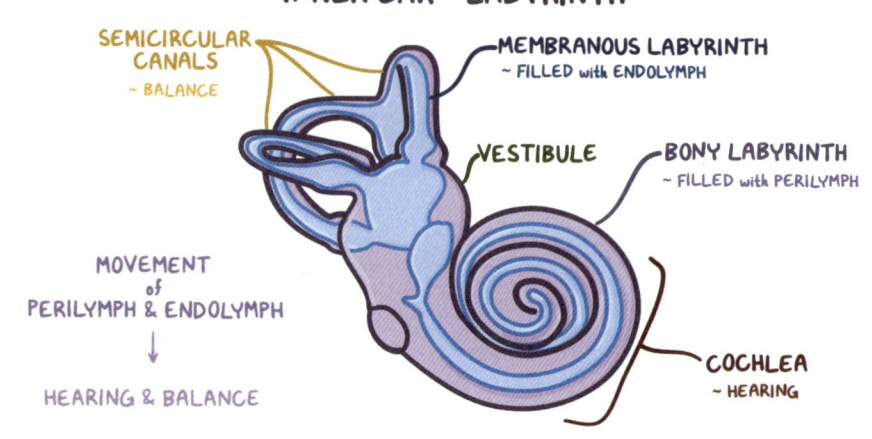

MOVEMENT of PERILYMPH & ENDOLYMPH ↓ HEARING & BALANCE

Figure 15.9

COCHLEA

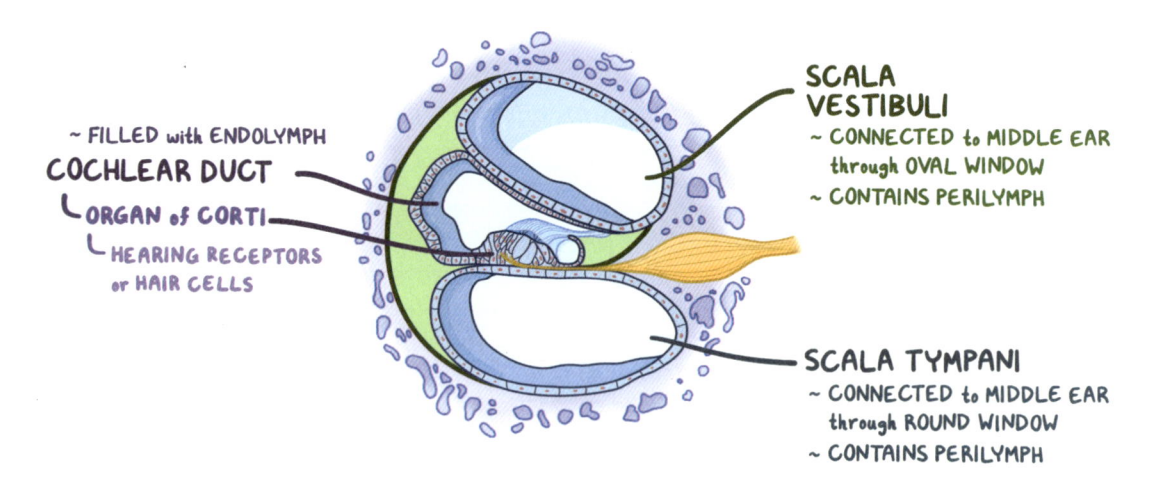

- COCHLEAR DUCT ~ FILLED with ENDOLYMPH
  - ORGAN of CORTI
    - HEARING RECEPTORS or HAIR CELLS
- SCALA VESTIBULI
  - ~ CONNECTED to MIDDLE EAR through OVAL WINDOW
  - ~ CONTAINS PERILYMPH
- SCALA TYMPANI
  - ~ CONNECTED to MIDDLE EAR through ROUND WINDOW
  - ~ CONTAINS PERILYMPH

Figure 15.10

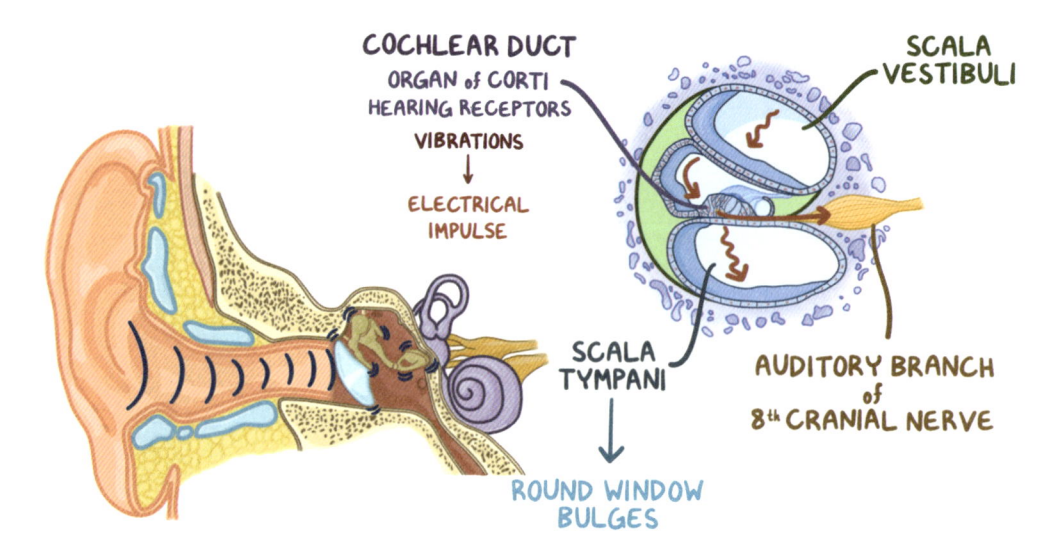

COCHLEAR DUCT
ORGAN of CORTI
HEARING RECEPTORS
VIBRATIONS ↓ ELECTRICAL IMPULSE

SCALA VESTIBULI

SCALA TYMPANI ↓ ROUND WINDOW BULGES

AUDITORY BRANCH of 8th CRANIAL NERVE

152 OSMOSIS.ORG

Chapter 15 The Ear

Figure 15.11

VESTIBULAR APPARATUS

- SEMICIRCULAR CANALS
- BALANCE
  - UTRICLE
  - SACCULE

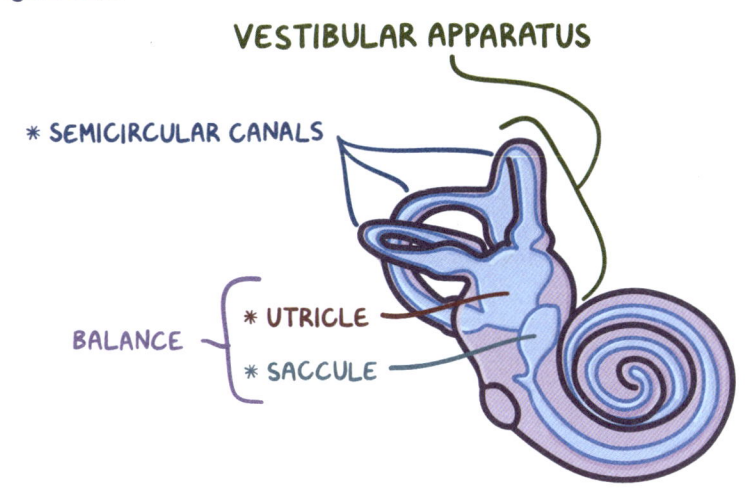

Figure 15.12

SEMICIRCULAR CANALS

ENDOLYMPH MOVES
↓
HAIR CELLS FIRE ELECTRICAL SIGNAL
↓
VESTIBULAR BRANCH of 8th CRANIAL NERVE
↓
BRAIN

POSTERIOR
ANTERIOR
LATERAL
90°
MEMBRANOUS SEMICIRCULAR DUCT
* CONTAINS ENDOLYMPH
UTRICLE
AMPULLA
~ DYNAMIC EQUILIBRIUM
HAIR CELLS

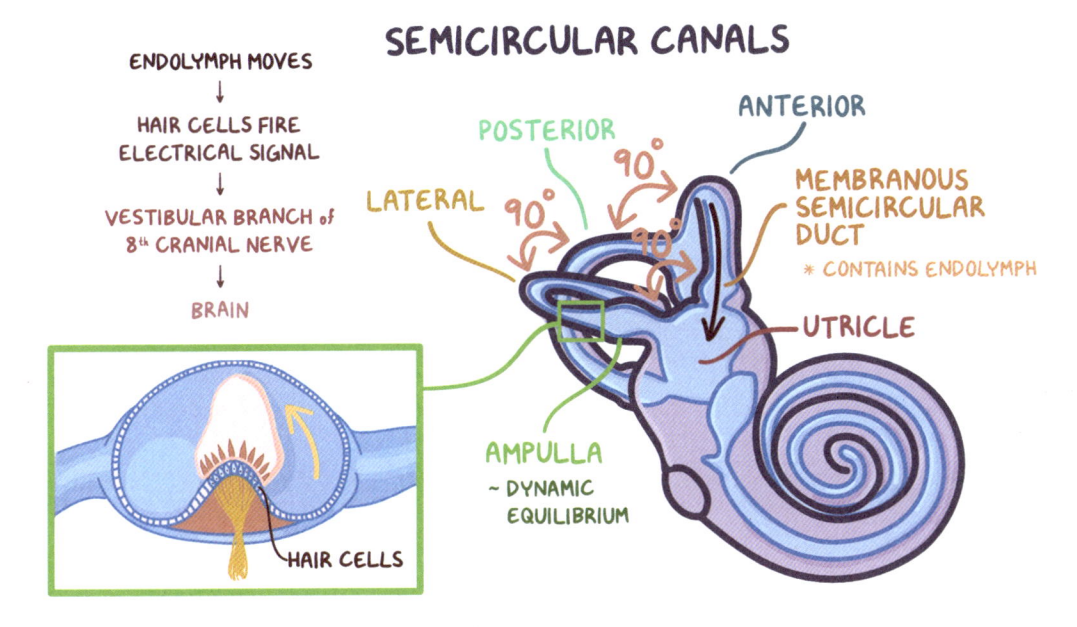

Figure 15.13

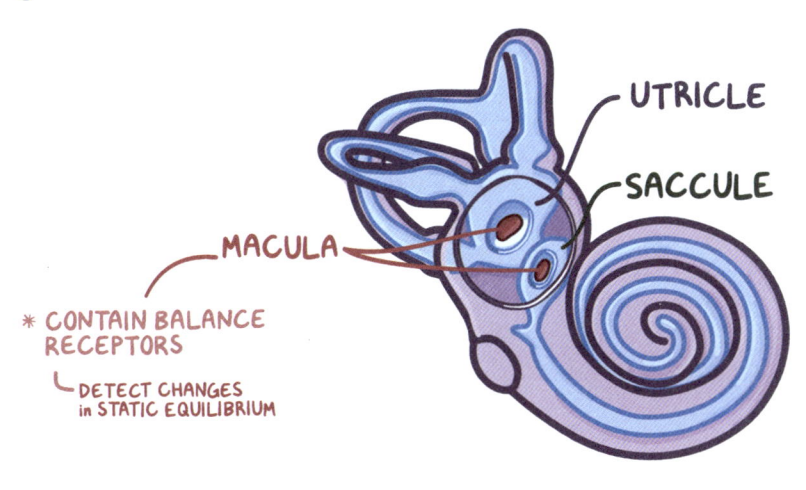

UTRICLE
SACCULE
MACULA
* CONTAIN BALANCE RECEPTORS
  - DETECT CHANGES in STATIC EQUILIBRIUM

The three semicircular canals are shaped like three letter Us—oriented in the three directions of space, with each of them forming a 90° angle with the other two. Think of a corner of your kitten's litter box, where the three sides meet. There's an anterior, posterior, and lateral semicircular canal, and inside each angle is a membranous semicircular duct. This duct contains endolymph and opens in the utricle. At one end of these canals, there is an enlarged portion called the ampulla. The ampula detects changes in our head rotation—our dynamic equilibrium. Inside the ampulla, there are balance receptors, also called hair cells. When we rise from bed to feed the cat, the endolymph inside the canals moves and the hair cells fire off an electrical signal. That signal's picked up by the vestibular branch of the cranial nerve VIII and is carried all the way up to the brain **(Figure 15.12)**.

Finally, we have the utricle and the saccule, which are also filled with endolymph. Both have a region called the macula, which contains sensory cells called balance receptors. Balance receptors detect changes in our head position in relation to horizontal or vertical acceleration—our static equilibrium. Think, for example, of being pushed backwards in the seat in a speeding car, or the sensation of being pushed downwards in a descending elevator **(Figure 15.13)**.

SUMMARY

All right, as a quick recap, the ear is the organ responsible for our sense of hearing and balance. Sound waves enter the outer ear and cause the eardrum to vibrate. Those vibrations are amplified by the tiny bones of the middle ear and eventually reach the inner ear. In the inner ear, the motion of perilymph and endolymph converts sound waves into electrical impulses, which are sent to the brain. The inner ear also houses the vestibular apparatus, which is made up of the three semicircular canals, which perceive rotational movement, and both the utricle and saccule, which detect our head position in relation to gravity **(Figure 15.14)**.

Figure 15.14

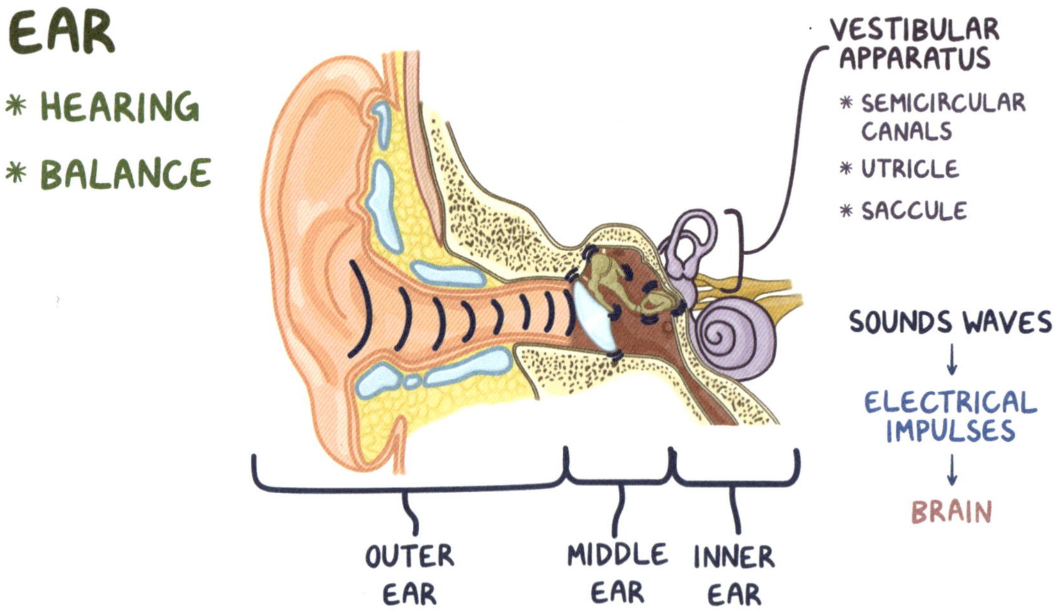

THE EYE

osms.it/eye_anatomy

Our eyes allow us to see the world around us. They make this possible by converting light waves into neural signals for our our brains to process. The eye itself is shaped like a sphere that is elongated horizontally, as opposed to being perfectly round. Only one-sixth of the eye, called the anterior, is visible **(Figure 16.1)**. The rest of the eye is contained within the orbit, or eye socket, of the skull **(Figure 16.2)**. In total, the eye consists of three layers: the outermost fibrous layer, which includes the sclera and cornea; the middle vascular layer, which includes the iris, pupil, choroid, and ciliary body; and the inner neural layer, which includes the retina and its own inner neural layer and outer pigmented layer.

Figure 16.1

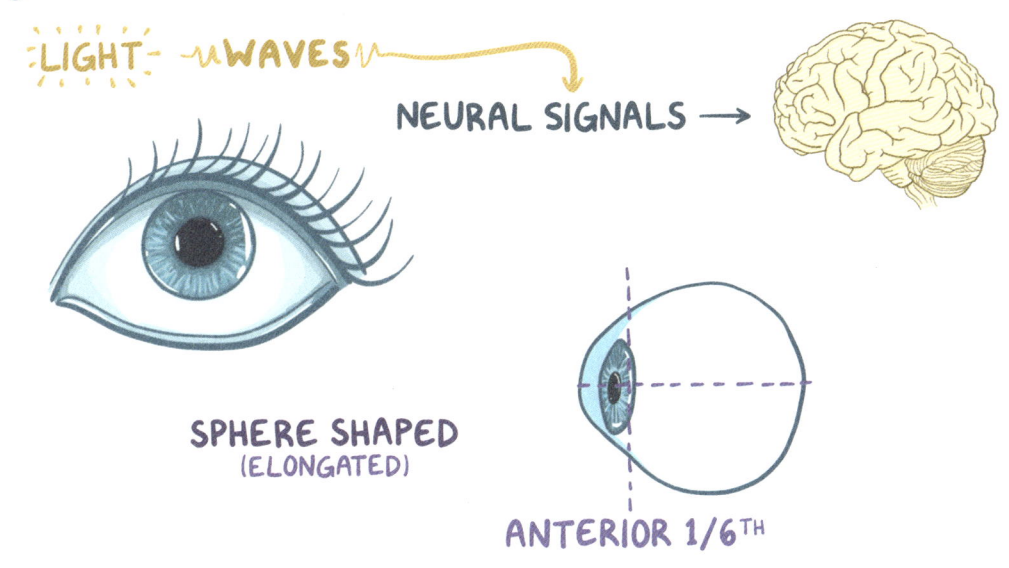

Figure 16.2

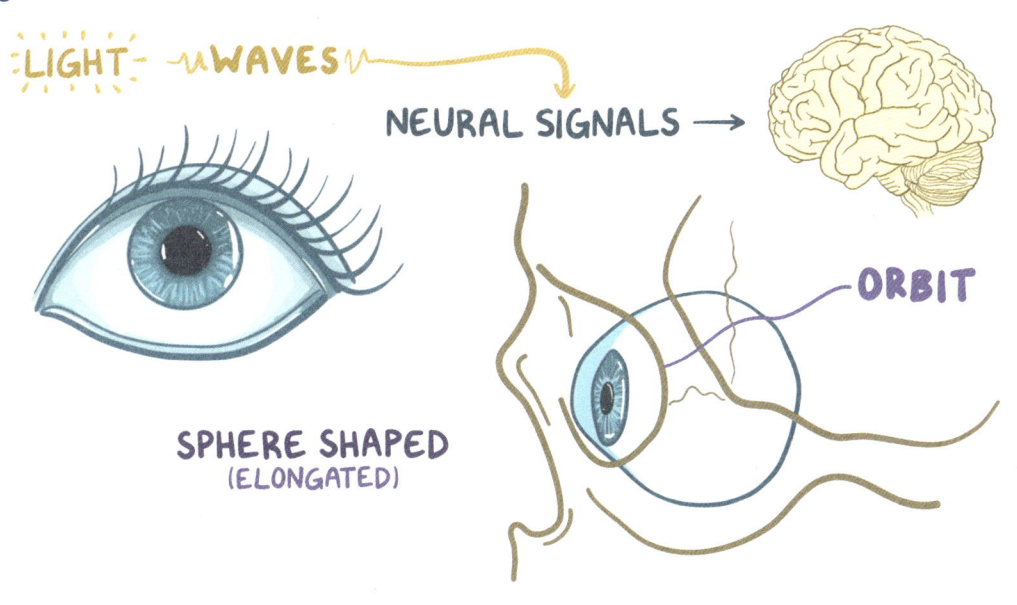

OUTER FIBROUS LAYER

The outer fibrous layer contains two main structures: the sclera and the cornea. The sclera makes up the majority of the outer layer and is the white portion of the eye. It's a tough fibrous covering that protects the more delicate structures within the eye. It is also an anchoring point to which the extrinsic eye muscles attach. The sclera is like a wall that's built around the eye. It has a tiny opening at the back, through which the optic nerve enters. As the sclera approaches the anterior portion of the eye, it reaches a transition point. This point is known as the corneal limbus and it is where the sclera becomes the cornea.

The cornea is a transparent, dome-shaped, clear layer that covers the iris and the pupil. It allows light to enter the eye and its curved shape helps focus light on the retina in the back of the eye. At the periphery of the cornea, there are stratified squamous epithelial cells, which continually divide and regenerate the cornea. These cells assist in healing after a corneal injury or abrasion. The cornea doesn't contain blood vessels; therefore, immune cells can't access the cornea. As a result, it's one of the few parts of the body that is "immune privileged." It can be transplanted without the fear of an immune response and organ rejection **(Figure 16.3)**.

MIDDLE VASCULAR LAYER

Moving inwardly from the fibrous layer, the next layer of the eye is the middle vascular layer, which is also called the uvea. Structures within this layer include the iris, pupil, choroid, and ciliary body **(Figure 16.4)**. The word *iris* derives from the Greek for "rainbow." The iris is, after all, the colorful part of the eye. Eye color is determined by the amount of melanin in the iris. People with a high concentration of melanin have dark brown eyes, those with medium amounts have green eyes, and those with low concentrations have blue eyes. The iris sits behind the cornea and is composed of two distinct muscle groups: the sphincter pupillae muscle, sometimes called circular muscle, and the dilator pupillae muscle, otherwise known as radial muscle. These muscles help control the the size of the pupil, the central opening at the center of the iris. The sphincter pupillae muscle surrounds the iris like a tiny circle. In bright light, this muscle tightens around the pupillary opening, reducing the pupil's size. In the dark, the dilator pupillae muscle pulls the iris radially, or outwardly, from the pupil. This increases the diameter of the pupillary opening, allowing more light to enter **(Figure 16.5)**.

After light passes through the cornea and pupillary opening of the iris, it reaches a biconvex transparent structure called the lens, which is located in a space called the posterior chamber. By biconvex, we mean the lens is curved on both sides. The lens itself can bend, allowing it to become flatter or rounder. This, in turn, bends the light entering the eye **(Figure 16.6)**.

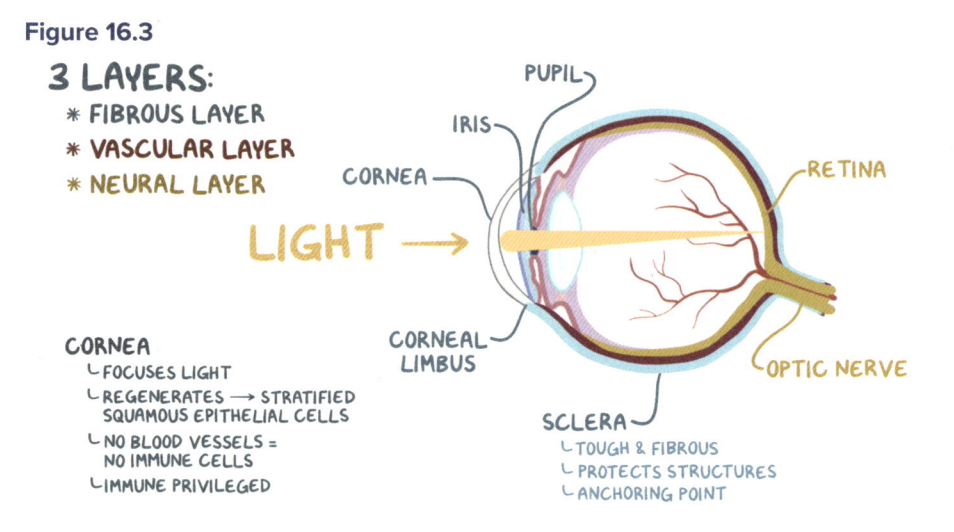

Figure 16.3

Chapter 16 The Eye

Figure 16.4

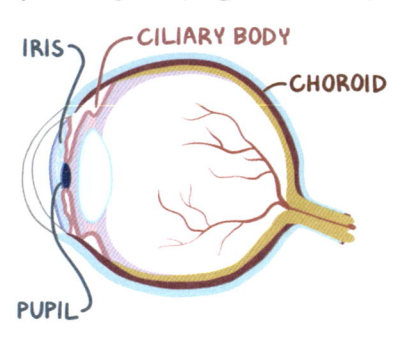

VASCULAR LAYER (UVEA)

- IRIS
- CILIARY BODY
- CHOROID
- PUPIL

Figure 16.5

VASCULAR LAYER (UVEA)

- PUPIL
- IRIS
- DILATOR PUPILLAE MUSCLE (RADIAL MUSCLE)
- SPHINCTER PUPILLAE MUSCLE (CIRCULAR MUSCLE)

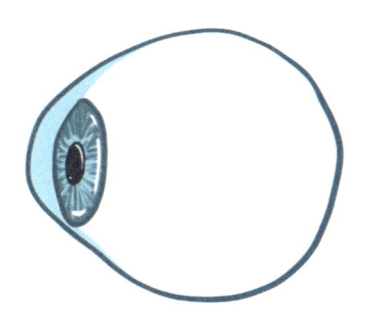

EYE COLOR: DETERMINED BY MELANIN
↑ CONCENTRATION OF MELANIN → DARK BROWN
MEDIUM → GREEN EYES
↓ CONCENTRATION → BLUE EYES

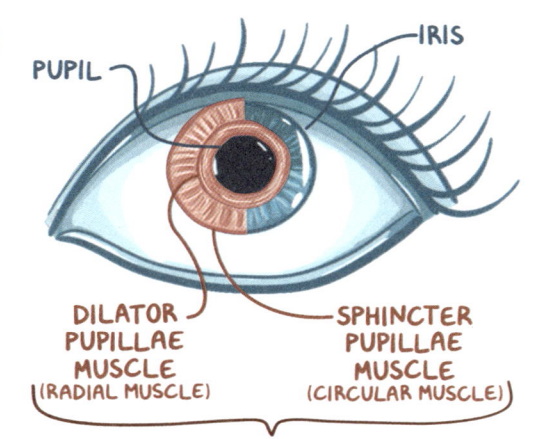

CONTROL PUPIL SIZE
↑ LIGHT → MUSCLE TIGHTENS → ↓ PUPIL SIZE
↓ LIGHT → MUSCLE PULLS IRIS RADIALLY → ↑ PUPIL SIZE

Figure 16.6

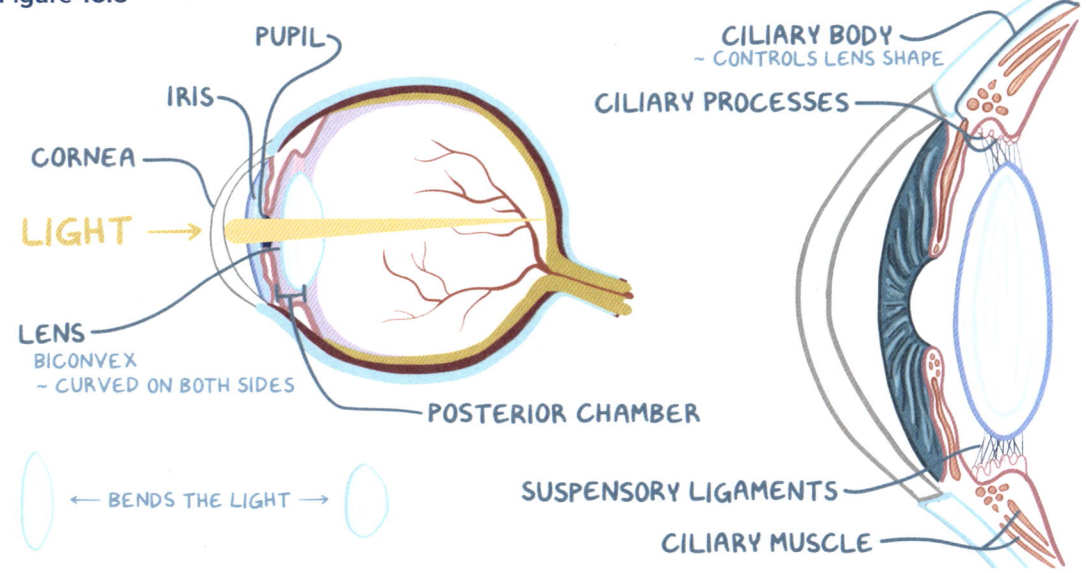

- PUPIL
- IRIS
- CORNEA
- LIGHT →
- LENS
  BICONVEX
  ~ CURVED ON BOTH SIDES
- POSTERIOR CHAMBER
- CILIARY BODY
  ~ CONTROLS LENS SHAPE
- CILIARY PROCESSES
- SUSPENSORY LIGAMENTS
- CILIARY MUSCLE

← BENDS THE LIGHT →

OSMOSIS.ORG 157

A structure called the ciliary body controls the degree to which the lens becomes flatter or rounder. The ciliary body includes the ciliary muscle and tiny projections from the ciliary muscle called ciliary processes. The ciliary processes connect to suspensory ligaments, which attach directly to the lens. They hold the lens in place behind the iris. They also help it change shape. When the ciliary muscles contract, the ciliary processes pull on the suspensory ligaments—like a taut rope—and the lens becomes flatter.

The final structure of the vascular layer is a membrane called the choroid, which is full of blood vessels that provide nutrients to most of the eye. The choroid is dark brown in color, and this allows it to absorb light. Without the choroid, light would be more likely to reflect and scatter within the eye, thereby preventing the light from being focused on the retina, which is necessary for visual processing **(Figure 16.7)**.

INNER NEURAL LAYER

The third and innermost layer of the eye is the retina. The retina includes an inner neural layer, which contains ganglion cells. These ganglion cells synapse with bipolar cells, which then synapse with the photoreceptors—both rods and cones. The retina also includes an outer pigmented layer, which consists of a one-cell-thick layer of pigmented epithelial cells. When light enters the eyes, it hits the retina, travels past the ganglion cells and bipolar cells, and, finally, hits the rods and cones. The light that doesn't hit the photoreceptors arrives at the pigmented layer, where the light is absorbed so that it doesn't scatter and bounce back to the photoreceptors **(Figure 16.8)**.

The rods are more numerous than the cones. Each eye has about 120 million rods. They are highly sensitive to light; even a single photon can cause them to activate. This means they are wonderfully equipped for seeing in low light conditions. The downside is that they only offer black and white vision.

In comparison, there are only about 6 million cones in each eye. Most of these are located in the macula—an oval spot in the middle of the posterior retina. At the center of the macula is the fovea, which contains the highest concentration of cones. The macula is the part of the retina that offers the highest visual acuity. Cones are less sensitive than rods to light, but each cone can detect one of the following: a red, green, or blue wavelength of light. For example, when you see a red apple, only the red cones are activated. When you see a purple flower, however, both the red and blue cones are activated **(Figure 16.9)**.

Figure 16.7

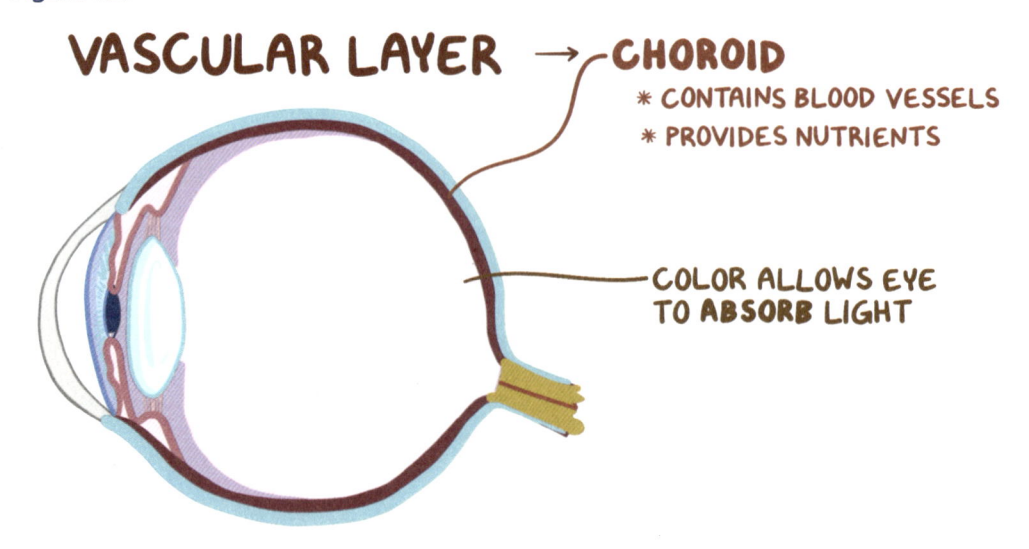

Chapter 16 The Eye

Figure 16.8

- RETINA ~ INNER NEURAL LAYER
- PHOTORECEPTORS
  - RODS & CONES
- PIGMENTED EPITHELIAL CELLS
  * LIGHT IS ABSORBED
- BIPOLAR CELLS
- GANGLION CELLS
- LIGHT

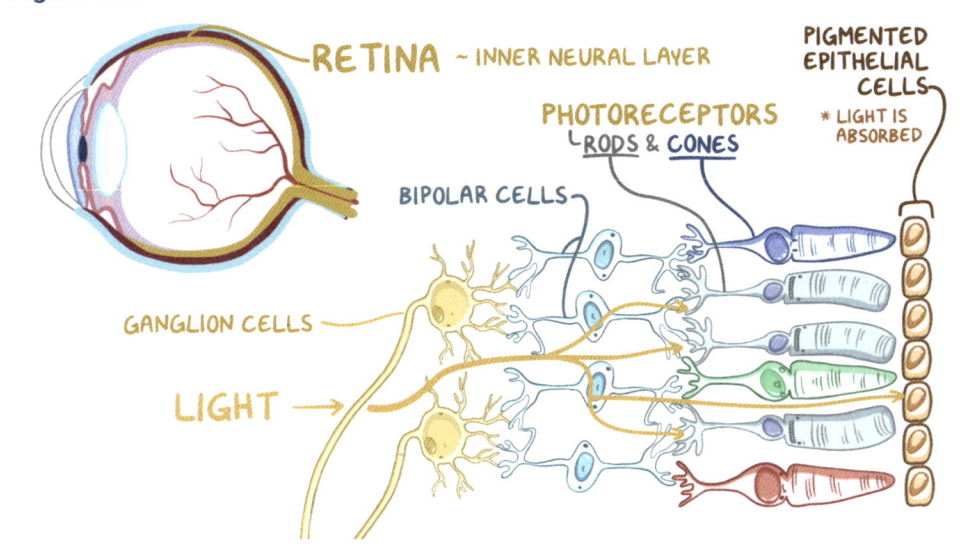

Figure 16.9

- MACULA
- OPTIC DISC (BLIND SPOT)
- OPTIC NERVE
- FOVEA
  * ↑ CONE CONCENTRATION
  * ↑ VISUAL ACUITY
- CONES
  - 6 MILLION / EYE
  - ↓ LIGHT SENSITIVE
  - DETECT RED, GREEN, OR BLUE LIGHT
- RODS
  - 120 MILLION / EYE
  - ↑ LIGHT SENSITIVE
  - BLACK & WHITE VISION

ACTION POTENTIAL
↓
DEPOLARIZATION
↓
VISUAL INFO
↓
BRAIN

ACTIVATED
FORMS OPTIC NERVE

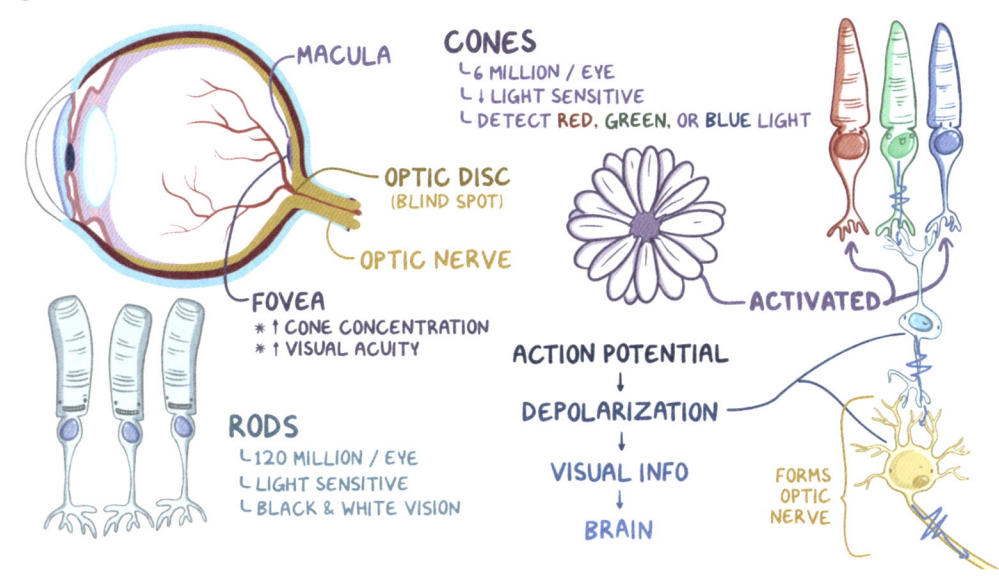

Figure 16.10

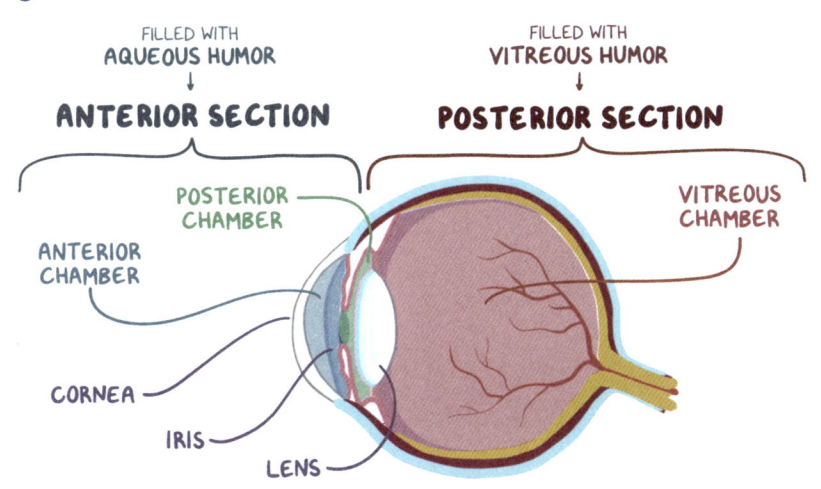

FILLED WITH AQUEOUS HUMOR
↓
ANTERIOR SECTION

FILLED WITH VITREOUS HUMOR
↓
POSTERIOR SECTION

- POSTERIOR CHAMBER
- ANTERIOR CHAMBER
- CORNEA
- IRIS
- LENS
- VITREOUS CHAMBER

OSMOSIS.ORG 159

When rods and cones are activated, they depolarize and create an action potential. This triggers the depolarization of the bipolar cells, which then triggers the depolarization of the ganglion cells. The action potential in the ganglion cells travels through their axons to the posterior portion of the retina to form the optic nerve, which leaves the eye through the optic disc medial to the macula. The optic disc doesn't have any photoreceptors, so it's known as the blind spot. The optic nerve then carries the visual information to the brain, where we process and recognize the visual information.

CHAMBERS OF THE EYE: ANTERIOR, POSTERIOR, & VITREOUS

Finally, let's zoom out and look at the eye as a whole. If we take a cross section of the eye, we can see that it's split up into different chambers: the anterior, posterior, and vitreous chambers. The anterior chamber includes the area from the cornea to the iris. Meanwhile, the posterior chamber is only a narrow space between the iris and the lens. The larger vitreous chamber includes the space between the lens and the back of the eye. Now, the following information may be a bit confusing: both the anterior and posterior chambers are located in the anterior section of the eye, and the vitreous chamber is located in the posterior section of the eye.

Typically, all of the chambers in the eye are filled with fluid. The anterior section—containing the anterior and posterior chambers—is filled with a liquid called aqueous humor. The posterior section—containing the vitreous chamber—is filled with vitreous humor. The aqueous humor is a transparent, watery fluid. It is secreted by the ciliary epithelium. In addition to secreting aqueous humor and providing nutrients to the lens and cornea, the ciliary epithelium provides structural support and helps to keep the shape of the eye.

The aqueous humor is secreted into the posterior chamber, then flows through a narrow space between the front of the lens and the back of the iris, and then through the pupil to the anterior chamber. From the anterior chamber, the fluid flows out of the eye through the trabecular meshwork, which is a spongy tissue that acts like a drain. This allows the fluid to enter a circular channel, called the canal of Schlemm, and, finally, the aqueous veins—part of the episcleral venous system, which are the veins around the sclera of the eye **(Figure 16.11)**.

Figure 16.11

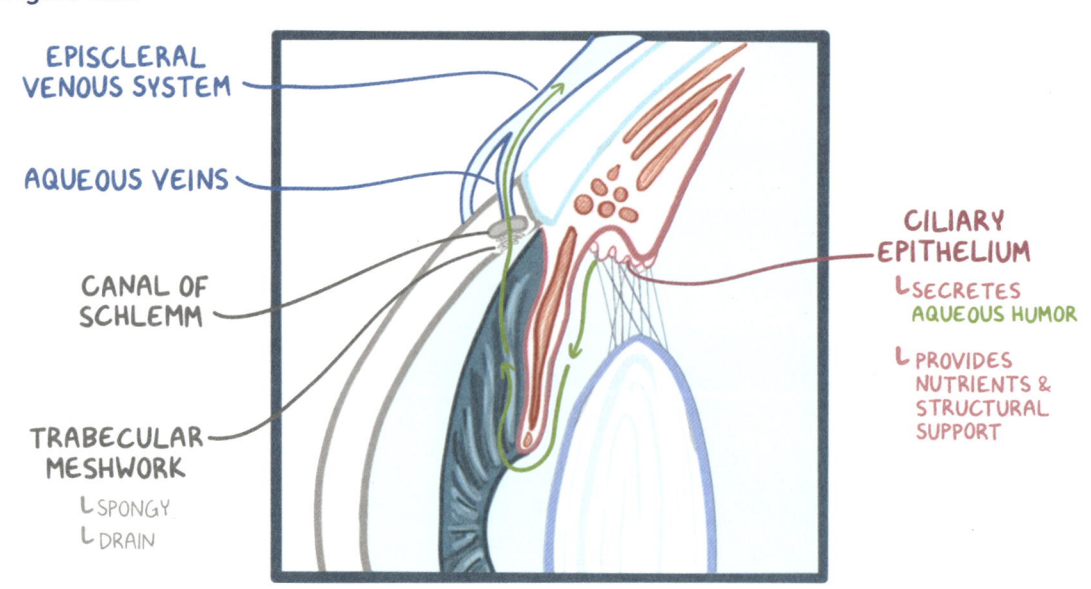

SUMMARY

All right, as a quick recap, the wall of the eye is made up of three major layers: the fibrous outer layer, which contains the cornea and sclera; the middle vascular layer, which contains the iris, pupil, choroid, and ciliary body; and, finally, the inner neural layer, which contains the retina with its own outer pigmented layer and inner neural layer. The inner neural layer of the retina is composed of photoreceptor cells that convert light into neural signals, which travel via the optic nerve to the brain for visual processing **(Figure 16.12)**.

Figure 16.12

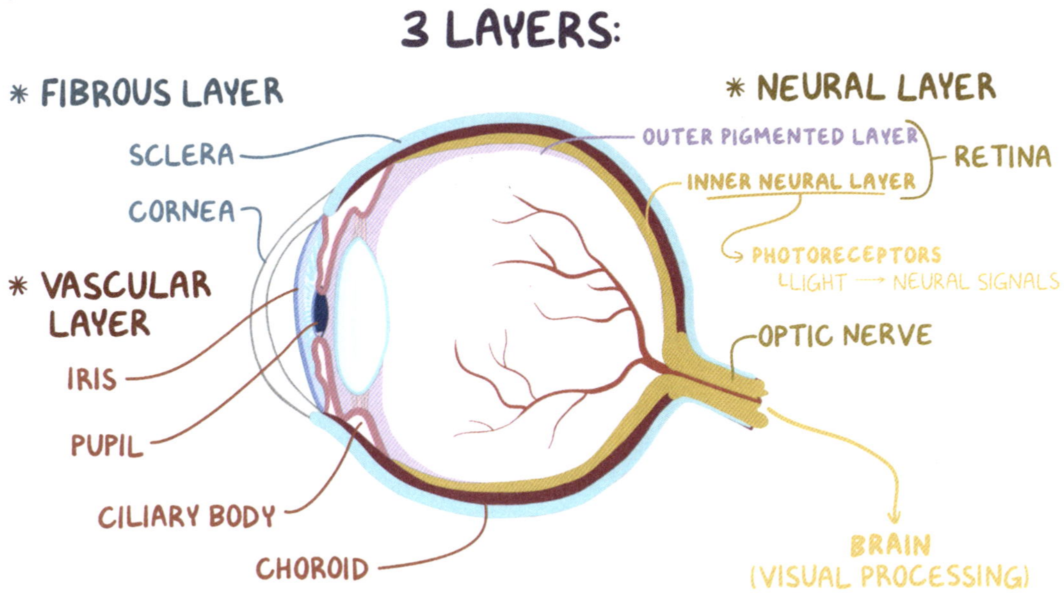

THE TONGUE

osms.it/tongue_anatomy

The tongue is a muscular organ in the mouth. It's the most flexible muscle in the body, and is used for many things like speech, chewing and swallowing food. Most important of all, it's involved in gustation—tasting delicious foods **(Figure 17.1)**!

TONGUE MUSCULATURE

The tongue's surface is covered by a mucus membrane called the mucosa. Below the mucosa, there's a combination of intrinsic and extrinsic muscles, all of which are innervated by cranial nerve 12, the hypoglossal nerve. Intrinsic muscles start and end within the tongue and help change its shape, while extrinsic muscles attach to structures outside the tongue and help guide its movement **(Figure 17.2)**.

Figure 17.1

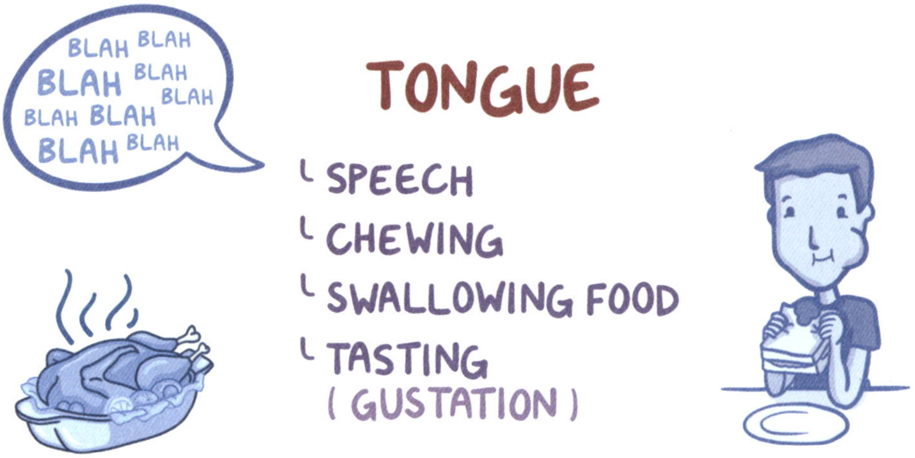

Figure 17.2

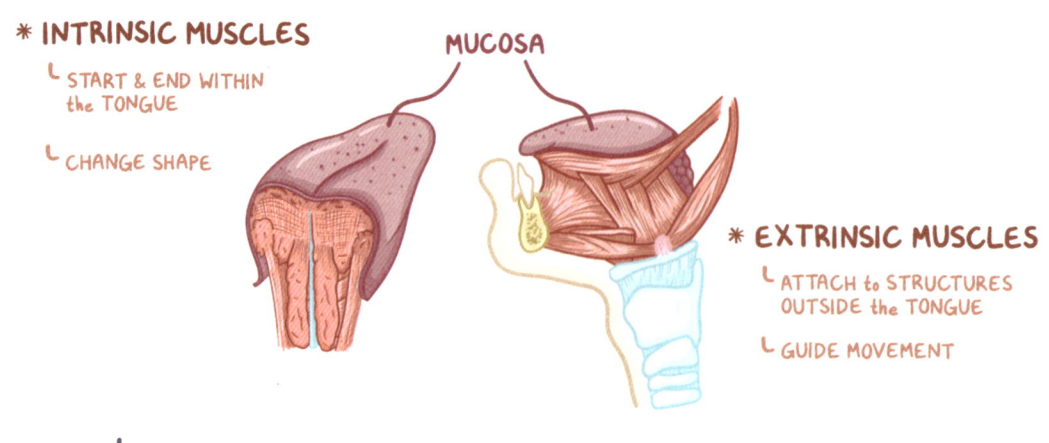

Chapter 17 The Tongue

PAPILLAE

There's a V-shaped groove on the tongue called the sulcus terminalis, which runs across its posterior portion and divides it into a posterior third and an anterior two-thirds. The posterior third of the tongue is covered in bumps made of lymphoid tissue called lingual papillae; these contain B and T cells that help fight off pathogens entering the mouth. The anterior two-thirds of the tongue is covered in smaller lumps called papillae, which help increase the tongue's surface area and give it a rough texture so food particles can stick to it **(Figure 17.3)**.

There are four types of papillae found across the different regions of the tongue. The most numerous are the thread-like filiform papillae which are scattered all over the anterior two-thirds of the tongue's dorsal surface. The filiform papillae are in charge of the tongue's sensation of touch—not taste. Next are the mushroom-shaped fungiform papillae; these are most commonly found at the tip of the tongue. The leaf-like foliate papillae are most common on the sides of the tongue. Finally, there are eight to 12 large, round circumvallate papillae located at the back of the anterior two-thirds of the tongue, just in front of the sulcus terminalis. The fungiform, foliate, and circumvallate papillae contain multiple taste buds, and each taste bud contains specialized epithelial cells called taste receptor cells which—yep, you guessed it!—detect taste **(Figure 17.4)**.

TASTE BUDS

Although taste buds are typically found on the tongue, some are also found on the soft palate, pharynx, epiglottis, larynx, and upper esophagus. Taste buds are oval-shaped, looking a bit like an orange **(Figure 17.5)**.

On the inside of each taste bud are specialized epithelial cells called taste receptor cells. These do the incredible work of detecting the flavors of different substances, like food. The taste receptor cells are arranged like orange wedges, with supporting cells lying in between each one. At the bottom of each taste bud are basal cells. These can differentiate into new taste receptor cells to replace the ones that die—this happens every two weeks or so. Taste receptor cells are chemoreceptors that respond to molecules found in foods and drinks, called tastants.

Figure 17.3

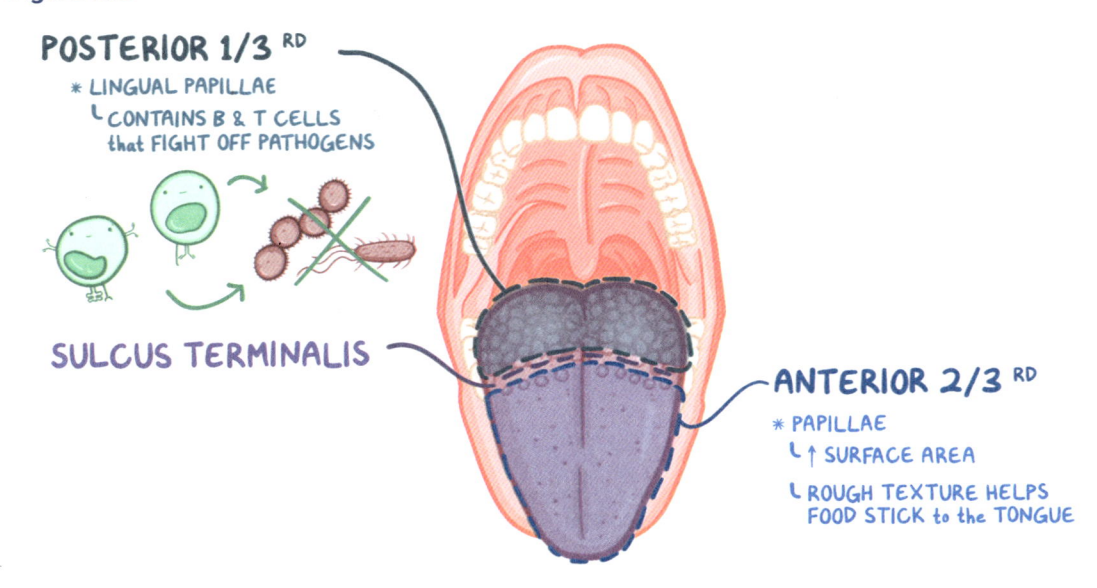

Figure 17.4

FOLIATE PAPILLAE

CIRCUMVALLATE PAPILLAE

FUNGIFORM PAPILLAE

FILIFORM PAPILLAE
- MOST NUMEROUS TYPE
- SENSATION of TOUCH (NOT TASTE)

* CONTAIN MULTIPLE **TASTE BUDS**
  - with TASTE RECEPTOR CELLS
    → DETECT TASTE

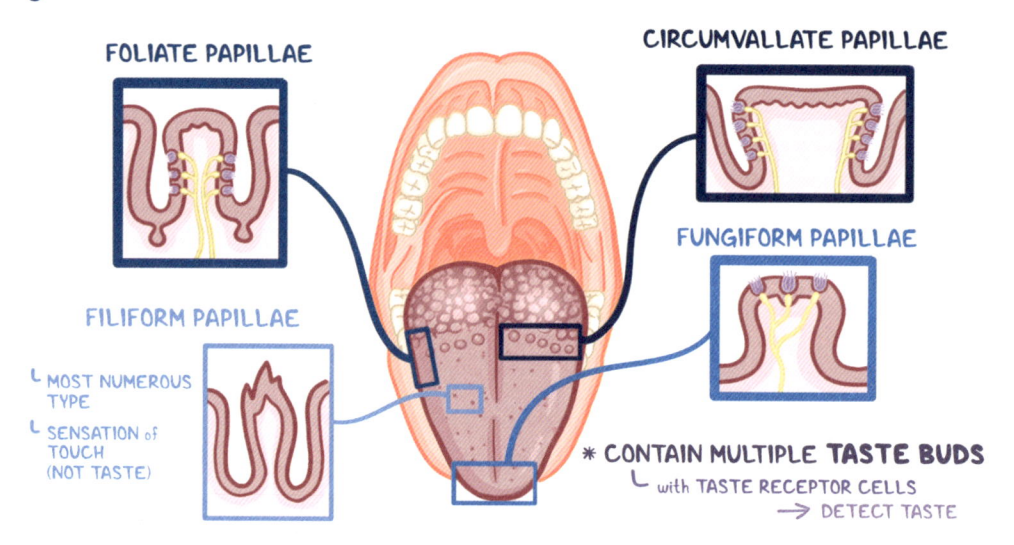

Figure 17.5

TASTE BUDS

* TYPICALLY on the TONGUE
* BUT ALSO:
  - SOFT PALATE
  - PHARYNX
  - EPIGLOTTIS
  - LARYNX
  - UPPER ESOPHAGUS

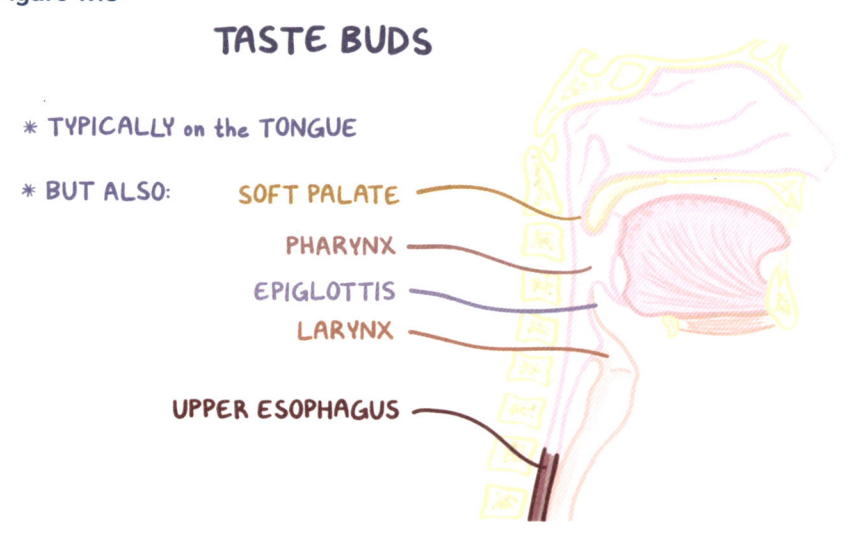

Figure 17.6

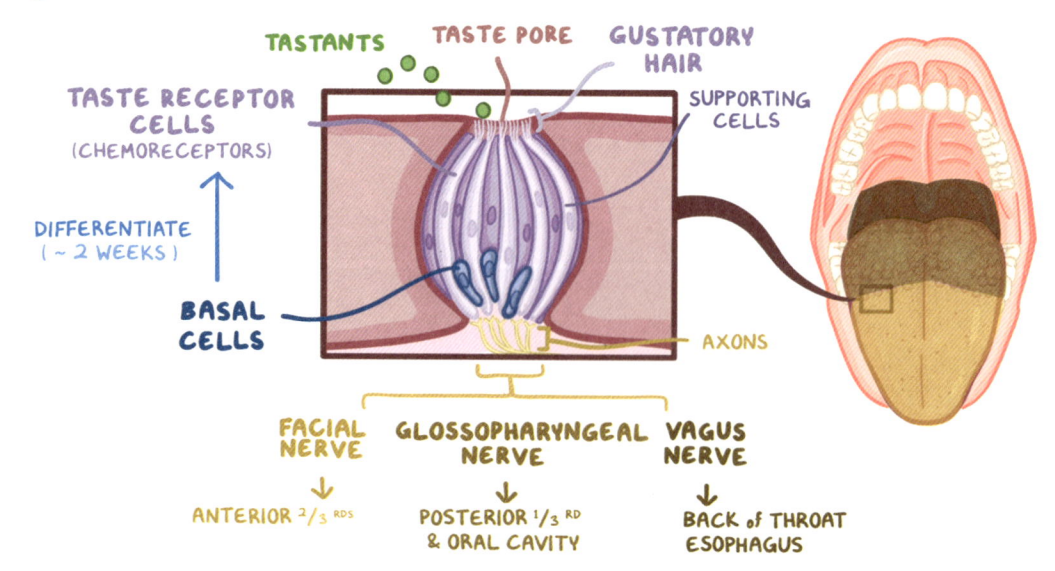

TASTANTS TASTE PORE GUSTATORY HAIR

TASTE RECEPTOR CELLS (CHEMORECEPTORS)

SUPPORTING CELLS

DIFFERENTIATE (~ 2 WEEKS)

BASAL CELLS

AXONS

FACIAL NERVE ↓ ANTERIOR 2/3 RDS

GLOSSOPHARYNGEAL NERVE ↓ POSTERIOR 1/3 RD & ORAL CAVITY

VAGUS NERVE ↓ BACK of THROAT ESOPHAGUS

The top of each taste receptor cell has a thin, hair-like microvillus called a gustatory hair, which sticks out of the taste pore, a small opening on the surface of each papillus. These hairs come into contact with tastants. Next are the cell bodies, the "orange wedges" lying within the capsule. Underneath the cell bodies are axons from one of the three nerves responsible for transmitting taste sensations to the brain: the facial nerve, which innervates taste buds from the anterior two-thirds of the tongue; the glossopharyngeal nerve, which innervates taste buds from the posterior third of the tongue and the rest of the oral cavity; and the vagus nerve, which innervates some taste buds at the back of the throat and esophagus **(Figure 17.6)**.

TASTE RECEPTOR CELLS

We have five primary tastes: bitter, salty, sour, sweet, and umami (a Japanese word describing the savory taste of meat). Each taste receptor cell is capable of detecting all five of these tastes, but responds most strongly to one of them. Taste receptor cells inside the fungiform papillae at the tongue's tip are more sensitive to sweet and umami, while the foliate papillae at the sides of the tongue are geared towards salty and sour tastes. The circumvallate papillae at the back of the tongue contain lots of bitter taste receptor cells. We sense more complex flavors like chocolate or coffee thanks to combinations of tastes receptors activating together **(Figure 17.7)**.

Now, when you eat, the chewed-up food particles get mixed up with saliva and travel to the papillae, where they make contact with the gustatory hairs poking out of the taste receptor cells. There are two mechanisms for converting a chemical signal from food into a neuron impulse. The first relates to salty or sour tastes, while the second relates to sweet, bitter, or savory tastes **(Figure 17.8)**.

Let's look at the first mechanism: let's say you eat something salty and sour, like french fries with ketchup. Sodium ions (Na$^+$) from the salty fries and hydrogen ions (H$^+$) from the sour ketchup come into contact with the gustatory hairs. The taste receptor cells contain ion channels that allow both Na$^+$ and H$^+$ ions into the cell, and the flow of ions causes the taste receptor cells' membranes to depolarize. The local depolarization raises the cells' resting membrane potential, triggering voltage-gated channels to open up, allowing extracellular calcium ions (Ca^{++}) to flow inside. The influx of Ca^{++} causes vesicles full of neurotransmitters like serotonin, acetylcholine, norepinephrine, and GABA to fuse with the cell membrane. When that happens, these neurotransmitters are released into the synaptic cleft near the neuron serving that region. Remember, the facial nerve innervates the anterior two-thirds of the tongue, the glossopharyngeal nerve innervates the posterior one-third of the tongue, and the vagus nerve innervates some taste buds at the back of the throat and esophagus. These nerves transmit the sensory information for taste to the brain.

Now, the second mechanism for converting a chemical signal into a neuron impulse relates to sweet, bitter, or savory tastes. Imagine that you're eating honey-glazed ham while drinking coffee. The gustatory hairs of the taste receptor cells that respond most strongly to these tastes have specific receptors: G protein-coupled receptors. When tastants reach the gustatory hairs, they bind to G protein-coupled receptors. This triggers a set of reactions within the taste receptor cell called a G protein-coupled receptor pathway. The G protein-coupled receptor pathway opens up Ca^{++} channels on the endoplasmic reticulum. The endoplasmic reticulum stores Ca^{++}, so when these gates open, intracellular Ca^{++} ions are released into the cell. As before, the increase in Ca^{++} ions causes vesicles full of neurotransmitters to fuse with the cell membrane, releasing neurotransmitters into the synaptic cleft. This taste information is then transmitted to the brain—just like with salty and sour tastes **(Figure 17.9)**.

Figure 17.7

5 PRIMARY TASTES

TASTE RECEPTOR CELLS DETECT ALL 5 TASTES
- BITTER
- SALTY
- SOUR
- SWEET
- UMAMI

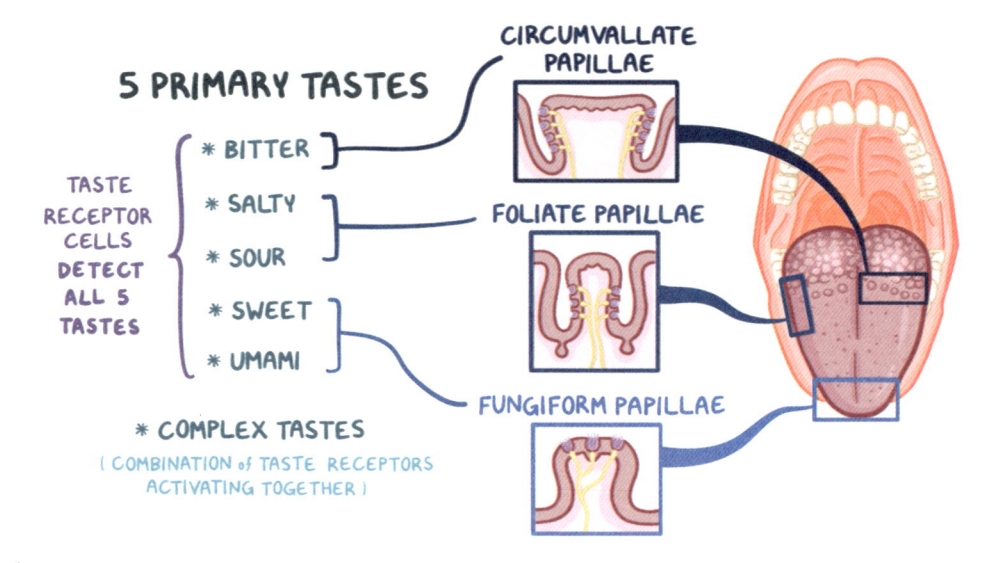

- CIRCUMVALLATE PAPILLAE
- FOLIATE PAPILLAE
- FUNGIFORM PAPILLAE

* COMPLEX TASTES
(COMBINATION of TASTE RECEPTORS ACTIVATING TOGETHER)

Figure 17.8

WHEN YOU EAT...

CHEWED UP PARTICLES → MIX with SALIVA → TRAVEL to PAPILLAE → GUSTATORY HAIRS → TASTE RECEPTOR CELLS

* CONVERTING a CHEMICAL SIGNAL → NEURON IMPULSE
  ① SALTY, SOUR TASTES
  ② SWEET, BITTER, SAVORY TASTES

Figure 17.9

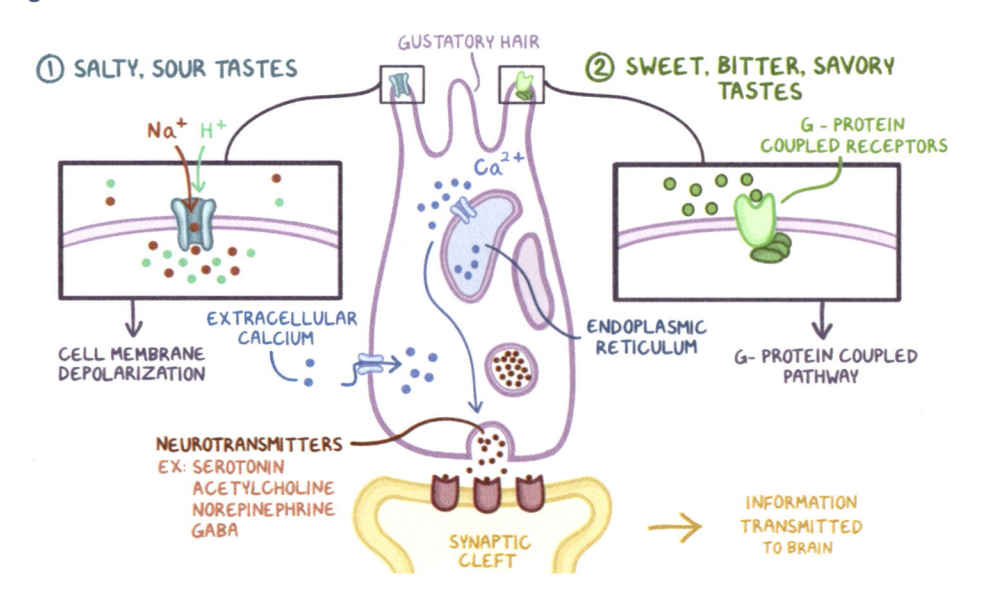

① SALTY, SOUR TASTES
- Na^+ H^+
- CELL MEMBRANE DEPOLARIZATION
- EXTRACELLULAR CALCIUM
- Ca^{2+}

② SWEET, BITTER, SAVORY TASTES
- G-PROTEIN COUPLED RECEPTORS
- ENDOPLASMIC RETICULUM
- G-PROTEIN COUPLED PATHWAY

GUSTATORY HAIR

NEUROTRANSMITTERS
EX: SEROTONIN
ACETYLCHOLINE
NOREPINEPHRINE
GABA

SYNAPTIC CLEFT → INFORMATION TRANSMITTED TO BRAIN

Chapter 17 The Tongue

FACTORS AFFECTING TASTE

So, we've established that taste receptor cells respond to tastants by transmitting taste signals through nerves to the brain. One interesting thing about taste is that when the taste receptor cells are exposed to the same levels of tastants over time, they start sending fewer and fewer signals, and eventually, they stop responding altogether. This is called adaptation, and it can start within just a few minutes of eating. This is one reason why the first bite is often the most delicious, and why some people keep adding salt or other seasonings to their food over the course of a meal **(Figure 17.10)**.

Besides adaptation, there are other factors affecting the intensity of our tasting experience. A big one is hunger, which makes taste receptor cells more sensitive to sweet and salty flavors. On the other end of the spectrum, people often have a weaker sense of taste when they have a viral infection or allergies, and that's because our sense of smell affects how we taste. The smell of food travels through the air in the form of small molecules called odorants, which stimulate smell receptors in the nose. Cranial nerve 1—the olfactory nerve—carries sensory information about smell to the brain, where it's processed alongside the sensation of taste, giving us the full sensory experience we call "flavor." Finally, age, affects taste: older people tend to have a poorer ability to taste because they don't replace taste receptors cells as quickly, and so there are fewer and fewer of these cells over time **(Figure 17.11)**.

Figure 17.10

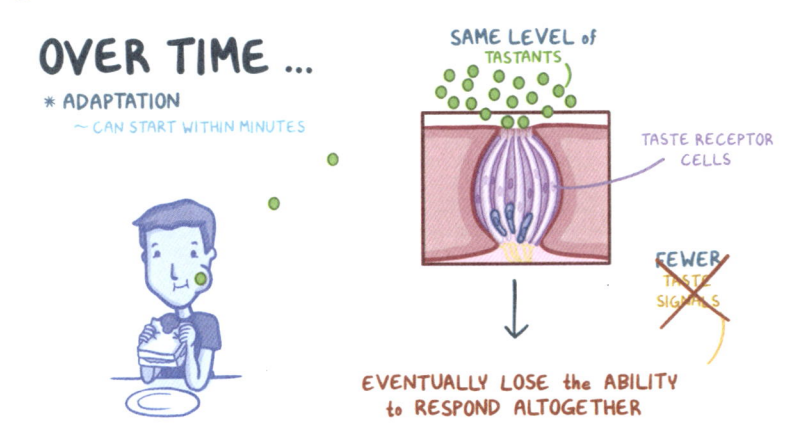

Figure 17.11

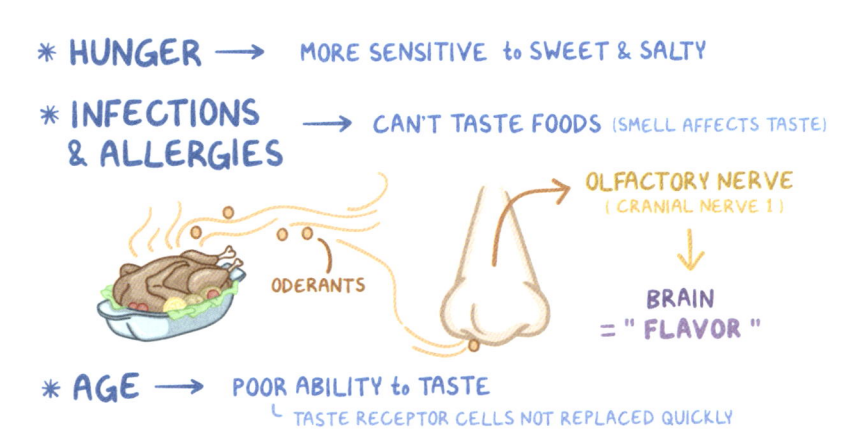

SUMMARY

Okay, as a quick recap... The tongue is covered by various types of papillae (circumvallate, foliate, filiform, and fungiform papillae) which contain different types of taste receptor cells. Each taste receptor cell can recognize all five of the major tastes (sweet, sour, salty, bitter, and umami) but is most sensitive to one of them. This sensory information is carried to the brain by the vagus, glossopharyngeal, and facial nerves. The sense of smell also plays a role in taste: the smell of the food is carried to the brain through the olfactory nerve, where it is processed together with taste information from the mouth. We recognize the final result as delicious (or disgusting) flavors **(Figure 17.12)**!

Figure 17.12

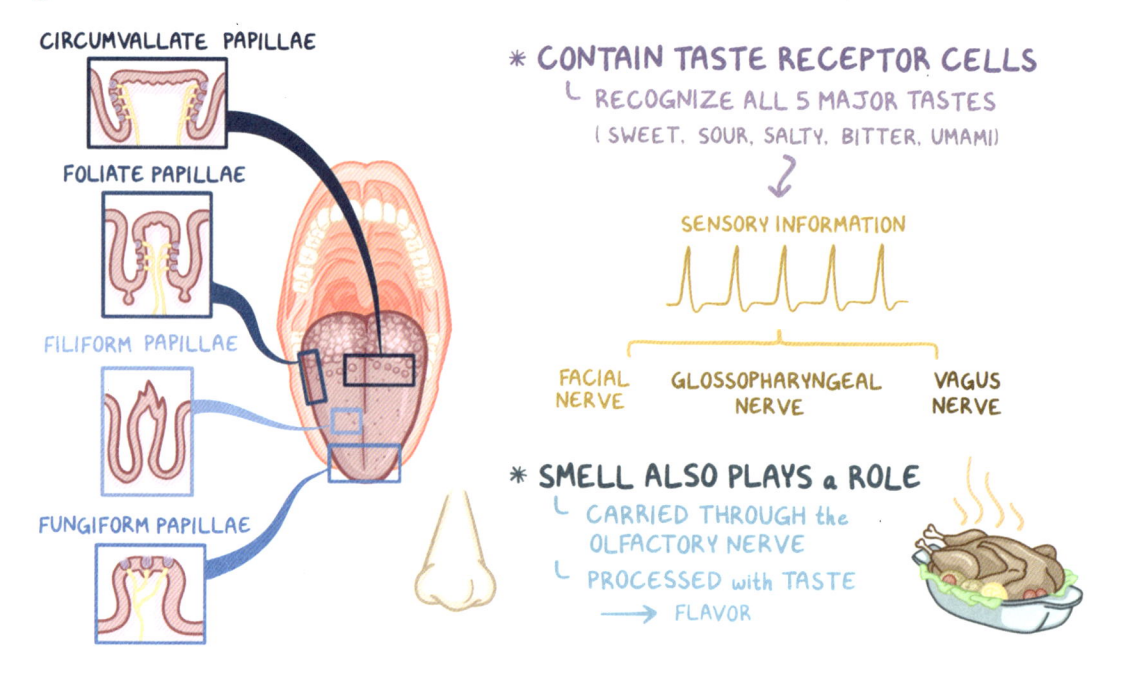

APPENDIX

CREDITS

THE CARDIOVASCULAR SYSTEM

Author: Andrea Day, MA

Editors: Fergus Baird, MA; Rishi Desai, MD; Jessica MacEachern, MA

Illustrator: Tanner Marshall, MS

THE RENAL SYSTEM

Author: Feiyang Pan

Editors: Rishi Desai, MD, MPH; Jessica MacEachern, MA; Vincent Waldman, PhD

Illustrator: Vincent Waldman, PhD

THE RESPIRATORY SYSTEM

Author: Debal Sinharoy, MBBS

Editors: Fergus Baird, MA; Rishi Desai, MD, MPH

Illustrator: Tanner Marshall, MS

THE GASTROINTESTINAL SYSTEM

Author: Antonia Syrnioti, MD candidate

Editors: Rishi Desai, MD, MPH; Jessica MacEachern, MA

Illustrator: Brittany Norton, MFA

THE ENDOCRINE SYSTEM

Author: Viviana Popa, MD candidate

Editors: Rishi Desai, MD, MPH; Jessica MacEachern, MA

Illustrator: Pauline Rowsome, BS

THE IMMUNE SYSTEM

Author: Maureen H. Richards, PhD

Editors: Rishi Desai, MD, MPH; Jessica MacEachern, MA

Illustrator: Tanner Marshall, MS

THE LYMPHATIC SYSTEM

Author: Andrea Day, MA

Editors: Rishi Desai, MD, MPH; Jessica MacEachern, MA

Illustrator: Vincent Waldman, PhD

THE HEMATOLOGIC SYSTEM

Author: Sean Watts, MD candidate

Editors: Rishi Desai, MD, MPH; Jessica MacEachern, MA

Illustrator: Brittany Norton, MFA

THE MUSCULAR SYSTEM

Author: Filip Vasiljevic, MS

Editors: Rishi Desai, MD, MPH; Jessica MacEachern, MA; Yifan Xiao, MD

Illustrator: Brittany Norton, MFA

THE SKELETAL SYSTEM

Author: Evode Iradufasha, MS

Editors: Rishi Desai, MD, MPH; Jessica MacEachern, MA; Yifan Xiao, MD

Illustrator: Brittany Norton, MFA

THE INTEGUMENTARY SYSTEM

Author: Sean Watts, MD candidate

Editors: Rishi Desai, MD, MPH; Jessica MacEachern, MA; Yifan Xiao, MD

Illustrator: Justin Ling, MD, MS

THE MALE REPRODUCTIVE SYSTEM

Authors: Viviana Popa, MD candidate

Editors: Rishi Desai, MD, MPH; Malorie Snider, MD

Illustrator: Brittany Norton, MFA

THE FEMALE REPRODUCTIVE SYSTEM

Author: Viviana Popa, MD candidate

Editors: Andrea Day, MA; Rishi Desai, MD, MPH; Malorie Snider, MD; Vincent Waldman, PhD

Illustrator: Vincent Waldman, PhD

THE NERVOUS SYSTEM

Author: Antonella Melani, MD candidate

Editors: Rishi Desai, MD; Jessica MacEachern, MA

Illustrator: Brittany Norton, MFA

THE EAR

Author: Viviana Popa, MD candidate

Editors: Rishi Desai, MD, MPH; Jessica MacEachern, MA

Illustrator: Kara Lukasiewicz, PhD, MScBMC

THE EYE

Author: Royce Rajan, MD, MBA

Editors: Fergus Baird, MA; Rishi Desai, MD, MPH; Jessica MacEachern, MA; Yifan Xiao, MD

Illustrator: Samantha McBundy, MFA

THE TONGUE

Author: Pavlos Pavlidis, M.Ost

Editors: Fergus Baird, MA; Rishi Desai, MD, MPH; Yifan Xiao, MD

Illustrator: Pauline Rowsome, BS

SOURCES

THE CARDIOVASCULAR SYSTEM

Costanzo, L. S. (2017). *Physiology* (6 edition). Philadelphia, PA: Elsevier.

Marieb, E. N. & Hoehn, K. (2013). *Human Anatomy & Physiology* (9 edition). London, UK: Pearson.

THE RENAL SYSTEM

Costanzo, L. S. (2017). *Physiology* (6 edition). Philadelphia, PA: Elsevier.

Kidney (n.d.). In *Wikipedia*. Retrieved April 9, 2018, from https://en.wikipedia.org/wiki/Kidney

Marieb, E. N. & Hoehn, K. (2013). *Human Anatomy & Physiology* (9 edition). London, UK: Pearson.

Renal corpuscle (n.d.) In *Wikipedia*. Retrieved April 9, 2018, from https://en.wikipedia.org/wiki/Renal_corpuscle

Tortora, G. J. (2014). *Principles of Anatomy & Physiology* (14 edition). Hoboken, NJ: Wiley.

Urethra (n.d.). In *Wikipedia*. Retrieved April 9, 2018, from https://en.wikipedia.org/wiki/Urethra

THE RESPIRATORY SYSTEM

Broadus, V. C., Mason, R. J., Ernst, J. D., King, T. E., Lazarus, S. C., Murray, J. F., Nadel, J. A., Slutsky, A., & Gotway, M. (2016). *Murray & Nadel's Textbook of Respiratory Medicine* (6 edition). Milton, ON: Elsevier Canada.

Costanzo, L. S. (2017). *Physiology* (6 edition). Philadelphia, PA: Elsevier.

Marieb, E. N. & Hoehn, K. (2013). *Human Anatomy & Physiology* (9 edition). London, UK: Pearson.

Weinberger, S., Cockrill, B., & Mandel, J. (2013). *Principles of Pulmonary Medicine*. Philadelphia, PA: Elsevier.

West, J. B. & Luks, A. M. (2015). *West's Respiratory Physiology: The Essentials* (10 edition). Philadelphia, PA: Wolters-Kluwer.

THE GASTROINTESTINAL SYSTEM

Agabegi, S. S. & Agabegi, E. D. (2016). *Step-Up to Medicine* (4 edition). Philadelphia, PA: Wolters Kluwer.

Boron, W. F., & Boulpaep, E. L. (2017). *Medical Physiology* (3 edition). Philadelphia: Elsevier.

Costanzo, L. S. (2017). *Physiology* (6 edition). Philadelphia, PA: Elsevier.

Fox, S. I. (2016). *Human Physiology* (14 edition). New York: McGraw-Hill Education.

Hall, J. E., & Guyton, A. C. (2010). *Guyton and Hall Textbook of Medical Physiology* (12 edition). Philadelphia, PA: Saunders.

Human digestive system (n.d.). In *Wikipedia*. Retrieved January 10, 2018, from https://en.wikipedia.org/wiki/Human_digestive_system

Kaplan Medical. (2017). *USMLE Step 1 Lecture Notes 2017–2018*. New York, NY: Kaplan Publishing.

Large intestine. (n.d.). In *Innerbody: Human Anatomy and Physiology*. Retrieved January 10, 2018 from http://www.innerbody.com/anatomy/digestive/large-intestine

Le, T., Bhushan, V., Sochat, M., & Chavda, Y. (2017). *First Aid for the USMLE Step 1 2017* (27 edition). New York, NY: McGraw-Hill Education / Medical.

Marieb, E. N. & Hoehn, K. (2013). *Human Anatomy & Physiology* (9 edition). London, UK: Pearson.

Small intestine. (n.d.). In *Innerbody: Human Anatomy and Physiology*. Retrieved January 10, 2018 from http://www.innerbody.com/image_digeov/dige10-new3.html

THE ENDOCRINE SYSTEM

Endocrine System, part 1 - Glands & Hormones: Crash Course A&P #23. (2015). *CrashCourse* [Video file]. Retrieved April 6, 2018, from https://www.youtube.com/watch?v=eWHH9je2zG4

Endocrine System, part 2 - Hormone Cascades: Crash Course A&P #24 (2015). *CrashCourse* [Video file]. Retrieved April 6, 2018, from https://www.youtube.com/watch?v=SCV_m91mN-Q

Hypothalamus. (n.d.) In *Wikipedia*. Retrieved April 6, 2018, from https://en.wikipedia.org/wiki/Hypothalamus

Oxytocin. (n.d.). In *Wikipedia*. Retrieved April 6, 2018, from https://en.wikipedia.org/wiki/Oxytocin

Posterior Pituitary. (n.d.). In *Wikipedia*. Retrieved April

6, 2018, from https://en.wikipedia.org/wiki/Posterior_pituitary

Vasopressin. (n.d.). In *Wikipedia*. Retrieved April 6, 2018, from https://en.wikipedia.org/wiki/Vasopressin

The Adrenal (Suprarenal) Glands. (n.d.) In *Boundless Anatomy and Physiology*. Retrieved April 6, 2018, from https://courses.lumenlearning.com/boundless-ap/chapter/the-adrenal-suprarenal-glands/

THE IMMUNE SYSTEM

Costanzo, L. S. (2017). *Physiology* (6 edition). Philadelphia, PA: Elsevier.

Le, T., Bhushan, V., Sochat, M., & Chavda, Y. (2017). *First Aid for the USMLE Step 1 2017* (27 edition). New York, NY: McGraw-Hill Education / Medical.

Marieb, E. N. & Keller, S. M. (2018). *Essentials of Human Anatomy & Physiology* (12 edition). London, UK: Pearson.

THE LYMPHATIC SYSTEM

Costanzo, L. S. (2017). *Physiology* (6 edition). Philadelphia, PA: Elsevier.

Khan Academy. (Sep 19, 2013). Why we need a lymphatic system | Lymphatic system physiology | NCLEX-RN | *Khan Academy* [Video file]. Retrieved April 9, 2018, from https://www.youtube.com/watch?time_continue=1&v=_GinTV94hUk

Lymph. (n.d.) In *Wikipedia*. Retrieved April 9, 2018, from https://en.wikipedia.org/wiki/Lymph

Lymphatic system (n.d.). In *Wikipedia*. Retrieved April 9, 2018, from https://en.wikipedia.org/wiki/Lymphatic_system

Marieb, E. N. & Keller, S. M. (2018). *Essentials of Human Anatomy & Physiology* (12 edition). London, UK: Pearson.

THE HEMATOLOGIC SYSTEM

Blood. (n.d.). In *Wikipedia*. Retrieved January 23, 2018, from https://en.wikipedia.org/wiki/Blood

Le, T., Bhushan, V., Sochat, M., & Chavda, Y. (2017). *First Aid for the USMLE Step 1 2017* (27 edition). New York, NY: McGraw-Hill Education / Medical.

Marieb, E. N. & Keller, S. M. (2018). *Essentials of Human Anatomy & Physiology* (12 edition). London, UK: Pearson.

Platelet. (n.d.). In *Wikipedia*. Retrieved January 23, 2018, from https://en.wikipedia.org/wiki/Platelet

Red blood cell. (n.d.). In *Wikipedia*. Retrieved January 23, 2018, from https://en.wikipedia.org/wiki/Red_blood_cell

THE MUSCULAR SYSTEM

Marieb, E. N. & Keller, S. M. (2018). *Essentials of Human Anatomy & Physiology* (12 edition). London, UK: Pearson.

Cardiac muscle. (n.d.). In *Wikipedia*. Retrieved January 15, 2018, from https://en.wikipedia.org/wiki/Cardiac_muscle

Skeletal muscle. (n.d.). In *Wikipedia*. Retrieved January 15, 2018, from https://en.wikipedia.org/wiki/Skeletal_muscle

Smooth muscle tissue. (n.d.). In *Wikipedia*. Retrieved January 15, 2018, from https://en.wikipedia.org/wiki/Smooth_muscle_tissue

THE SKELETAL SYSTEM

Khan Academy. (May 5, 2014). Cellular structure of bone | Muscular-skeletal system physiology | NCLEX-RN | *Khan Academy*. Retrieved April 10, 2018, from https://www.youtube.com/watch?v=q1LIWexoKks

Khan Academy. (May 5, 2014). Skeletal structure and function | Muscular-skeletal system physiology | NCLEX-RN | *Khan Academy*. Retrieved April 10, 2018, from https://www.youtube.com/watch?v=-IrKDRAbP38

List of bones of the human skeleton. (n.d.) In *Wikipedia*. Retrieved April 10, 2018, from https://en.wikipedia.org/wiki/List_of_bones_of_the_human_skeleton

Marieb, E. N. & Keller, S. M. (2018). *Essentials of Human Anatomy & Physiology* (12 edition). London, UK: Pearson.

Warren, Andrew. (2018). Human skeletal system. In *Encyclopædia Britannica*. Retrieved April 10th, 2018, from https://www.britannica.com/science/human-skeletal-system

Sources

THE INTEGUMENTARY SYSTEM

Bolognia, J. L., Schaffer, J. V., Cerroni, L. (2018). *Dermatology* (4 edition). Milton, ON: Elsevier.

Elastic fibers. (n.d.). In *Wikipedia*. Retrieved January 15, 2018, from https://en.wikipedia.org/wiki/Elastic_fibers

Fibroblast. (n.d.). In *Wikipedia*. Retrieved January 15, 2018, from https://en.wikipedia.org/wiki/Fibroblast

Integumentary system. (n.d.). In *Wikipedia*. Retrieved January 15, 2018, from https://en.wikipedia.org/wiki/Integumentary_system

Le, T., Bhushan, V., Sochat, M., & Chavda, Y. (2017). *First Aid for the USMLE Step 1 2017* (27 edition). New York, NY: McGraw-Hill Education / Medical.

Marieb, E. N. & Keller, S. M. (2018). *Essentials of Human Anatomy & Physiology* (12 edition). London, UK: Pearson.

Thibedeau, G. A., & Patton, K. T. (2006). *Anatomy & Physiology* (6 edition). St. Louis, MO: Elsevier Health Sciences.

THE MALE REPRODUCTIVE SYSTEM

Androgen-binding protein. (n.d.). In *Wikipedia*. Retrieved January 8, 2018, from https://en.wikipedia.org/wiki/Androgen-binding_protein

Armandohasudungan. (2013). Reproductive system—male overview [Video file]. Retrieved January 8, 2018, from https://www.youtube.com/watch?v=k1aFBOy6dDI

Costanzo, L. S. (2017). *Physiology*. Philadelphia, PA: Elsevier.

Erection. (n.d.). In *Wikipedia*. Retrieved January 8, 2018, from https://en.wikipedia.org/wiki/Erection

Inguinal canal. (n.d.). In *Wikipedia*. Retrieved January 8, 2018, from https://en.wikipedia.org/wiki/Inguinal_canal

Leydig cell. (n.d.). In *Wikipedia*. Retrieved January 8, 2018, from https://en.wikipedia.org/wiki/Leydig_cell

Marieb, E.N. & Hoehn, K. (2013). *Human Anatomy & Physiology* (9 edition). San Francisco, CA: Pearson Benjamin Cummings.

OpenStax. (2013). Anatomy and physiology of the male reproductive system. *Anatomy and Physiology*. Retrieved January 8, 2018, from https://opentextbc.ca/anatomyandphysiology/chapter/27-1-anatomy-and-physiology-of-the-male-reproductive-system/

Slomianka, Lutz. (2009). Male reproductive system. In *School of Anatomy and Human Biology - The University of Western Australia*. Retrieved January 8, 2018, from http://www.lab.anhb.uwa.edu.au/mb140/corepages/malerepro/malerepro.htm

Spermatogenesis. (n.d.). In *Encyclopædia Britannica*. Retrieved January 8, 2018, from https://www.britannica.com/science/spermatogenesis

Spermatogenesis. (n.d.). In *Wikipedia*. Retrieved January 8, 2018, from https://en.wikipedia.org/wiki/Spermatogenesis

THE FEMALE REPRODUCTIVE SYSTEM

Costanzo, L. S. (2017). *Physiology*. Philadelphia, PA: Elsevier.

Follicular phase. (n.d.). In *Wikipedia*. Retrieved January 8, 2018, from https://en.wikipedia.org/wiki/Follicular_phase

Folliculogenesis. (n.d.). In *Wikipedia*. Retrieved January 8, 2018, from https://en.wikipedia.org/wiki/Folliculogenesis

Hypothalamic-pituitary-gonadal axis. (n.d.). In *Wikipedia*. Retrieved January 8, 2018, from https://en.wikipedia.org/wiki/Hypothalamic-pituitary-gonadal_axis

Marieb, E.N. & Hoehn, K. (2013). *Human Anatomy & Physiology* (9 edition). San Francisco, CA: Pearson Benjamin Cummings.

Ovary. (n.d.). In *Wikipedia*. Retrieved January 8, 2018, from https://en.wikipedia.org/wiki/Ovary

Thackray, V. G., Mellon, P. L., & Coss, D. (2010). Hormones in synergy: Regulation of the pituitary gonadotropin genes. *Molecular and Cellular Endocrinology*, 314(2), 192–203. Retrieved January 8, 2018, from http://europepmc.org/abstract/med/19747958

Young, J. M., & Mcneilly, A. S. (2010). Theca: the forgotten cell of the ovarian follicle. *Reproduction*, 140(4), 489–504. Retrieved January 8, 2018, from https://www.ncbi.nlm.nih.gov/pubmed/20628033

THE NERVOUS SYSTEM

Brain. (n.d.). In *Wikipedia*. Retrieved April 11, 2018,

from https://en.wikipedia.org/wiki/Brain

Brainstem. (n.d.). In *Wikipedia*. Retrieved April 11, 2018, from https://en.wikipedia.org/wiki/Brainstem

Cerebellum. (n.d.). In *Wikipedia*. Retrieved April 11, 2018, from https://en.wikipedia.org/wiki/Cerebellum

Costanzo, L. S. (2017). *Physiology* (6 edition). Philadelphia, PA: Elsevier.

Cranial nerves. (n.d.) In *Wikipedia*. Retrieved April 11, 2018, from https://en.wikipedia.org/wiki/Cranial_nerves

Marieb, E. N. & Hoehn, K. (2013). *Human Anatomy & Physiology* (9 edition). London, UK: Pearson.

Nervous system. (n.d.). In *Wikipedia*. Retrieved April 11, 2018, from https://en.wikipedia.org/wiki/Nervous_system

Peripheral nervous system. (n.d.). In *Wikipedia*. Retrieved April 11, 2018, from https://en.wikipedia.org/wiki/Peripheral_nervous_system

Somatic nervous system. (n.d.). In *Wikipedia*. Retrieved April 11, 2018, from https://en.wikipedia.org/wiki/Somatic_nervous_system

Spinal cord. (n.d.). In *Wikipedia*. Retrieved April 11, 2018, from https://en.wikipedia.org/wiki/Spinal_cord

Spinal nerve. (n.d.). In *Wikipedia*. Retrieved April 11, 2018, from https://en.wikipedia.org/wiki/Spinal_nerve

THE EAR

Helicotrema. (n.d.) In *ScienceDirect*. Retrieved April 11, 2018, from https://www.sciencedirect.com/topics/neuroscience/helicotrema

Marieb, E. N. & Hoehn, K. (2013). *Human Anatomy & Physiology* (9 edition). London, UK: Pearson.

Pujol, R., Nouvian, R., & Lenoir M. (2016). Hair cells: overview. *Journey into the World of Hearing*. Retrieved April 11, 2018, from http://www.cochlea.eu/en/hair-cells

Stereocilia (inner ear). (n.d.). In *Wikipedia*. Retrieved April 11, 2018, from https://en.wikipedia.org/wiki/Stereocilia_(inner_ear)

THE EYE

Costanzo, L. S. (2017). *Physiology* (6 edition). Philadelphia, PA: Elsevier.

Khan Academy. (Sep 13, 2017). The structure of the eye | Processing the Environment | MCAT | *Khan Academy* [Video file}. Retrieved December 17, 2017, from https://www.youtube.com/watch?v=cTZl2qnzifc

Marieb, E. N. & Hoehn, K. (2013). *Human Anatomy & Physiology* (9 edition). London, UK: Pearson.

Tortora, G. J. (2014). *Principles of Anatomy & Physiology* (14 edition). Hoboken, NJ: Wiley.

THE TONGUE

Berne, R. & Levy, M. (2000). *Principles of Physiology* (2 edition). St. Louis, MO: Mosby.

Costanzo, L. S. (2017). *Physiology* (6 edition). Philadelphia, PA: Elsevier.

Finger, T. E. (2005). Cell types and lineages in taste buds. *Chemical Senses*, 30(Suppl. 1)., i54—i55. Retrieved April 12, 2018, from https://academic.oup.com/chemse/article/30/suppl_1/i54/270027

Institute for Quality and Efficiency in Health Care (2016). How does our sense of taste work? In *PubMed Health*. Retrieved April 12, 2018, from https://www.ncbi.nlm.nih.gov/pubmedhealth/PMH0072592/

Medler, K. (2015). "Calcium signaling in taste cells." *Biochimica et Biophysica Acta (BBA) - Molecular Cell Research*, 1853(9), 2025–2032. Retrieved April 12, 2018, from https://www.sciencedirect.com/science/article/pii/S0167488914004029

Porter, R. (2011). *The Merck Manual of Diagnosis and Therapy* (19 edition). Rahway, NJ: Merck & Company, Inc.

Purves, D., Augustine, G. J., Fitzpatrick, D., et al. (2001). *Neuroscience* (2 edition). Sunderland, MA: Sinauer Associates.

Reiter, S., Campillo Rodriguez, C., Sun, K., & Stopfer, M. (2015). "Spatiotemporal coding of individual chemicals by the gustatory system." *J. Neurosci*, 35(35), 12309–12321. Retrieved April 12, 2018, from http://www.jneurosci.org/content/35/35/12309.long

Tortora, G., Derrickson, B., & Tortora, G. (2011). *Principles of Anatomy and Physiology* (13 edition). Hoboken, NJ: Wiley.

INDEX

Numbers in red indicate the terms are defined on those pages.

A

abducens nerve 144
ABP. *See* androgen-binding protein
absorption **43**, **49**
accessory nerve 144
acetylcholine 96, 165
acinar cell 48
acrosome **121**
ACTH. *See* adrenocorticotropic hormone
actin filament **96**
action potential **99**, **138**, 160
activin **129**
adaptation (taste) **167**
adaptive immune response 67, **68**, **89**
adenoid tonsil **86**
ADH. *See* antidiuretic hormone
adipocyte **108**, **117**
adipose capsule **26**
adrenal gland 52, 55, **63**
adrenaline. *See* epinephrine
adrenal medulla **63**
adrenocorticotropic hormone **57**
adventitia (bladder) **32**
adventitia (gastrointestinal) **44**
afferent arteriole 27, 30
afferent division (nervous system) **137**
afferent fiber 138, **142**
airway 39–42
albumin 78, **90**
aldosterone **63**
allergy 70, 89, 167
alpha cell **63**
alpha globulin **90**
alveolar duct **41**
alveolar macrophage **41**
alveolar wall **41**
alveolus **16**, **41–42**
ampulla (ductus deferens) 123
ampulla (ear) **154**
ampullar region (fallopian tube) **133**
anal canal **43**
androgen-binding protein **120**
androstenedione **127**, 129
anterior chamber (eye) **155**, **160**
anterior hard palate **43**

anterior horn (spinal cord) **142**, 144
anterior leaflet **16**
anterior lobe (pituitary gland) **55**, 57, 141
anterior wall (ear) **149**
antibody **74**, 77, 83–84, 89
antidiuretic hormone **57**
antigen **68**
antigen presentation **72–77**
antrum **127**
anus 43
aorta **16**, 22, 27
aortic valve **16**, 18
apoptosis **73**
appendicular skeleton **100**
appendix (large intestine) **50**
aqueous humor **160**
arachnoid mater **142**
arcuate artery **27**
arcuate vein 27
armpit 83
aromatase **127**
arteriole 22, 78
artery 78
ascending colon **50**
asthma 70
astrocyte **138**
atrioventricular valve **14**
auditory receptor 137
Auerbach's plexus. *See* myenteric plexus
auricle. *See* pinna
autonomic nervous system 22, 34, 39, 137, **147**
axial skeleton **100**
axon **138–147**

B

basal cell (tongue) **163**
basal ganglia **140**
basal layer. *See* stratum basale
basal metabolic rate **61**
basophil **69–70**, 77, **89**
B cell **73–77**, 77, **83**, 89, 163
belly (muscle) **93**
beta-2 adrenergic receptor 39
beta cell **63**
beta globulin **90**
bicarbonate 91
biceps brachii **93**
bile 48
bile duct 48

bipolar cell **158–160**
bladder **32**, 35, 99, 123, 133
blind spot. *See* optic disc
blood 69, 72, **87–92**
blood-brain barrier **138**
blood clot **90**
blood-gas barrier **41**
blood osmolarity **91**
blood pressure **142**, 147
blood sugar 63
blood-testis barrier **120**
blood vessel **11–25**, 99, 104, 106, 115, 117
body (stomach) **46**
bolus **43**
bone marrow 69–70, 88, **108**
bone matrix **106**
bone metabolism **61**
bone remodeling **106**
bony labyrinth **151**
Bowman's capsule **30**
brain 20, 102, 137, 154, 160, 165
brainstem 51, 138, **142**
breast 57
breastbone. *See* sternum
breastfeeding 57
breast milk 57
broad ligament **126**
bronchial artery 39
bronchiole **39**
bronchomediastinal trunk **81**
brush border enzyme **49**
brush border (intestine) **49**
buffy coat 87, **88**
bulb (corpus spongiosum) **124**
bulbourethral gland **123**

C

calcitonin 61
calcium **90–91**, 96, 99, 111
calcium metabolism **61**
canal. *See* meatus
canal of Schlemm **160**
cancer 73, 89, 111
capillary 22, 78
carbon dioxide 11–25, 88, 91
cardia **46**
cardiac muscle 93, **96–98**
cardiac output **18**
cardinal ligament **133**
cardiomyocyte **96–98**
cardiovascular system. *See* circulatory

system
carina **37**
carpal bone 101
caudate nucleus **140**
caveolae **99**
cavity (bone) **105**
C cell **61**
CD3+CD4+ T cell. *See* helper cell
CD3+CD8+ T cell. *See* cytotoxic T cell
CD4 T cell **74–77**
CD4+ T cell. *See* helper cell
CD8 T cell **74–77**
CD8+ T cell. *See* cytotoxic T cell
cecum **50**
cell body (tongue) **165**
cell-mediated immunity **74**
central nervous system **137**
centrifuge **87**
cerebellum **138**, **141**
cerebral cortex **138–141**
cerebrospinal fluid **142**
cerebrum **138**
cerumen **149**
ceruminous gland **149**
cervical nerve **144**
cervix 57, **126**, **133**
chemoreceptor 137, 163
chest cavity. *See* thorax
chloride **91**
cholecystokinin **48**
cholesterol precursor molecule 111
chordae tendineae **14**
choroid **155–161**
chylomicron **83**
chyme **46**, 50–51
ciliary body **155–161**
ciliary muscle **158**
ciliary process **158**
ciliated columnar cell 39, 40, 67
circadian rhythm **61**, 141
circular muscle. *See* sphincter pupillae muscle
circulatory system **11–25**
circumcision **124**
circumvallate papillus **163**, 168
clitoral hood **136**
clitoris 34, 126, **136**
clonal deletion **68**
clonal expansion **68**, 77
clotting factor protein 90
club cell **40**
coccygeal nerve **144**
coccyx 102
cochlea **148**, **151**
cochlear duct **151**

collagen 14, **115**, 117
collection duct **30**
colon. *See* large intestine
complete immune response **77**
conducting bronchiole **39**
cone **158**
contractility (muscle) **93**
cornea **155–161**
corneal limbus **156**
coronary sinus **14**
coronary vessel **14**
corpora cavernosum **124**
corpus albicans **131**
corpus luteum **131**
corpus spongiosum **124**
cortex (adrenal gland) **63**
cortical bone **106**, 108
cortical radiate artery **27**
cortical radiate vein **27**
cortical zone **27**
corticotropin-releasing hormone 55, **57**
cortisol **63**
cranial nerve I. *See* olfactory nerve
cranial nerve II. *See* optic nerve
cranial nerve III. *See* oculomotor nerve
cranial nerve IV. *See* trochlear nerve
cranial nerve IX. *See* glossopharyngeal nerve
cranial nerve V. *See* trigeminal nerve
cranial nerve VI. *See* abducens nerve
cranial nerve VII. *See* facial nerve
cranial nerve VIII. *See* vestibulocochlear nerve
cranial nerve X. *See* vagus nerve
cranial nerve XI. *See* accessory nerve
cranial nerve XII. *See* hypoglossal nerve
CRH. *See* corticotropin-releasing hormone
CSF. *See* cerebrospinal fluid
cusp **14–25**
cystic duct 48
cytokine **72–77**
cytotoxic granule **73**
cytotoxic T cell **74–77**, 77

D

dandruff **113**
defecation reflex **51**
deltoid muscle **103**
deltoid tuberosity **103**
dendrite **138–140**
dendritic cell 69, **72**, 74, 83, **111**

descending colon **50**
detrusor muscle **32**, 34
diapedesis **90**
diaphragm **11**, 36, 48, 84, 93
diastole **18**
diastolic pressure **18**, 22
diencephalon **138**, **141**
diffuse lymphoid tissue **83**
digestion **43**, 63, 142, 147
digestive tract **57**
dilator pupillae muscle **156**
distal convoluted tubule **30**, 31
dominant follicle **131**
dopamine **57**
dorsal horn (spinal cord) **142**
duodenum **47**, 63
dura mater **142**
dynamic equilibrium **154**

E

ear **148–154**
ear canal **148–149**
eardrum 104. *See* tympanic membrane
ear lobe **149**
earwax. *See* cerumen
efferent division (nervous system) **137**
efferent fiber **138**, **142**
efferent nerve **144**
ejaculation 34, 118, 121, 125
ejaculatory duct **123**, 125
elastic artery **22**
elasticity (muscle) **93**
elastin 20, **115**
endocardium **14**
endocrine gland **52–66**, **63**
endocrine system **52–66**, 141
endolymph **151**, 154
endometrium **133**
endomysium **94**
enteroendocrine cell **48**
eosin **70**
eosinophil **69–70**, 77, **89**
epicardium **11**, 14
epidermis **110–116**
epididymis **119**, 121, 123, 125
epiglottis 37, **43**, 163
epimysium **93**
epinephrine **53**, 63
episcleral venous system **160**
epitympanic recess **149**
erection **124**
erythrocyte. *See* red blood cell
esophageal sphincter **44**

Index

esophagus 43, **43–51**, 163, 165
estradiol **127**
estrogen 57, **129–131**
ethmoid sinus 37
eustachian tube **149**
excitability (muscle) **93**
excretion **43**
exhalation **36**
exocrine gland **63**
extensibility (muscle) **93**
external acoustic meatus. *See* ear canal
external urethral orifice **123**
external urethral sphincter **34**
extrinsic muscle (tongue) **162**
eye **155–161**
eye socket **155**

F

facial nerve 144, **165**, 168
fallopian tube **126**, **133**
fascicle **94**
fat 90, 108
fatty acid **90**
fecal matter **51**
female reproductive system **126–136**
femur 101, 108
fertilization **131**
fiber **50**
fibrinogen **90**
fibroblast **115**, 117
fibrous cardiac skeleton **14**
fibrous layer (eye) **155–156**
fibrous pericardium **11**
fibula **101**
fight-or-flight response **147**
filiform papillus **163**, 168
filtrate **30**
filtration slit **30**
fimbriae **133**
fingerprint **115**
flat bone **101–102**
floating rib **26**
floor (ear) **149**
foliate papillus **163**, 168
follicle-stimulating hormone **57**, **120–121**, **129**, 131
follicle-stimulating hormone receptor **129**
follicular development **126–127**
follicular phase **129**
foramen **104**
foramen magnum **104**
foreskin **124**

fossa **105**
fovea **158**
frontal lobe **140**
frontal sinus 37
fructose 49, **123**
FSH. *See* follicle-stimulating hormone
fundus **46**, **133**
fungiform papillus **163**, 168

G

GABA. *See* gamma-aminobutyric acid
galactose **49**
gallbladder 43, **48**
gamete **57**, 126
gamma-aminobutyric acid **165**
gamma globulin **90**
ganglion **137**
ganglion cell **158–160**
gap junction **99**
gastric gland **46**
gastric pit **46**
gastric secretion **46**
gastrointestinal system 20, **43–51**
gastrointestinal tract **43–51**, 83
generation (bronchus) **37**
GHIH. *See* growth hormone-inhibiting hormone
GHRH. *See* growth hormone-releasing hormone
glans penis **123–125**
glial cell **137**
globulin **90**
glomerulus **27**, 30
glossopharyngeal nerve 144, **165**, 168
glucagon 53, **63**
glucose 49, **91**
glycogen **63**
glycolipid **111**, 113
glycosaminoglycan **40**
GnRH. *See* gonadotropin-releasing hormone
goblet cell **39**
gonad **52**, 118
gonadotropin-releasing hormone 55, **57**, **120**, **129**
G protein-coupled receptor **165**
G protein-coupled receptor pathway **165**
graafian follicle **127**
granule **89**
granulocyte **69**, **89**
granulosa cell **127**
grey column. *See* grey horn

grey horn **142**
grey matter **142**. *See* cerebral cortex
groin **83**
growth hormone-inhibiting hormone **57**
growth hormone-releasing hormone **55**
gustation **162–169**
gustatory hair **165**
gut **67**
gut microbiome **50**

H

hair cell (ear) **151**, 154
hair follicle **115**
haversian canal **106**
hearing **151**
hearing receptor. *See* hair cell
heart **11–25**, 78, **96**, 102
heart rate **147**
heart string. *See* chordae tendinae
helper cell **74**, 77
hematocrit **88**
hematologic system **87–92**
hematopoiesis **69**
hematopoietic stem cell 69
hematoxylin **70**
heme chain **84**
hemoglobin 16, **84**
Herring body **57**
homeostasis **52**
hormone 83, 91
humerus 101, 103
humoral immunity **74**
hymen **136**
hypodermis **117**
hypoglossal nerve 144, **162**
hypophyseal fossa. *See* sella turcica
hypotension **31**
hypothalamic gonadotropin-releasing hormone **131**
hypothalamic hormone **55**
hypothalamic-pituitary axis **141**
hypothalamo-hypophyseal-portal system **55**
hypothalamus 55, 57, **120**, **129**, **141**
hypovolemia **31**

I

ileocecal sphincter **50**
ileum **47**
immune privilege **156**
immune response **67–77**
immune surveillance 78, 83

immune system **67–77**
immunoglobulin. *See* antibody
immunologic memory **68**, **89**
incus **148–149**
inferior vena cava **14**, 27
infundibulum **133**
ingestion **43**
inhalation **36**, 86
inhibin **121**, **131**
inhibitory hypothalamic hormone **57**
innate immune response **67**
inner ear 148, **151–154**
insertion (muscle) **94**
insulin 53, 63
integumentary system 20, **110–117**
intercalated disc **99**
intercostal muscle 36
interlobar artery **27**
interlobar vein 27
intermediate urethra **34**
internal anal sphincter 51
internal capsule **140**
internal urethral orifice 34
internal urethral sphincter **34**
internal wall. *See* medial wall (ear)
interstitial fluid. *See* lymph
intestinal microvillus **47**
intestinal trunk **81**
intestinal villus **47**
intestinal wall 83
intrinsic muscle (tongue) **162**
iris **155–161**
iron 84
irregular bone **101**
isthmus region **133**

J

jejunum **47**
jugular trunk **81**
jugular vein 149
juxtaglomerular cell **30**, 31
juxtaglomerular complex **30**
juxtamedullary zone **27**

K

Kegel exercise **34**
keratin **111**
keratinization **113**
keratinocytes **111–113**
keratin precursor protein 113
keratohyalin granule **113**
kidney 20, **26–35**, 52, 63

L

labia 126
labia majora **136**
labia minora 34, **136**
labyrinth. *See* inner ear
lactase 49
lacteal **83**
lacuna (osteocyte) **106**
lamellar granule **113**
lamina propria **44**
large intestine 43, **50**, 99
laryngopharynx **37**
larynx **37**, 163
lateral horns **142**
lateral horn (spinal cord) 147
left atrium 25
left cerebral hemisphere **138**
left lobe (thyroid gland) **61**
left lung 37
left main stem bronchus 37
left renal artery 27
left renal vein 27
left ventricle 18, 25
lens **156–161**
leukocyte. *See* white blood cell
leukocytes. *See* white blood cell
Leydig cell **120**
LH. *See* luteinizing hormone
lingual papillus **163**
lingual tonsil **86**
liver 43, **48**, 90
lobule (testicle) **119**
long bone 57, **101**
loop of Henle **30**
lower lobe (left lung) 37
lower lobe (right lung) 37
lumbar nerve 144
lumbar trunk **81**
lumen (blood vessel) **20**, 22
lumen (intestine) 48
lumen (seminiferous tubule) **120–121**
lung 11, 25, **36–42**, 77, 102
luteal phase **129**, 131
luteinizing hormone **57**, **120–121**, **129**, 131
luteinizing hormone receptor 129
lymph 72, **78–86**
lymphatic capillary **79**, 83
lymphatic duct **81**
lymphatic system 49, **78–86**, 117
lymphatic trunk **81**
lymphatic vessel 26, **79–86**, **81**, 83, 115
lymph node 72, 77, **83–86**
lymphocyte **89**

lymphoid cell **73**
lymphoid progenitor cell 69, **73**
lymphoid system. *See* lymphatic system
lysozyme **36**, 67

M

macrophage **69–77**, **115**, 117
macula **158–161**
macula densa cell **30**, **31**
macula (ear) **154**
main stem bronchus **37**
major calyx **27**
major histocompatibility complex **72**
male reproductive system **118–125**
malleus **148–149**
maltase **49**
mandible 102
mast cell **69–70**, 77
mastication **43**
mastoid antrum **149**
mastoid cavity 149
maxilla **105**
maxillary bone **105**
maxillary sinus 37, 105
meatus **104**
mechanoreceptor **106**
medial wall (ear) **149**
mediastinum **11**
mediastinum testis **119**
medulla **142**, 144
megakaryocyte **88**
meiosis I 121, **126–127**
meiosis II 121, 131
Meissner corpuscle **115**
Meissner's plexus. *See* submucous plexus
melanin **111**, 156
melanocyte **111**
melanosome **111**
melatonin **61**
membranous labyrinth **151**
membranous semicircular duct **154**
memory cell **68**, 77
meninges. *See* meninx
meninx **142**
menstrual cycle 127, **129–131**
menstruation **133**
mesangial cell **30**
mesometrium **133**
mesosalpinx 133
metacarpal **101**
metacarpal phalangeal joint 102
metarteriole **24**
metatarsal 101

Index

metatarsal phalangeal joint 102
MHC. *See* major histocompatibility complex
MHC II 74, 77
micelle **48**
micturition center **35**
micturition reflex **35**
midbrain **142**, 144
middle ear **148–149**
middle lobe (right lung) 37
minor calyx **27**, 30
mitochondrion 121
mitosis 121
mitral valve **16**
monocyte 69, **72**, **89**
monosaccharide **49**
mons pubis 126, **136**
motor cortex **142**
motor fiber. *See* efferent fiber
motor nerve. *See* efferent nerve
motor neuron 96
mouth 43
mucociliary escalator **39**, 41
mucosa (stomach) **44**
mucosa (tongue) **162**
mucus (nasal) **36**
mucus (stomach) **46**
muscarinic receptor 39
muscle cell **94–99**
muscle fiber **94**
muscle memory **141**
muscularis externa **44**, 46
muscularis interna. *See* muscularis mucosa
muscularis mucosa **44**
muscular system **93–99**
myelin **138**
myeloid cell **69**
myeloid progenitor cell **69**
myenteric plexus **44**
myocardium **14**
myocyte. *See* muscle cell
myofibril **96**
myometrium **133**
myosin filament **96**

N

nasal bone 105
nasal cavity 36, **105**
nasopharynx **37**, 149
natural killer cell. *See* NK cell
neck 83
nephron **30**, 31
nephron loop. *See* loop of Henle
nerve 26, 104, 115, 117

nerve ending 115
nervous system 35, **137–147**
neural layer (eye) **155**, 158
neural layer (retina) 155
neuromuscular junction **144**
neuron **137**
neurotransmitter **138**
neutrophil 69, **69–70**, **77**, **89**
NK cell **73**, 77, 89
nocturnal penile tumescence **124**
nonspecific immune cell **67**
nonsteroid hormone **53**
noradrenaline. *See* norepineprhine
norepinephrine **53**, 63, 165
nose hair **36**
nostril 36
nucleus (neuron) **137**

O

oblique smooth muscle 46
occipital bone 104
occipital lobe **140**
oculomotor nerve 144
odorant **167**
oil gland 110, 115
olfactory nerve 144, **167**, 168
oligodendrocyte 138
oligosaccharide **49**
oncotic pressure **90**
oocyte 57, **121**, 123
optic canal **104**
optic disc **160**
optic nerve 104, 144, 156, 160
orbit. *See* eye socket
organ of Corti **151**
origin (muscle) **94**
oropharynx **37**
osteoblast **106**
osteoclast **106**
osteocyte **106**
osteon **106**
outer ear **148–149**
oval window **149**
ovarian artery 126
ovarian cortex **126**
ovarian follicle 126
ovarian ligament **126**
ovarian medulla **126**
ovarian nerve plexus 126
ovarian vein 126
ovary 52, 57, **126–136**
ovulation 57, **129–131**
oxidative burst **70**
oxygen 11–25, 88, 91
oxytocin 57

P

pacemaker cell **99**
Pacinian corpuscle **115**
palatine bone 105
palatine tonsil **86**
pallidum **140**
pancreas 43, **48**, 63
pancreatic amylase **48**
pancreatic duct cell 48
pancreatic lipase **48**
papillary layer **115**
papillary muscle **14**
papillus **115**, **163**
parafollicular cell. *See* C cell
paranasal sinus **37**, 105
parasympathetic nerve **39**
parasympathetic nervous system **147**
parasympathetic neuron 51
parathyroid hormone **61**
paraventricular nucleus 57
parietal lobe **140**
parotid gland **43**
patella bone 102
pelvic floor 34
pelvic girdle **100**
pelvis 34, 100
penile urethra **123**, 125
penis 34, 118
pepsin **46**
peptidase **49**
peptidic hormone **53**
perilymph **151**
perimetrium **133**
perimysium **94**
perineum 124
periosteum **106**
peripheral nervous system **137**, **144**
peristalsis (gastrointestinal) **44**, 51
peristalsis (testicle) **121**
peritoneal membrane **26**
peritoneal space 133
peritoneum 34, 133
peritubular capillary 27, 30
Peyer's patch **83**
phagocytosis **70**, 72–77, 89
phagolysosome 70
phagosome **70**
phalange 101
pharynx **37**, 39, 41, 43, 163
phosphate metabolism 61
photoreceptor **158**
pia mater **142**
pigmented layer (retina) 155
pineal gland **61**

OSMOSIS.ORG **181**

pinealocyte **61**
pinna **148–149**
pisiform bone 102
pituitary follicle-stimulating hormone **129**
pituitary gland **55**, 105, **120–121**, 129, 131, **141**
pituitary stalk **57**
placenta 131
plasma 87, **90–92**
plasma cell **74**, 77, 83
platelet 69, 84, **87–92**, 108
platelet plug **90**
plexus **44**
PMN. *See* polymorphonuclear cell
pneumocyte **41**
podocyte **30**
polymorphonuclear cell **69**, **69–70**
pons 35, **142**, 144
pontine micturition center **35**
pontine storage center **35**
posterior **142**
posterior chamber (eye) **156**, **160**
posterior horn (spinal cord) 144
posterior leaflet **16**
posterior lobe (pituitary) **141**
posterior lobe (pituitary gland) **55**, 57
posterior soft palate **43**
posterior wall (ear) **149**
postganglionic neuron **147**
potassium 63, 91
preganglionic neuron **147**
pregnancy 32
primary follicle **127**
primary oocyte **126–131**
primary spermatocyte **121**
priming **72**
primordial follicle **126–127**
progesterone 57, 129, 131
prolactin-inhibiting factor. *See* dopamine
prostate 34, **123**
prostatic fluid 123
prostatic urethra **34**
proximal convoluted tubule 30
puberty 86, 125, 129
pubic hair **136**
pulmonary arteriole 16
pulmonary artery **14**, 41
pulmonary capillary 16
pulmonary valve 18
pulmonary vein 16
pupil **155–161**
putamen 140

pyloric antrum **46**
pyloric sphincter **46**

R

radial muscle. *See* dilator pupillae muscle
radius (arm bone) 101
rectum 32, **50**, 133
red blood cell **16**, 69, 78, 84, **87–92**, 108
red marrow **108**
red pulp **84**
reflex **142**
releasing hormone. *See* stimulatory hormone
renal artery 26
renal capsule **26**
renal column 27
renal corpuscle **30**
renal cortex **27**
renal fascia **26**
renal hilum **26**
renal lobe **27**
renal medulla **27**
renal papilla 27
renal pelvis **27**
renal pyramid 27
renal system **26–35**
renal tubule **30**
renal vein 26
renin **31**
respiratory bronchiole 40, **41**
respiratory system **36–42**
respiratory tract 83
rete testis **119**, 121
reticular layer **115**
retina 155
rib 100, 102
ribcage 11
right atrium 14
right cerebral hemisphere **138**
right jugular vein 81
right lobe (thyroid gland) **61**
right lung **37**
right lymphatic duct **81**
right main stem bronchus 37
right renal artery 27
right renal vein 27
right subclavian vein 81
right ventricle 14, 25
rod **158**
round ligament **133**
round window **149**
ruga 32

S

S1 **18**
S2 **18**
saccule 151, 154
sacral nerve 144
sacrum 102
saliva 43, 165
salivary amylase **43**
salivary gland 43
sarcolemma **96**
sarcomere **96**
sarcoplasm **96**
sarcoplasmic reticulum **96**
scala tympani **151**
scala vestibuli **151**
scapula 100, **102**
Schwann cell 138
sclera **155–161**
scrotal raphe **118**
scrotum **118**
secondary follicle **127**
secondary oocyte **131**
secretin **48**
segmental artery 27
self-antigen **86**
sella turcica **105**
semen 34, 123
semicircular canal **148**, **151**, **154**
seminal fluid **123**
seminal vesicle **123**
seminiferous tubule **119–125**
sensory cortex **142**
sensory fiber. *See* afferent fiber
septa (testicle) **119**
serosa **44**
serotonin 165
serous pericardium **11**
Sertoli cell **120–121**
serum **74**, 90
sesamoid bone **101–102**
sex chromosome 121
sex hormone **57**
short bone **101**
shoulder blade. *See* scapula
sigmoid colon **50**
sinus (bone) **105**
skeletal muscle 20, 81, **93–96**, 137, 142, 144
skeletal system **100–109**
skin 67, 93, **110–117**, 144
skull 100, 102, 104
small intestine 43, **43–51**, 63, 83, 99
smooth muscle 93, **99**, 124, 133, 137

Index

sodium 91
soft palate **37**, 163
somatic nervous system 137, **144**
somatosensory receptor **137**
somatostatin. *See* growth hormone-inhibiting hormone
sperm 57, **118–125**, 125, 131
spermatic cord 123
spermatocyte **120**
spermatogenesis **120–121**
spermatogonium **120**, 121
spermiogenesis **121**
sphenoid bone 104–105
sphenoid sinus 37
sphincter pupillae muscle **156**
spinal cord 35, 51, 96, 137, **142**
spinal nerve 144
spiral artery **133**
spleen **84**
spongy bone. *See* trabecular bone
spongy urethra **34**
stapes **148–149**
static equilibrium **154**
sternum **11**, 100, 102
steroid hormone **52**
stimulatory hormone **55**
stomach **43–51**, 67, 84
stratified squamous epithelium (eye) **156**
stratum basale **111**, 115
stratum corneum **113**
stratum granulosum **113**
stratum lucidum **113**
stratum spinosum **111**
striated muscle **96–99**
striatum **140**
subarachnoid space **142**
subcutaneous tissue. *See* hypodermis
subendothelial basement membrane 24
sublingual gland **43**
submandibular gland **43**
submucosa **44**
submucous plexus **44**
sucrase 49
sulcus terminalis **163**
superficial inguinal ring 123
superior vena cava **14**
supraoptic nucleus 57
surfactant **41**
suspensory ligament **126**, **158**
sweat gland 110, 115
sympathetic nerve **39**
sympathetic nervous system **147**
synapse **138–147**

systemic artery 20
systemic capillary 20
systemic circulation **18**, 25
systemic vein 20
systole **18**
systolic blood pressure **18**
systolic pressure 22

T

T3. *See* triiodothyronine
T4. *See* thyroxine
tarsal bone 101
tastant **163**
taste bud **163–169**
taste pore **165**
taste receptor cell **163–169**
T cell **72–77**, **84**, 89, 163
temporal bone 104, 149
temporal lobe **140**
tendon 93, 102
terminal bronchiole **40**
tertiary. *See* graafian follicle
testicle 52, 57, **118**
testis. *See* testicle
testosterone 57, 120
thalamus 51, **141**
theca cell **127**, 129
thermoregulation **22**, **115**, 141
thoracic duct **81**, 83
thoracic nerve 144
thorax **11**
throat 86, 165. *See* pharynx
thymus **86**
thyroid follicle **61**
thyroid gland 55, **61**
thyroid-stimulating hormone **55**
thyrotropin-releasing hormone 55
thyroxine **61**
tibia 101
tongue 43, **162–169**
tonsil **86**
tooth 43
touch **115**
trabecula **108**
trabecular bone **106**, **108–109**
trabecular meshwork **160**
trachea **37**
transverse colon **50**
transverse tubule **96**
TRH. *See* thyrotropin-releasing hormone
tricuspid valve **14**
trigeminal nerve 144
trigone region **32**
triiodothyronine **61**

trochlear nerve 144
trypsin **48**
T tubule. *See* transverse tubule
tubal tonsil **86**
tubercle **103**
tuberosity **103**
tunic **20**
tunica albuginea **119**, **124**
tunica externa **20**
tunica intima **20**, 24
tunica media **20**
tympanic membrane **149**
type I collagen 106
type II pneumocyte **41**
type I pneumocyte **41**
tyrosine **53**
tyrosine-derived hormone **53**

U

ulna 101
upper lobe (left lung) **37**
upper lobe (right lung) 37
ureter 26, **27–35**, 31
ureterovesical junction **31**
urethra **34**
urinary system. *See* renal system
urination **35**, 142
urination center. *See* micturition center
urine 123
uterine body **133**
uterine isthmus 133
utero-sacral ligament **133**
uterus 32, 99, **126–136**
utricle 151, 154
uvea. *See* vascular layer (eye)
uvula **37**, **43**

V

vagina 32, **126–136**
vaginal mucosa **136**
vaginal urethra **136**
vagus nerve 144, **165**, 168
vasa vasorum **22**
vascular layer (eye) **155–158**
vas deferens **123**, 125
vasoconstriction **22**, 57
vasodilation **22**
vasopressin. *See* antidiuretic hormone
venous return **18**
vertebra 100
vertebral column 11, 142
vestibular apparatus **154**
vestibule 151

vestibulocochlear nerve 144, 151, 154
virus 73, 77, 89
visual receptor 137
vitamin D **111**
vitreous chamber **160**
vitreous humor **160**
voice box. *See* larynx
Volkmann's canal **106**
voluntary muscle **93**
vulva 126
vulval vestibule 34
vulvar vestibule **136**

W

white blood cell **69, 88–92**, 108
white matter **138–140**, 142
white pulp **84**
windpipe. *See* trachea

Y

yellow marrow **108**

Z

zona fasciculata **63**
zona glomerulosa **63**
zona reticularis **63**
zygote 133

READ OUR OTHER BOOKS!

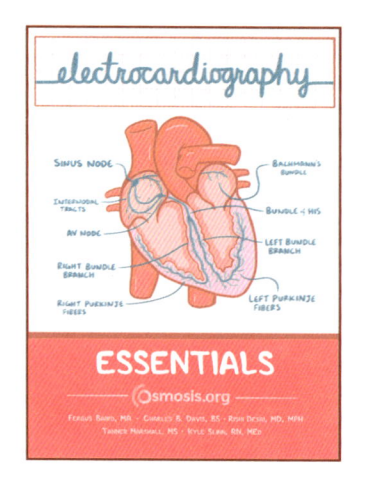

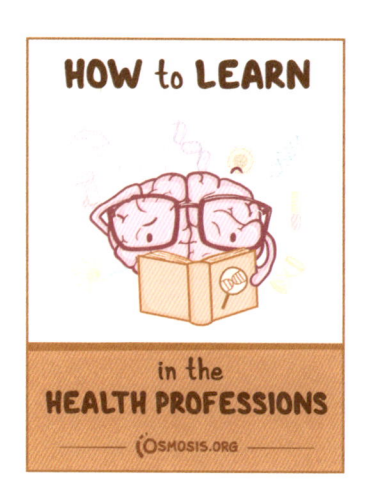

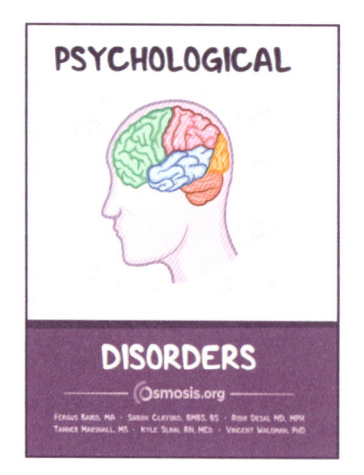

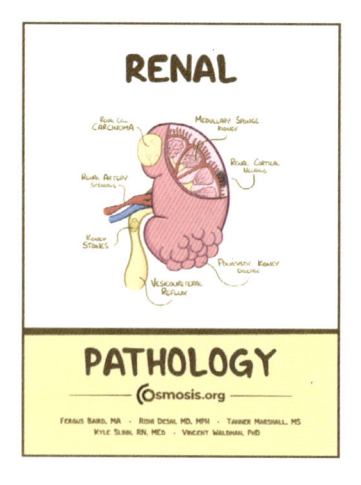

BUY THESE AND MORE AT

books.osmosis.org

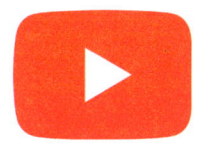

Watch our new videos every week:
www.youtube.com/osmosis

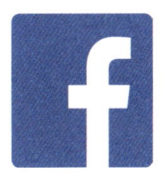

Follow us on Facebook:
@osmoseit

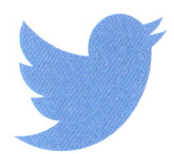

Follow us on Twitter:
@osmoseit

Follow us on Instagram:
@osmosismed